Acknowledgment

We would like to thank our teachers, Professors and colleagues who have been very supportive to us throughout our career.

Thanks to our teachers who taught us effectively during our PACES examination.

Special Thanks to our consultants.

Also we would like to thank our families who encouraged us in every way.

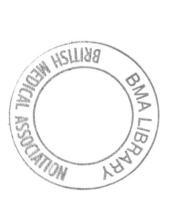

III

Disclaimer

Every effort has been made in preparing this book to provide up to date information in accord with the accepted standards, guidelines and practice at the time of the publication. The authors can make no warranties that the information contained herein is totally free from errors, not least because clinical standards are constantly changing. The authors therefore disclaims all liability for direct or consequential damage resulting from the use of material within this book. Readers are recommended to check all drug doses, indications, contraindications and interactions used with British National Formulary or drug data sheet prior to use. If a reader is unsure what to do, then they should seek help from a senior medical adviser. Patient should seek help from health care professionals.

If you have any comments please email us @ our
email: TheLastSecondMRCPPACES@outlook.com

The Last Second MRCP PACES

Fady Zakharious   MRCP (UK)
Senior Clinical Fellow Geriatrics Medicine
Frimley Health NHS Foundation Trust
Wexham Park Hospital
Slough
UK

Mahmoud Montasser   MD, MRCP (UK), SCE
Specialist Registrar Renal Medicine
East Kent Hospitals University Foundation Trust
Kent & Canterbury Hospital
Canterbury
UK

Copyrights

Table Of Contents

The Last Second MRCP PACES 4th Edition

This book provides comprehensive and valuable materials for candidates sitting the MRCP PACES examination.

The book introduces the history and the relevant examination that should be done in station V.

This book teaches you how to pass station V easily and with high marks.

The book introduces a full practical history taking skills from A to Z.

The book provides you with a specific Scheme for history taking; you will not miss any point during history taking anymore.

The book introduces Templates for ethical and communication skills issues (Station IV), Don`t worry about the communication skills station any more.

The book provides you with a Broad range of abilities to manage the patients concern easily and safely.

This Book provides full clinical examination skills for each station.

This book is for MRCPUK PACES candidates, and for every Internist, medical student going to sit a Clinical examination.

This book is very concise yet, very comprehensive for candidates not having time to study all the available MRCP PACES books.

This book is a savior for every candidate working and studying at the same time.

In the Fourth edition we introduced a special history taking scheme, communication skills scheme exclusive to the Last Second MRCP PACES.

In the Fourth edition we added examination findings & Cases for examination skills stations which are very helpful tools for you to pass your clinical examination stations easily.

The Fourth edition has a better formatting and a more convenient interface than the previous electronic editions.

Introduction To The MRCP PACES

MRCP PACES is five stations

STATION I

Abdomen

- 10 minutes (6 minutes' examination, 4 minutes' discussion with examiners).
- The examiner will tell you at 5 mins that 1 minute is left.

Chest

- 10 minutes (6 minutes' examination, 4 minutes' discussion with examiners).
- The examiner will tell you at 5 mins that 1 minute is left.

STATION II

History taking skills

20 minutes:

- 14 minutes for taking the history.
- 1 minute for reflection.
- 5 minutes' discussion with examiners.
- The examiner will tell you when there are 2 minutes left from the 14 minutes (ask for the concern; don't miss it).

STATION III

Cardiology

- 10 minutes (6 minutes' examination, 4 minutes' discussion with examiners).
- The examiner will tell you at 5 mins that 1 minute is left.

Neurology

- 10 minutes (6 minutes' examination, 4 minutes with examiners).
- The examiner will tell you at 5 mins that 1 min is left.

STATION IV

Communication skills

20 minutes:

- 14 mins for communicating with your patient.
- 1 min for reflection.
- 5 minutes discussion with examiners.
- The examiner will tell you when there are 2 minutes left of the 14 mins (ask for the concern; don't miss it).

STATION V

Brief clinical consultation

Two cases for each you have:

10 minutes:

- 8 minutes for history, examination, and managing concern.
- 2 minutes' discussion with examiners.
- The examiner will tell you when 2 minutes are left of the 8 minutes (ask for the concern, don't miss it)

You have 5 mins between each Station to read instructions carefully.

Important Instructions:

Marking in MRCP PACES is for Clinical examination skills, physical findings skills, differential diagnosis, clinical judgment, maintaining the patient welfare, communication skills, patient`s concern.

In station I, III, V while examining the patient think about:

- Examination findings.
- Diagnosis.
- Complications.
- Possible causes.
- Associated conditions the patient may have.

Respect the patient dignity and welfare.

Don't hurt the patient always ask if he feels any pain.

Address patients as this lady, this gentleman.

Give yourself time to **Read instructions carefully** and See the patient as a whole, don't rush to examination, **Bed side clues** & other clues in the patient especially in neurology case are very important (e.g.: flexed adducted upper limb in a case of examination of lower limbs = Hemiplegia)

Maintain eye contact with **both examiners.**

Hold your hands together behind your back, don`t point to your body, don`t turn your head to the patient.

Always hold your stethoscope in your hands, don't put it over your shoulders.

When presenting the case ... Comment on the signs observed or bed side clues first before commenting on the system examined....... at the end say, I would like to complete my examination by (important other bedside examinations) e.g.: Doing fundoscopy if suspecting infective endocarditis.

If asked what your diagnosis is: say;

- "This Young Lady, Gentleman Is Having...... As Evidenced By (Your Comment)"

Never to say what you omitted in examination; the examiner might not have noticed it e.g.: don't say "I should have examined the radiation of the murmur to the neck" but be humble and accept what the examiner says.

In discussion say everything. Don't let the examiner to drag information from you; if asked what tests you want to do for this patient with pulmonary fibrosis answer "Chest X-Ray Which Will Show Reticular Shadow"

If asked what is your differential diagnosis? Answer with:

- The most probable diagnosis
- Other differentials and reasons for exclusion.

If asked how will you investigate this patient?

- Investigations to confirm the diagnosis.
- Investigations to Rule out differential diagnoses.
- Investigations for complications.
- Investigations for the etiology.

If asked how will you treat this patient?

- Non pharmacological (Patient education, Psychological & Social support)
- Pharmacological
- Surgical

Sleep well the day before the examination.

Please read the marking process for the MRCP PACES examination on the following link: https://www.mrcpuk.org/sites/default/files/documents/Marking%20of%20PACES%2020 15.pdf.

Please be familiar with the marking sheets of the MRCP PACES examination; to know how the examiners are assessing you on the following
link: https://www.mrcpuk.org/sites/default/files/documents/PACES-marksheets.pdf

30 Seconds General Survey Of The Patient

We would recommend that you spend 30 seconds in all clinical scenarios to do a general survey of the patient and his surroundings to:

1. **Read Instructions Carefully**
2. **Look For Any Bedside Clues**
- Inhalers → **Obstructive lung disease.**
  - Asthma
  - COPD
- Sputum pots → **Bronchiectasis, Chest infection, T.B.**
- Oxygen masks/NIV machine
- Chest drain or its scar → **Pleural effusion, Pneumothorax** (COPD, Asthma, Marfan`s syndrome)
- Walking aids, Wheel chair
- ECG Monitor → Arrhythmias, Ischemic heart disease.
3. **Any Clues Within The Patient Himself**
- Flexed adducted Upper limbs in **Hemiplegia**
- Myotonia grip during greeting him → **Myotonia**
- Excessive coughing with sputum production →**Bronchiectasis**
- Staccato speech → **Cerebellar disease.**
- Medic Alert bracelet / Necklace → **Read it please**
- **Marfanoid features** (Tall, Span > height, Thumb sign (Steinburg sign), Wrist sign (Walker-Murdoch sign)) look for:
  - Pneumothorax
  - Mitral valve prolapse (MVP), Mitral regurgitation (MR)
  - Aortic regurgitation (AR)
4. **Face**
- Plethoric, Rounded with fullness, acne, hirsutism → **Cushing syndrome**
- Expressionless, infrequent blinking → **Parkinson disease**
- Unlined face, with drooping of mouth →**Myopathy, Myasthenia gravis**
- **Facial nerve palsy** (loss of nasolabial fold, deviation of mouth to opposite side)
- Loss of hair → **SLE, Hypothyroid, Alopecia** areata/totalis
- **Acromegalic** (wrinkled forehead, prominent supraorbital ridge, prognathism, large nose and lips)
- **Hypothyroid** (puffiness around eyes, loss of outer 1/3 of the eye brow, coarse hair, goiter, obese)
- **Myotonic Facies** (frontal baldness, Bilateral ptosis)
- **Down Syndrome** (upward slanting of eyes, low set ears, silky hair)
- **Noonan Facies** (epicanthal folds, hypertelorism, low set ears)
- **Turner Syndrome** (webbed neck, shield chest, short stature)
- **SLE Butterfly Rash** sparing the nasolabial fold
- Lupus Pernio (violaceous papules not respecting the nasolabial fold resembling frost bite) → **Sarcoidosis**
- Malar Flush in **Mitral Stenosis**
- Facial flushing with telangiectasia in **Carcinoid syndrome.**
- Prominent Zygoma & Maxilla with widely spaced teeth & muddy complexion in **Chronic Hemolytic anemia.**
5. **Eyes**
- Prominent supra-orbital ridge →**Acromegaly**
- Starring look → **Grave`s disease**
- Xanthelasma → **Ischemic heart disease, hypercholesterolemia**
- Puffiness around eye lids Might be **Nephrotic syndrome.**
- Loss of outer 1/3 eye brow → might be **Hypothyroidism.**
- Horner`s (Ptosis, Miosis) → **Lateral Medullary Syndrome, Carotid Artery Dissection, Cluster Headache, Pancoast's Tumor.**

- 3rd nerve palsy (Ptosis, Mydriasis, Eye down & out) → **Mid brain stroke, Posterior communicating artery aneurysm, Mono-neuritis Multiplex, Multiple Sclerosis**
- Nystagmus → could be **Cerebellar/Vestibular disease.**

6. Ears
- Low set ears → **Down syndrome**
- Large ears → **Acromegaly**
- Hearing Aid + Renal disease →**Alport`s Disease**
- Diagonal lobular Crease in the ear lobule → **Ischemic heart disease**

7. Nose
- Large might be due to **Acromegaly.**
- Butterfly rash might be **SLE.**
- Tipped nose → **Systemic sclerosis**
- Depressed nasal bridge/Saddle nose could be Vasculitis e.g. **Granulomatosis with Polyangiitis.**

8. Lips
- Large lips → **Crohn's disease, Acromegaly**
- Oral Ulcers → **Behcet`s, SLE, Crohn`s disease, Coeliac disease**
- Multiple telangiectasia → **Hereditary Hemorrhagic telangiectasia (HHT), Systemic Sclerosis**
- Brownish freckles around the lips → **Peutz Jeghers syndrome**

9. Mouth (ask patient to open mouth & look with a torch)
- Dark pigmentations in oral mucous membranes →**Addison`s disease**
- High Arched palate → **Marfan`s syndrome, Friedreich`s ataxia**
- Fetor hepaticus → Chronic liver disease(CLD)
- Uremic fetour → Chronic kidney disease (CKD)
- Skin puckering around the mouth with microstomia → **Systemic sclerosis**

10. Temporalis Wasting → Myotona,Chronic liver disease & Terminal Malignancies

11. Parotid Enlargement → Chronic liver disease, Sarcoidosis, Sjogran, Pleomorphic adenoma.

12. Neck
- Using accessory muscles of respiration → **Respiratory distress.**
- Enlarged Thyroid
- Enlarged L.Ns.
- Skin Color
- Tattoos.
- Webbed neck → **Turner, Noonan.**
- Pulsations → Aortic regurgitations (AR).
- Central lines → Hemodialysis, ITU Admission.
- Raised JVP → **Heart failure, fluid overload, Pulmonary hypertension, tricuspid regurgitation, SVCO.**
- Tracheostomy Scar → Prolonged Invasive ventilation.
- Medic alert necklace

13. Chest
- Skin (Color & Rash)
- Gynecomastia → **Chronic liver disease, Amiodarone, Digoxin, Spironolactone, klinefelter`s disease.**
- Scars
  - Mid line sternotomy scar = **CABG, Valve replacement.**
  - Left sub-mammary = **Mitral valve repair.**
  - Lateral thoracotomy scar → **Pneumonectomy, Lobectomy.**
  - Chest drain scars → **Pleural effusion, Pneumothorax.**
- Central lines
- Spider nevi → **Chronic liver disease (CLD)**
- Hair → **Sparse hair in CLD**
- Tattoos, Radiation tattoos
- Intercostal in drawing → **Obstructive airway disease.**
- Tachypnea

- Asymmetry
  - Unilateral fibrosis.
  - Unilateral collapse.
  - Pneumonectomy.
  - Lobectomy.
  - Pleural effusion.
  - Pneumothorax.

14.   Abdomen
- Distension:
  - Fluid = Ascites/ blood.
  - Fat.
  - Flatus (could be intestinal obstruction or simple distension)
  - Fetus.
  - Feces = constipation.
  - Fibroid.
- Flank fullness probably **Ascites**
- Shift of umbilicus downwards →Increased intra-abdominal pressure
- Scars
  - Laparotomy could it be **Crohn`s disease**.
  - Laparoscopy
  - Left subcostal → **Splenectomy**
  - Right iliac fossa → Appendectomy, Renal transplant.
  - Left iliac fossa → **Renal transplant.**
  - Mercedes Benz scar → **Liver transplantation**.
- Dilated Veins → Portal hypertension, Inferior vena cava obstruction
15.   Arms
- Medic alert bracelet
- Tattoos increase risk of **HBV, HCV, HIV**.
- Nails
  - Pitting & onycholysis → **Psoriasis**, ? associated auto-immune disease
  - Koilonychia → **Iron deficiency**
  - Half & Half nail → **CKD**
  - Leuconychia → **Hypoalbuminemia, CLD**
  - Tar staining could the patient has **COPD, CA lung**
  - Splinter hemorrhage → **Infective endocarditis (IEC),** traumatic.
  - Jane way/Osler nodules → **IEC**
  - **Clubbing**
    - Chronic liver disease (CLD)
    - Infective endocarditis (IEC).
    - Familial adenomatous polyposis (FAP).
    - Coeliac disease,
    - Inflammatory bowel disease (IBD).
    - CA lung.
    - Bronchiectasis.
    - Empyema.
    - Lung abscess.
    - Idiopathic pulmonary fibrosis (30% only).
    - Thyroid acropachy.
    - Cyanotic heart disease (Blue clubbing).
- Scars → Venous harvest graft for CABG.
- Purpura/Ecchymosis.
  - Cushing.
  - On warfarin for AF or valve replacement.
  - Myelofibrosis.
  - Steroids use.
- A-V fistula/Graft.
- Amputations

16. Legs

- Unilaterally Swollen
    - DVT
    - Baker cyst
    - Trauma
    - Lymphoedema
    - Varicose veins
- Bilaterally swollen
    - Heart failure
    - CLD
    - CKD (chronic kidney disease)
    - Hypo-albuminemia
    - Tricuspid regurgitation
    - Varicose veins
    - Nephrotic syndrome
    - Calcium channel blockers use.
- Erythema nodosum
    - Sarcoidosis
    - IBD
    - Streptococcal infection
    - Oral contraceptive pills (OCPs)
- Necrobiosis Lipoidica / diabetic dermopathy = **DM**.
- Pyoderma Gangrenosum
    - Inflammatory bowel disease
    - Rheumatoid arthritis
    - Vasculitis.
- Nails

STATION I

Respiratory System Examination
Abdominal Examination

Station I Respiratory Examination

1. **Scrub Your Hands with Antiseptic liquid.**

Antiseptic liquid is provided to you in the station.

2. **Greet The Patient, Introduce Yourself And Take Permission.**
3. **Position The Patient 45 Degrees In Bed.**
4. **Expose The Patient From Head To Mid Abdomen.**
5. **Stand At The End Of The Bed, Take Your Time To Observe:**

Ask The Patient to Breath in & Cough; "Can You Take A Deep Breath In For Me Please; Can You Cough For Me Please?" And note:

- The patient`s type of **Cough**, is it productive?
- **Bed side clues:**
  o Sputum pots
  o Excessive Coughing of patient
  o Inhalers
  o Chest drains
  o Oxygen Masks, Nasal Cannula, BIPAP/CPAP machine.
- **Age:**
  o Young= Asthma, Bronchiectasis, Pneumonia, Pneumothorax.
  o Old = COPD, Fibrosis, CA (cancer), Pneumonia, Effusion, Lobectomy, Pneumonectomy, Pneumothorax.
- **Comfortable** vs Tachypnea
- **Built**
  o <u>Overweight</u>: OSA (obstructive sleep apnoea), OHS (Obesity hypoventilation syndrome).
  o <u>Cachexia:</u> COPD, Bronchiectasis, Cancer.
- Any Audible **wheeze**
  o COPD
  o Asthma
  o Carcinoid
  o Acute bronchitis
  o Cardiac Asthma
  o Anaphylaxis
- **Face and Neck**
  o Use of Accessory muscles = Respiratory Distress
  o Horner`s ? CA Lung
  o Radiation burn → CA Lung → Collapse, Cavity, Fibrosis, Consolidation.
  o Amiodarone pigmentation? Fibrosis
  o SLE Rash → Fibrosis, Effusion.
  o Tipped nose, Skin Puckering around mouth, Sclerodactyly, Telangectasia = Systemic Sclerosis → Fibrosis, PH
  o Cushingoid face = Steroid use → Sarcoidosis, Asthma, COPD, Wegner`s granulomatosis (granulomatosis with polyangiitis)
  o Lupus Pernio = Sarcoidosis → look for Fibrosis if present.
  o Heliotrope rash = Dermatomyositis → Look for Lung fibrosis.
- **Chest** "Take A Deep Breath For Me Please"
  o Asymmetry:
    ▪ Increased A-P diameter → COPD
    ▪ Bulge → Pneumothorax, Pleural effusion
    ▪ Retraction → Fibrosis, Collapse ,Lobectomy, Pneumonectomy
    ▪ You will note the diseased side by decreased expansion on that side.
  o Pectus Excavatum
  o Pectus Carinatum
  o Limited chest expansion on both sides or 1 side
  o Intercostals indrawing = Hoover sign → COPD / Obstructive Lung Disease
  o Scars
    ▪ Lateral thoracotomy scar → Pneumonectomy/Lobectomy
    ▪ Chest drain scar → Effusion / Empyema / Pneumothorax

- o Dilated veins over the chest with congested face and congested arms = SVCO → CA Lung
- o Radiation tattoos
- o Radiation burn
- o Cardiac apex beat site, if on Rt. → Kartagner`s syndrome = Bronchiectasis
- **Hands**
  - o RA (Z deformity, ulnar deviation, buttoniere, swan neck) → Basal Lung Fibrosis, Effusion, Bronchiolitis Obliterans.
  - o Sclerodactyly ,Thin stretched shiny skin, Curling of Fingers = Systemic Sclerosis → Lung Fibrosis, PH (Pulmonary HTN)
  - o Clubbing = Bronchiectasis, ILD , CA , Empyema , Abscess
  - o Yellow nails = Yellow Nail Syndrome → Effusion, Bronchiectasis
  - o Cyanosis
  - o Tar staining
- **Arms**
  - o Purpura ? Steroid use → COPD, Fibrosis
- **Legs**
  - o Lower limb swelling
    - ▪ Unilateral ? DVT
    - ▪ Bilateral ? L.L edema ? Core pulmonale
  - o Clubbing of nails
  - o Cyanosis
  - o Erythema Nodosum → T.B, Sarcoid, Streptococcal Infection
  - o Erythema Multiform → Mycoplasma infection
  - o Purpuric Eruptions ? Steroid use → Fibrosis or COPD

6. <u>Ask The Patient To Extend His Hands And Examine Dorsum Of Hands for:</u>
- Clubbing
- Peripheral Cyanosis
- Yellow nail syndrome
- Tar staining
- Purpura
- Wasting of small muscles of the hands → Lung CA, RA.
- Fine tremors = B2 agonist → COPD
- Feel For Thinning Of Skin = steroids use → Fibrosis, COPD, Asthma.

7. <u>Ask Patient To Turn His Hands Up And Examine Palms for</u>
- Palmar erythema = CO_2 retention
- Feel Radial Pulse → If Collapsing → CO_2 retention.
- Count respiratory rate in 15 secs x 4 whilst feeling the pulse.
- Look for signs of ABG sampling signs.

8. <u>Ask The Patient To Pull His Wrist Back And Examine For Flapping Tremors</u> Flapping = CO_2 retention → respiratory failure.

9. <u>Examine Both Eyes Same Time</u> For
- Pallor :"Can You Look Up For Me Please"
- Horner`s (Ptosis & Miosis)

10. <u>Examine Mouth</u> For:
- Central Cyanosis at the dorsal surface of the tongue.
- Fish mouth (Narrow with Skin puckering around mouth and telangiectasia → Systemic Sclerosis → Look for PH, Fibrosis.

11. <u>Ask The Patient To Turn His Neck And Examine JVP</u>
- Elevated JVP (Pulsating)
  - o PH (Pulmonary HTN)
  - o Core Pulmonale
  - o Pulmonary embolism (PE)
  - o Heart failure
- Prominent A wave = PH
- Non-Pulsating raised JVP → SVCO.

12. <u>Ask The Patient To Sit Forward And Examine The Trachea From The Front for:</u>
- Position (Central or Deviated)
- Tracheal tug = COPD

- Cricoid Sternal distance (Normal >3 fingers breadths) if < 3 =COPD

Signs Of Tracheal Shift

- Inspection of the neck (Unequal grooves on both sides)
- Palpation with index finger In the grooves (Don't push hard in grooves)
- Palpation with middle finger to the trachea with index & ring over sterno-clavicular joints & note the position of your middle finger in accordance of the other fingers.

13. **Inspect The Back Of The Chest** For
- Symmetry
- Shape (Kyphosis, Scoliosis)
- Scars
- Limited chest expansion

14. **Palpate Chest Expansion From The Back**
- Ask Him To Cross His Arms Over Shoulders & To lean forward.
- Confirm symmetry
- Confirm Chest expansion
- TVF (You can do vocal resonance instead while you auscultate)

15. **Percuss The Back Of Chest With Heavy Percussion And Take Your Time Don`t Rush It, Listen And Feel Carefully**
- Suprascapular
- 3 Interscapular spaces
- 3 Subscauplar spaces & look for:
  - Resonance (Equal on both sides)
  - Hyperresonance bilaterally =COPD
  - Hyperresonace unilaterally = Pneumothorax
  - Impaired note=Fibrosis , Bronchiectasis , Collapse ,Consolidation, Lobectomy
  - Stony dullness= Pleural effusion

16. **Auscultate Breath Sounds at Same Sites of Percussion** For
- **Breath sounds** (Air entry) → Normal or Diminished.
- **Type of breathing**
  - Vesicular → Normal
  - Bronchial
    - Consolidation
    - Mass
    - Cavitation
  - Vesicular with prolonged expiration:
    - COPD
    - Asthma
    - Obstructive lung disease.
- **Added sounds**
  - *Wheezing:*
    - COPD
    - Asthma
    - Anaphylaxis
    - Carcinoid
    - Cardiac Asthma
  - *Fine Crackles* (Late Inspiratory)
    - Lung Fibrosis → Fine end inspiratory crackles
    - Pulmonary edema
  - *Coarse crackles* (May be early inspiratory or expiratory)
    - Bronchiectasis
    - Pneumonia
    - Secretions
  - Pleural Rub
    - Pleurisy

17. **If You Find Any Crackles Ask The Patient To Cough & Re-auscultate**
- Crackles of secretions disappear by coughing
- Bronchiectasis Crackles change in character by coughing but doesn't disappear.
- Lung fibrosis crackles doesn't change in character or disappear by coughing.
18. **Ask The Patient To Say 99 Each Time You Put Your Stethoscope Over His Back And Listen For Increased Vocal Resonance**
19. **If You Find Increased Vocal Resonance Ask Him To Whisper 99 For Positive Whispering**
- + ve whispering =Bronchial breathing
- Causes of Increased Vocal Resonance
  - Consolidation
  - Bronchiectasis
  - Cavitation
  - Mass
  - Lung collapse with mediastinal shift to the side of the lesion.
  - Dense Lung fibrosis
- Causes of decreased Vocal resonance
  - Pleural effusion
  - Pneumothorax
  - Lung fibrosis
  - Lobectomy
  - Pneumonectomy
20. **Ask The Patient To Lie On His Back**

21. **Inspect The Front Of Chest for:**
- Symmetry.
- Limited expansion.
- Shape.
- Scars.
- Apex of the Heart.
- Intercostal in drawing.
- Dilated veins (usually with facial plethora, dilated arm veins) = SVCO = CA Lung
22. **Palpate The Front Of The Chest For:**
- Expansion & TVF
- Palpable Rhonchi
- Palpate Heart Apex = Shifted Or Not
- Palpate Lt. Sternal Edge For Lt. Parasternal Heave = RVH (Right Ventricular hypertrophy) → PH (Pulmonary HTN)
- Palpate Pulmonary Area For Palpable P2 (Diastolic Shock)= PH
23. **Percuss The Chest**
- Apex of the Lungs (Kronig`s Isthmus)
- Clavicles
- 2 Supra-mammary areas
- Mammary area
- 2 infra-mammary areas
- 2 Axillary areas
24. **If You Find Hyper-Resonance Bilaterally Percuss For:**
- Hepatic dullness.
- Cardiac dullness (3rd , 4th Lt. ICS)

If these areas are resonant not dull this means hyper-inflated chest

25. **Auscultate The Front in same sites as for Percussion As You Have done in the Back.**
26. **Auscultate for Vocal resonance**
27. **Ask If He Has Any Pain In The Legs and Examine The Patient Legs for:**
- Feel for L.L edema
- Clubbing of nails
- Purpura of skin
- Erythema nodosum

28. **Examine L.Ns** (Carcinoma , T.B , Sarcoidosis , Lymphoma)
- Cervical
- Supraclavicular
- If you couldn`t examine the L.Ns because of the time, mention it to the examiner that you would like to complete your examination by examining L.Ns.

29. **Formulate Your Comment And Diagnosis**
- **The Diagnosis** (COPD , Bronchiectasis , Fibrosis , Effusion)
- **Possible Cause** (Smoking)
- **Possible Complications** (Pulmonary HTN)

30. **Thank The Patient And Greet Him**
31. **Cover The Patient**
32. **Scrub Your Hands Again**

Respiratory Case Presentation

This Gentleman / Lady Is Lying Comfortable At Rest With Average Built, He Has No L.L Edema, He Has Tar Staining Of The Nails But No Clubbing, No Pallor Or Cyanosis, Trachea Is Central, With Decreased Cricoid Notch Distance, And Positive Tracheal Tug, He Has Intercostal In Drawing On Inspiration, Chest Exp

ansion Is Bilaterally Limited With Increased Resonance On Percussion Bilaterally Encroaching Over The Hepatic And Cardiac Dullness, Breath Sounds Are Diminished Bilaterally, Breathing Is Vesicular With Prolonged Expiration, There Are Widespread Expiratory Rhonchi Scattered Over The Chest

I Would Like To Complete My Examination By Examining Sputum Pots, Flow Rate, Patient's Observation Charts, Doing Pulse Oximetry & Examining L.Ns (If You Didn`t Examine The L.Ns During Your Examination).

N.B:

The Anterior Part Of The Chest Is Mainly Formed Of The Upper Lobe, And The Posterior Part Of The Chest Is Mainly Formed Of The Lower Lobe (Base Of The Lung)

Respiratory Examination Common Pitfalls

1-A lot of candidates forget to count the respiratory rate which is very important in a chest case examination

2-Many candidates fail to examine the position of the Trachea which is a very powerful diagnostic sign.

3-Some candidates are hesitant with chest Auscultation, as a result; they take a lot of time listening to the back and do not have enough time to complete the examination of the chest for which they lose marks.

4-Most of the chest signs will be more evident on the back.

5-Train yourself to finish the examination completely within 6 mins.

6-Some candidates are in a hurry to complete the whole examination to demonstrate to the examiners their skills in clinical examination, but they do not pay good attention to the signs for which they do not reach a diagnosis.

7-Some Candidates go directly to examine the chest without spending 30 seconds for a general survey of the patient, as a result they could miss precious obvious signs in the patient.

8-Some candidates start auscultation without warming the stethoscope diaphragm, as a result the patient would tell them it is very cold, and they would lose time and confidence in the exam & may be some marks as well (Patient's Welfare)

9-A lot of candidates miss to palpate the pulmonary area and left parasternal area, as a result they could miss an evident pulmonary hypertension.

Respiratory Cases

Chronic Obstructive Pulmonary Disease

Clinical Examination

- Tar staining
- ? COPD Cachexia.
- No clubbing unless complicated.
- May be signs of CO2 retention
  - Collapsing pulse
  - Warm peripheries
  - Flapping tremors
  - Palmar erythema
- Decreased cricoid Sternal distance.
- Tracheal tug.
- Central trachea unless complicated
- Intercostal in drawing.
- Hyper inflated chest.
- Increased A-P diameter.
- Hyper resonance B/L (Bilateral) on Percussion.
- Decreased breath sounds B/L
- Breathing is Vesicular with prolonged expiration
- Wheezing B/L

Look for complications:

- *Pulmonary HTN:* Raised JVP, accentuated P2, palpable 2nd heart sound
- *Core Pulmonale:* Pulmonary HTN signs + Lt.Parasternal heave + ? L.L edema & enlarged tender liver if Rt. Sided heart failure developed.
- *Bronchiectasis:* See later

Quick Discussion:

What Are The Causes of COPD?

- Smoking (Tar staining)
- Macleod syndrome (Childhood bronchiolitis)
- Coal dust
- Alpha 1 antitrypsin deficiency

How Would You Confirm your diagnosis?

1) Clinically
- Coughing on most of the days > 3 months for 2 successive years.

2) Investigations To Confirm Diagnosis
- *CXR:* Hyperlucency, Horizontal ribs, depressed Copulae of diaphragm, Ribbon shaped heart
- *Pulmonary Function tests:* FEV1 < 80%, FEV1/FVC < 70%

3) Investigastion For Complications
- *Bloods:*
  - Raised CrP & WBCs if infection exacerbation of COPD
  - Polycythemia due to hypoxia
- *CXR:* looking for consolidation if pneumonia develops.
- *ABG:* Type II RF either compensated or decompensated.
- *Spirometry:* Obstructive pattern, TLCO is decreased.
- *Sputum MC&S*
- *ECG:* Right ventricular hypertrophy if PH
- *Echo-cardiogram:* If Core-pulmonale
- *CT chest:* if Lung Ca or Bronchiectasis suspected

4) Investigations for Alpha 1 Antitrypsin deficiency

What Is The Treatment of COPD?

1) Non-Pharmacological
- Vaccines

- Chest physiotherapy
- Stop smoking

2) **Pharmacological**
- Antibiotics to treat infections.
- Controlled O2 therapy.
- Bronchodilators.
- Steroids & Nebs in exacerbations
- BIPAP if in acute Type II RF not responding to medical therapy.
- LTOT if PO2 < 7.3 KPa or between 7.3-8 Kpa with Pulmonary HTN, Polycythemia, Nocturnal hypoxia.

3) **Surgical**
- Bullectomy & Lung resection to increase compliance
- Chest drain for pneumothorax

What Are The Complications Of COPD?

- 2ry Polycythemia.
- Respiratory failure
- Recurrent chest infections.
- Core-Pulmonale.
- Heart failure.
- Bronchiectasis.
- Pneumothorax.

> ### Causes of Clubbing in a COPD Case
> - **Bronchiectatic Changes**
> - **Fibrosis** (Not all cases of Fibrosis are associated with Clubbing)
> - **Lung Cancer**
> - **Empyema**
>
> **N.B:** COPD itself is not a cause of Clubbing

What Is The Definition Of Pulmonary HTN?

- Mean Pulmonary Blood Pressure > 25 mmhg at rest.

How Can You Assess Severity Of COPD?

- FEV1 (Mild > 80, Moderate 50-80, Severe < 30-50, Very Severe < 30)

How Can You Differentiate between Asthma & COPD?

1) Clinically
- *Asthma:* Young age, occurs in attacks, Completely reversible, usually non-Smoker, History of Atopy
- *COPD:* Usually Smoker, Middle or old age, Usually symptomatic between attacks, chronic cough for most of the days > 3 months for 2 successive years.

2) Investigations
- *Asthma*: Challenge test (Methacoline test) Obstructive pattern with reversibility on Treatment with bronchodilators & Steroids
- *COPD*:Reversibility is limited.

Bronchiectasis

Clinical Examination

- Under weight.
- Sputum pots on bedside.
- Patient might be on oxygen mask.
- Clubbing.
- Trachea is central
- Excessive coughing during examination.
- Limited chest expansion on the affected side
- Palpable Rhonchi.
- May have Increased TVF.
- Heterogeneously impaired note of percussion on the affected side.
- Decreased breath sounds.
- Coarse inspiratory crackles which change in character by coughing.

Look for a Cause:

- *Kartagner's syndrome* : Examine Cardiac apex site & feel the liver if dextrocardia specially if a young patient .
- *COPD signs*
- *Yellow nails*
- *Cystic Fibrosis:* Young, Short stature, May be signs of Diabetes.
- *Lung CA signs:* ? Tar staining, radiation burns, SVCO signs, Palpable Lymphadenopathy.

Look for Complications:

- *Respiratory failure:* flapping tremors, disturbed LOC, Palmar erythema, Collapsing pulse, Warm peripheries.
- *Pulmonary HTN:* see below

Quick Discussion:

What Are The Causes of Bronchiectasis?

- T.B , Whooping cough , Measles , ABPA
- COPD
- Lymphoma
- Yellow nail syndrome
- Hypogamaglobulinema
- Cystic fibrosis
- Kartagner's (Dextrocardia)
- Lung fibrosis (you will find fine and coarse crackles)
- Lung Cancer

What Is The Differential Diagnosis of Bronchiectasis?

- Lung Fibrosis
- Lung CA
- Chronic Lung abscess

What Are The Complications Of Bronchiectasis?

- Core-Pulmonale
- Respiratory Failure
- Amyloidosis
- Recurrent chest infections
- Hemoptysis

How Would You Like To Diagnose This Case?

1) Investigations To Confirm Diagnosis
- *CXR:* Honey-comb appearance, Tram lines
- *HRCT:* Signet ring appearance & dilated varicose bronchioles

2) Investigations For The Cause:

- *T.B:* T Spot, X-Ray, Sputum for AFBs/Culture.
- *Lung CA*: CT chest/ CT CAP
- *ABPA*: Aspergillus precipitans
- *Cystic fibrosis:* Sweat teats, CFTR gene
- *Bronchoscopy :* localized malignancy

5) Investigastion For Complications

- *Bloods:*
  - Raised CrP & WBCs in infection
  - Polycythemia due to hypoxia
- *ABG:* Type II RF
- *Spirometry:* Obstructive pattern.
- *Sputum MC&S*
- *ECG :*Right ventricular hypertrophy
- *Urine Dip* for proteinuria (Amyloidosis)
- *Echo-cardiogram:* if Core-pulmonale

What Is The Treatment of Bronchiectasis:

1) Non-Pharmacological

- Vaccines,
- Chest physiotherapy
- Stop smoking

2) Pharmacological

- Antibiotics to treat infections and long term Azithromycin for prophylaxis if needed.
- Bronchodilators.
- Steroids.
- Treatment of the cause.

3) Surgical

- Pneumonectomy, Lobectomy If Failed Medical Treatment)
- Lung Transplantation.

What Are The Common Organisms found In Bronchiectasis?

- Streptococcus Pneumonie
- H.Influenza
- Moraxella Catarrhalis
- Staphylococcus
- Pseudomonas
- Mycoplasma
- Legionella

What Do You Know About Yellow Nail Syndrome?

- It Is A Disorder Of Lymphatics Characterized By:
  - Pleural Effusions
  - Bronchiectasis
  - Sinusitis
  - Yellow Nails Especially in L.Ls

How Can You Differentiate Between Lung Fibrosis And Bronchiectasis Clinically?

- By The Type Of Crackles
  - Fine crackles in Lung fibrosis
  - Coarse crackles in bronchiectasis
- Changeability With Coughing
  - Crackles in Bronchiectasis Change in character after coughing
  - Crackles in Lung Fibrosis doesn't change in character by coughing
- And The Presence Productive Cough In Bronchiectasis

Pulmonary Fibrosis

Clinical Examination

- Clubbing in 30% of cases of idiopathic Pulmonary fibrosis.
- ? Central cyanosis.
- Limited chest expansion on the affected side
- Trachea deviated to the side of the lesion unless B/L
- Retraction of the chest
- Impaired note of percussion
- Decreased breath sounds
- Fine end inspiratory crackles which doesn't change in character by coughing

Look for a cause:

- *RA*: Rheumatoid hands.
- *SLE:* Rash, mouth ulcers, alopecia.
- *Scleroderma:* Hand and face signs.
- *Amiodarone:* Slate grey Pigmentations
- *Idiopathic Pulmonary fibrosis*: Clubbing + No obvious cause
- *Sarcoidosis:* HSM (Hepatosplenomegaly), Lupus Pernio, red eyes, Large parotids.
- *Dermatomyositis:* Heliotrope rash, Gottron`s papules.
- *Extrinsic allergic alveolitis (Hypersensitivity pneumonitis):* Might get the clue from information given e.g. Please Examine this Farmer`s chest.
- *Polymyositis:* Examine for proximal muscle weakness (If you Can not find any obvious cause for B/L Basal Lung Fibrosis please examine the patient for proximal muscle weakness & Tenderness)

Look for complications

- *Pulmonary HTN*
- *Complications of the cause accordingly*
- *Respiratory failure*

Quick Discussion:

What Are The Causes of Pulmonary Fibrosis?

1) **Bilateral Fibrosis** :
- Idiopathic Pulmonary Fibrosis (? Clubbing, No Obvious Cause)
- Extrinsic Allergic Alveolitis (Hypersensitivity Alveolitis)
- Asbestosis (Shipyard worker)
- Sarcoidosis
- Bronchiectasis
- RA
- SLE
- Systemic Sclerosis
- Polymyositis
- Dermatomyositis
- Ankylosing spondylitis (Kyphosis + Apical fibrosis)
- Good pasture
- Wegner`s granulomatosis (Granulomatosis Polyangiitis)→ Saddle nose, May be signs of renal replacement therapy.
- Amiodarone
- Bleomycin
- Methotrexate
- Nitrofurantoin (UTI prophylaxis)
- Kyphoscoliosis

2) **Unilateral Fibrosis:**
- T.B
- Lung Abscess
- ABPA

- Post-Radiation
- Post-Traumatic
- Post-infectious

3) Upper Lobes Fibrosis :
- Ankylosing spondylitis
- T.B
- Sarcoidosis
- EAV (Extrinsic Allergic Alveolitis)= Hypersensitivity pneumonitis
- Silicosis (Glass workers)
- Amiodarone induced
- Radiation.

4) Lower Lobes Fibrosis:
- ILF (Idiopathic interstitial fibrosis)
- SLE
- RA
- Systemic Sclerosis
- Asbestosis
- Drugs except amiodarone.
- Aspiration Pneumonia

> **Differences Between Lung Collapse And Fibrosis Clinically**
> - In Collapse Homogenous Dullness While In Fibrosis Hetregenous Area Of Dullness And Impaired Note
> - In Collapse There Is Absent Breath Sounds While In Fibrosis There Are Breath Sounds But Diminished.
> - Note That In Dense Unilateral Fibrosis You Will Find Bronchial Breathing.
> - In Collapse There Are No Crackles While In Fibrosis There Is Fine End Inspiratory Crackles

How Would You Like To Diagnose This Case?

1) Investigation to Confirm diagnosis
- *CXR*: Reticulonodular shadows
- *HRCT*: is diagnostic shows ground glass appearance
- *PFTs*: Restrictive pattern; decreased FVC, FEV1/FVC > 70%, decreased TLCO

2) Investigations for complications
- ABG: Type I RF
- Echo: Pulmonary HTN

3) Investigations for the Cause
- Bronchoalveolar lavage in EAA, Sarcoidosis if lymphocytosis = good prognosis
- ANA, RF, Anti CCP
- Serum Ca & Serum ACE → Sarcoidosis …etc

What Is The Treatment of Pulmonary Fibrosis?

1) Non Pharmacological
- Stop Smoking
- Vaccines
- Chest Physiotherapy

2) Pharmacological
- Steroids
- Azathioprine
- Cyclophosphamide
- Treatment of the cause
- Treatment of exacerbations.
- Treatment of infection.
- Oxygen

3) Surgical
- Unilateral Lung Transplant

What Do You Know About Hamman-Rich Syndrome?

It is a rapidly progressive Cryptogenic Lung fibrosis with a very poor prognosis.

Consolidation:

Clinical Examination

- Decreased chest expansion on affected side
- Trachea is central
- Impaired note of percussion/ dullness
- Decrease breath sounds
- Bronchial breathing
- +ve whispering
- Coarse crackles
- May be signs of SIRS
- May be signs of pleural effusion.
- May be signs of Malignancy

Quick Discussion:

What Are The Causes of Consolidation?

- Pneumonia
- Lung Abscess
- Cavitation
- Lung Mass

How Would You Like To Diagnose This Case?

1) Investigations to Confirm Diagnosis
- *CXR*: Consolidation with air-bronchograms if pneumonia, Cavitation, Mass, Abscess
- *CT chest*: will show consolidation & air-bronchograms if pneumonia, Mass, Cavitation, Abscess

2) Investigations for the cause
- *Sputum Mc&S*
- *Urine* for Legionella, Streptococcal antigen
- *Klebsiella serology*
- *CT chest* for Lung CA & Abscess

3) Investigations for complications
- *ABG*: Type I RF
- *Investigation for Complications of the cause*
  - Hyponatraemia & deranged LFTs if legionella
  - Metsatsasis if Lung CA.
- *CT chest*: if Localized Lung fibrosis suspected.

What Is The Treatment of Pneumonia?

- *Antibiotics* (Please Follow Your Hospital Local Protocols)
  - *CAP*: Amoxicillin + Clarithromycin (Be familiar with your hospital local protocols)
  - HAP: Amoxicillin + Metronidazole / Co-amoxiclav
  - Aspiration Pneumonia: Amoxicillin + Metronidazole
- Oxygen if needed
- Stopping smoking
- Treat complications.

How does aspiration Pneumonia present?

- Usually Consolidation On The Right Middle Or Lower Lobes
- Usually in a patient with swallowing problems or PEG fed.

What Are The Causes Of Cavitary Lung Lesions?

- T.B
- Staphylococcus aureus
- Klebsiella
- Granulomatosis with Polyangiitis
- Lung Abscess

What Is The Treatment Of T.B?

- Intensive phase (2 months : Rifampicin, INH, Ethambutol, Pyrazinamide)
- Continuation phase (4 months :Rifampicin & INH)

How Would You Assess Pneumonia Severity?

- CURB -65 Score
  - o Confusion
  - o Urea>7
  - o B.P < 90/60
  - o R.R >30
  - o Age 65
- A score of 1 or less is low risk; consider home treatment
- A score of 2 might need short inpatient hospitalization or closely supervised OP treatment
- A score of 3 or more indicates severe pneumonia and needs hospital admission.

Lung Cancer

Clinical Examination

- Tar staining
- Any chest signs/Findings
- Clubbing
- L.Ns
- Cachexia
- ? SVCO

Quick Discussion:

How Would You Like To Diagnose This Case?

1) Investigations to Confirm the diagnosis
- CT Scan of the Chest: diagnostic
- CT CAP: for staging
- Tapping of effusion
- Trans-bronchial Biopsies

2) Investigations for Complications
- *Blood tests*:
  - o *FBC*: Anemia, raised inflammatory markers if infection
  - o LFTS: Deranged LFTs if metastasis
- *CXR:* for new consolidation if infection suspected.

What Is The Treatment of Lung CA?

1) Surgery
- Lobectomy if FEV1>1.5
- Pneumonectomy if FEV1> 2L

2) Chemotherapy
3) Palliative Treatment If Metastatic
4) Treatment of complications
- Stenting & Radiotherapy for SVCO.
- Oxygen for Respiratory failure.
- Antibiotics for Chest infections.

Pleural Effusion

Clinical Examination

- Trachea might be deviated to the opposite side.
- There might be a bulge of the chest on the affected side.
- There might be chest drain or its scar.
- Limited chest expansion on the affected side.
- Stony dullness on affected side.
- Decreased breath sounds on the affected side.
- Decreased Vocal Resonance.
- Might have bronchial breathing at the apex of the effusion.

Look for a Cause:

- *Malignancy:* Cachexia, Old age, L.Ns, Clubbing, Tar staining of nails, ? SVCO signs, ? Horner`s syndrome ,any chest finding
- *Infection:* Consolidation signs, SIRS.
- *Cardiac failure:* Bilateral effusion, raised JVP, L.L. edema, Gallop rhythm, Pulsus alternans, ? Ascites, Regurgitation murmur of mitral/tricuspid valve, Enlarged Tender Liver.
- *SLE:* Butter fly rash, Oral ulcers, Alopecia
- *RA:* RA Changes in the hands
- *Chronic Liver disease:* B/L effusion, Stigmata of chronic Liver disease, Ascites.

Quick Discussion:

What Are The Causes of Pleural effusion?

1) Exudates
- Parapneumonic Effusion
- T.B.
- Empyema
- Malignancy
- RA
- SLE
- Acute Pancereatitis
- Yellow Nail Syndrome
- Hypothyroidism

2) Transudates
- Hypoalbuminemia
- Renal Failure
- Nephrotic Syndrome
- Heart Failure
- Meigs Syndrome (Ovarian Fibroma)
- Mal-Absorption Syndrome
- Hypothyroidism

3) Chylous Effusion → thoracic duct obstruction

How Would You Like To Diagnose This Case?

1) Investigations To Confirm The Diagnosis
- *CXR:* Obliteration of costo-phrenic angle rising to axilla
- *U/S of the Thorax*
- *CT Chest*

2) Investigations To Search For A Cause
- *Diagnostic tap to apply Light`s Criteria*
  - Exudates
    - LDH>2/3 normal
    - LDH >0.6 of serum
    - Pleural Fluid Proteins > 0.5 of serum
  - Transudates

- LDH < 2/3 normal
  - LDH < 0.6
  - Pleural proteins < 0.5 of the serum
- *T.B* (adenosine de-aminase +ve in the pleural fluid)
- *Sputum MC&S & AFBs*

3) <u>Investigations For Complications</u>

- *ABG* for Respiratory failure

How Can You Diagnose Empyema?

- Turbid Fluid On Thoracocentesis
- Pleural Fluid Ph < 7.2
- Positive Gram Stain Of Pleural Fluid
- U/S Scan Showing Loculated Effusion (Not All Loculated Effusions Are Empyema)

What Is The Treatment of Pleural effusion?

- Therapeutic aspiration if medium size effusion with symptoms.
- Chest drain if empyema or affecting Gas exchange
- Treatment of the cause
- Pleurodesis for recurrent effusions

What is the differential diagnosis of dullness at Lung bases on percussion?

- Pleural Effusion (Vocal Resonance Is Decreased)
- Pleural Thickening (Vocal Resonance Is Normal)
- Raised Copula Of Diaphragm (Abdominal Distension)
- Fibrosis
- Bronchiectasis
- Collapse
- Consolidation

What Are Rheumatoid Arthritis Effects On Lungs?

- Pulmonary nodules
- Obliterative bronchiolitis
- Lung fibrosis (basal fine end inspiratory crackles)
- Pleurisy
- Pleural effusion (<u>HIGH</u>: protein , LDH , RF , <u>LOW</u> : Glucose,C3,C4 , never blood stained)

SVCO

Clinical Examination

- Dilated chest veins
- Congested non pulsating neck veins
- Dilated arm veins
- Congested face
- U.Ls edema
- Any chest finding
- Findings consistent with Lung CA

Look for a cause:

- *Lung CA*: as above
- *Lymphoma:* L.Ns generalized, HSM
- *End stage renal disease on hemodialysis with multiple failures of vascular access:* eg thrombosed fistulas, scars of previous neck lines or tunneled lines for hemodialysis.

Quick Discussion:

How Would You Like To Diagnose This Case?

CT Chest with Contrast Is Diagnostic

What Is The Treatment of SVCO?

- Dexamethasone.
- Stenting
- Anticoagulation
- Radiotherapy
- Oncology R/V
- Respiratory R/V

Pneumonectomy/Lobectomy

Clinical Examination

- Lateral Thoractomy scar
- Depression of the chest on the affected side
- Decreased chest expansion on the affected side
- Shift of Trachea to the affected side

	Upper Lobe Lobectomy	Lower Lobe Lobectomy	Pneumonectomy
Lung Expansion	Limited chest expansion	Limited chest expansion	No Chest movement on the affected side
Tracheal Shift	Severely shifted	Mildly shifted	Mildly or severely shifted
Percussion Posteriorly	Resonant	Dullness	Resonant in upper zone , dull in lower zone
Percussion Anteriorly	Dullness	Resonance	Resonant in upper zone , dull in lower zone
Breath Sounds Post.	Present	Diminished	Present upper zone , absent lower zone
Type of breathing	Vesicular /Bronchial	Vesicular	Vesicular/Bronchial + Crackles of the Stump due to its fibrosis
Breath Sounds Ant.	Diminished	Present	Present in upper zone , absent lower zone
Vocal Resonance Posteriorly	Normal	decreased	Absent in lower zones
Vocal Resonance Anteriorly	Decreased	Normal	Absent in lower zones

Quick Discussion:

What Are The Causes of Lobectomy/Pneumonectomy?

- Lung cancer (NSLC)
- Solitary pulmonary nodule of unknown cause
- Pulmonary adenoma causing hemoptysis
- Emphysema
- Bronchiectasis resistant to treatment Or localized
- T.B in old times
- Abscess
- ABPA
- Pulmonary infarcts

How Would You Like To Diagnose This Case?

- *CXR:* White out on the affected side with mediastinal shift

What Do Yo Know About Post Pneumonectomy Syndrome?

- Cough, Dyspnea, Inspiratory Stridor And Pneumonia After Pneumonectomy Of The Rt. Lung
- Due To Extrinsic Compression Of Trachea & Main Stem Bronchus Due To Mediastinal Shift And Hyperinflation Of Other Lung

How Can You Differentiate Between Lung Collapse & Pneumonectomy Clinically?

- Both have the same signs clinically
- The Only difference is By the presence of lateral thoracotomy scar in Pneumonectomy

What Are The Causes Of Lung Collapse?

- Post-surgical
- Pneumothorax
- Pleural effusion
- Enlarged L.Ns (Lymphoma)
- Bronchial Carcinoma
- Mucous Plug

Pneumothorax

Clinical Examination

- Limited chest expansion on affected side.
- Bulge of the affected side of the chest.
- There might be chest drain scars of previous pneumothoracis.
- Trachea deviated to the opposite side
- Hyper resonance on percussion
- Decreased breath sounds on affected side
- Decreased vocal resonance.

Look for a cause:

- *Idiopathic*: Young, tall, fit (Rupture Bleb)
- *Marfan Syndrome*: Tall, Span > height, high arched palate, thumb sign, Wrist sign
- *COPD:* Hyperinflated chest, Increased A-P diameter, Tar staining, Wheezing B/L, decreased Crico-Sternal distance, Tracheal tug (Rupture emphysematous bulla)
- *Asthma:* Young, wheezy
- *Central Lines, Ventilators, Chest Aspiration Scar, Trauma*

N.B: In Pneumothorax the trachea may be shifted away from lesion (tension) or towards lesion (if pneumothorax causing atelectasis of the lung)

Quick Discussion:

How Would You Like To Diagnose This Case?

1) Investigations To Confirm Diagnosis
- *CXR:* Jet Black at the affected side with collapsed lung, wide Ribs.

2) Investigations For The Cause & Underlying condition
- *CT chest:* Looking for bullae

3) Investigations For Complications
- ABG to assess oxygenation

What Are The Types Of Pneumothoracis?

1) Primary → Young age with no underlying lung disease
2) Secondary → More than 55 age with underlying lung disease

What Is The Treatment of Pneumothorax?

1) Primary
- If < 2 cm → No treatment required
- If > 2cm → Aspiration

2) Secondary
- If < 2 cm → Aspiration
- If > 2 cm → Chest drain

Cystic Fibrosis

Clinical Examination

- Short Stature
- Bronchiectasis
- Signs of diabetes (Necrobiosis Lipoidica, Diabetic Dermopathy, Peripheral Neuropathy)

Quick Discussion

What Other Symptoms & Signs Associated With Cystic Fibrosis?

- Infertility
- Chronic Pancereatitis (D.M, Malabsorption)

What Is The Cause Of Cystic Fibrosis?

- Autosomal recessive
- Chloride channel abnormality

How Can You Diagnose It?

- CFTR gene on chromosome 7
- Sweat test → Chlorine > 60 mmol

How would you Treat it?

- Supportive
- Treat complications (See Bronchiectasis)

Kartagner`s syndrome

Clinical Examination

- Dextrocardia
- Bronchiectasis

Quick Discussion

What Other Symptoms & Signs Associated With Cystic Fibrosis?

- Infertility
- Recurrent Sinusitis

How Can You Diagnose It?

- Electron Microscopy to Visualize Ciliary Ultra-Structure
- Investigations for Bronchiectasis
- Investigations for other complicatuons.

Tuberculosis

Clinical Examination

- ? Cervical Lymphadenopathy
- ? Erythema nodosum
- Consolidation, Cavitation, Bronchiectasis, Apical fibrosis , pleural effusion signs
- Most Signs are in the Upper Lobes.
- T.B is a cause of unilateral Lung fibrosis

Quick Discussion

How Will You Diagnose It?

- Diagnosed by 3 sputum analysis with Zeil Neilson for acid fast bacilli
- Culture with Bactic or Lovenstien Jensen
- QUANTIFERON
- T-Spot

How Would You Treat him?

- Admission to hospital if Open T.B.
- Isolation
- Treatment with anti-tuberculous medications

What Is Phrenic Nerve Crush?

Supraclavicular scar for T.B treatment in old times

Obesity Related Lung Disease (OSA,OHS)

Clinical Examination

- Obesity
- Pulmonary HTN signs
- ? Core-Pulmonale
- Diminished breath sounds bilaterally

Quick Discussion

What Are The Cause of Morbid Obesity?

- Cushing
- Laurance moon Biedl
- Acromegaly
- Down syndrome
- Hypothyroidism
- PCO
- Eating disorders

What Other Symptoms & Signs The Patient Might have?

- Early morning headaches
- Day time Somnolence
- Apnea during night
- HTN
- Diabetes
- Pulmonary HTN
- Polycythemia
- Type II RF

What Investigations Should You Do For This Patient?

- Restrictive defect on PFTs
- Sleep studies are diagnostic (Polysomnography)
- ABG might show Type II RF

What is the Treatment for This Patient?

- Wt. Loss
- CPAP/ BIPAP
- Mandibular Advancement Devices

Summary Of Respiratory Cases

	Vocal Resonance	Added Sounds	Type Of Breathing	Breath Sounds	Percussion	Trachea	Clubbing
Fibrosis	+/-	Fine End Inspiratory Crackles	Vesicular	Decreased	-	To	+ (30%)
Collapse	-/+	Absent	Absent/Bronchial	Absent	-	To	-
Pleural Effusion	-	Absent/Pleural Rub	Vesicular	Decreased	Stony Dull	Away	-
Consolidation	+	Crackles	Bronchial	Decreased	-	Central	-
Bronchiectasis	+	Early Coarse Crackles Change In Character By Coughing	Vesicular	Decreased	-	Central	+
COPD	-	Expiratory Rhonci	Vesic With Prolonged Expiration	Decreased	+	Central	-
Pneumothorax	-	Absent/Pleural Rub	Vesicular	Decreased	+	To/Away	-
Lobectomy	-	Absent	Vesicular	Decreased	-	To	-

Station I Abdominal Examination

1. <u>Scrub Your Hands</u>
2. <u>Greet The Patient, Introduce Yourself And Take Permission</u>
3. <u>Position The Patient 45 Degrees In Bed.</u>
4. <u>Expose Him From Chest (Nipples) To Inguinal Area And Read Instructions.</u>
5. <u>Stand At The End Of The Bed Take Your Time And Observe</u>

- **Built**
- **Age**
- **Comfortable** Or Not
- **Face** And **Neck**
  - *Parotid Enlargement*
    - CLD (Chronic Liver Disease)
    - Sarcoidosis
  - *Temporalis Wasting* → CLD
  - *Cushingoid Face*
    - Steroids Use →AIH (Auto-Immune Hepatitis) , Sarcoidosis , Renal Transplant
    - Cushing`s Syndrome
  - *Lipoatrophy/Hearing Aid* → Mesangiocapillary G.N
  - *SLE Rash* → AIH, Renal Failure, Renal Transplant
  - *Jaundice* → CLD , Chronic Hemolytic Anemia (CHA)
  - *Spider Nevi* → CLD
  - *Tattoes* → CLD
  - *Purpra* → Steroids/Myelofibrosis
  - *Central Lines* →Renal Failure
  - *Xanthelasma* → Nephrotic / PBC (Primary Biliary Cirrhosis)
  - *Muddy Complexion* → Chronic Hemolytic Anemia
  - *Thalassemia Facies*
  - *Facial Plethora + Conjunctival Injection* → PRV (Polycythemia Rubra Vera)
  - *Lupus Pernio* → Sarcoidosis
  - *Systemic Sclerosis Face*
- **Chest**
  - Gynecomastia → CLD/Spironolactone
  - Sparse Hair → CLD
  - Spider Nevi →CLD
  - Purpura
- **Abdomen**
  - Distension
  - Scars
  - Dilated Veins
  - Moving Organs
  - Flank Fullness → Ascites
  - Umbilicus Shifted Down → Organomegaly/Ascites
- **Hands**
  - *Clubbing*
    - CLD
    - FAP (Familial Adenomatous Polyposis)
    - IBD (Inflammatory bowel disease)
  - Leuconychia → Hypo-albuminema → CLD, Nephrotic syndrome
  - A-V Fistula
  - *RA changes* look for
    - Splenomegaly →Felty`s
    - HSM → If Amyloidosis
  - Tattoes → HCV,HBV
- **Legs**
  - Clubbing
  - L.L Edema

6. <u>Ask Him To Extend His Arms And Examine The Dorsum</u> For:

- Clubbing
- Leuconychia
- Half And Half Nails → Renal Failure
- Koilonychia → Iron Deficiency
- Purpura
- RA
- Systemic Sclerosis
  - Renal Failure
  - AIH
- Splinter Hemorrhage Look For Speelomegaly → IEC (Infective Endocarditis)

7. Ask Him To Turn His Hand Up And Examine The Palms For
- Palmar Erythema (Erythema Sparing The Center Of The Palm)=CLD
- Jane Way & Osler Nodules = IEC
- Carpal Tunnel Scar = Amyloidosis

8. Feel For Dupuyterin`s Contracture Or Its Scar → CLD

9. Ask Him To Pull His Wrist Back with The Patient Arms Unsupported And Examine For Flapping Tremors = CLD

10. Inspect The Patient`s Arms
- Purpra, Eccymosis
- *A-V Fistula* note if
  - It is Functioning → Thrill felt, Bruit Heard
  - Recently Used→ Needle mark signs
- Spider Nevi

11. Inspect Axilla
- Scars Of L.N. Biopsy → Lymphoprolefrative disorder
- Sparse Hair = CLD

12. Examine Eyes
- Jaundice = CLD, Hemolytic Anemia, PBC, Cancer Pancreas
- Pallor
- Xanthelasma → PBC, Nephrotic Syndrome

13. Examine Mouth
- Ulcers → IBD / Celiac Disease
- Lip Hyperplasia → Crohn`s Disease, Acromegaly
- HHT (Hereditary Hemorrhagic Telangiectasia)
- Gum Hypertrophy
  - Cyclosporine = Renal Transplant
  - AML (Acute Myeloid Leukemia)
  - Phenytoin Use
- Large Tongue = Amyloidosis

14. Ask Him To Turn His Head And Examine Neck for
- **JVP**
  - Elevated JVP with Prominent V wave + L.L Edema + Enlarged Tender Pulsatile Liver = Tricuspid Regurgitation
- **Spider Nevi**

15. Examine His Chest
- Gynecomastia → CLD
- Spider Nevi → CLD
  - Dilated Capillaries with branches which blanches on compression
  - Found in the distribution of SVCO (Arms, Face, Neck & Chest)
- Sparse Hair → CLD
- Lung Biopsy Scars could it be Sarcoidosis?
- Permcath or its scar → Hemo-dialysis

16. Ask Him To Sit Forward

17. Examine Cervical Lymph Nodes & Lt. Supraclavicular L.Ns
- If you find Enlarged Cervical L.Ns look for
  - Enlarged spleen
  - Inguinal & Axillary L.Ns

18. **Inspect The Back For Scars & Spider Nevi**
- Renal Scars:
  - o Nephrectomy= ADPKD
  - o Stones → Look for Lympho-Prolefrative Disorders
19. **Ask If He Has Any Pain In His Back And Examine For Sacral Edema**
20. **Take Permission To Lower The Bed Flat and lay the patient flat on bed.**
- You May Ask Him To Bend His Knees To Lax The Abdominal Muscles
21. **On Your Knees Inspect The Abdomen And Ask Him To Take Deep Breath**
- **Scars** (Stretch The Abdomen Skin If The Patient Is Obese To See The Scars)
  - o Lt. Subcostal = Splenectomy= Cr.H.A (Chronic Hemolytic Anaemia)
  - o Rt.Subcostal = Cholecystectomy = Cr.H.A
  - o Laparoscopy = Cholecystectomy = Chr.H.A, Crohn`s disease
  - o Ascites Tapping scars
  - o Peritoneal Dialysis (Tenchkoff Catheter)
  - o Rt. Illiac Fossa Scar = Renal Transplant /Appendectomy
  - o Mid Line Scar/Multiple Scars =Crohns
  - o Mercedes Benz Scar → Liver Transplantation
- **PEG Tube**
  - o If you find a PEG tube look for a neurological problem affecting swallowing
- **Dilated Veins**
  - o *Caput Madusa*
    - Portal HTN → CLD
    - Filling Away Of the Umblicus
  - o *IVCO* (Filling Towards the Umbilicus)
  - o Do Milking Test On the Dilated Veins Below Umbilicus, Feel For Thrill, Auscultate For Hum
22. **Ask If He Has Any Pain In The Abdomen**
- "Do You Have Any Pain In Your Tummy?"
23. **On Your Knees Superficially Palpate The Abdomen And Look To The Patient`s Face For Any Tenderness**
- If The Patient has Pain in an area start palpating away from the Site of Pain.
- The Rule is to start from the Right Iliac Fossa & to Palpate all the nine quadrants of the abdomen.
- Note Any Masses In Rt./Lt. Iliac Fossae
- Note Epigastric Masses
- Note Liver Mass , Note Splenic Mass
24. **Palpate For The Liver Lower Border** from Rt. Iliac Fossa upwards **asking the patient to breath in during palpating** And **Percuss For It** & **Feel Its Edge** & **Measure How Many Cm.... Below Costal Margin & Note:**
- **Consistency**
  - o *Firm*
    - CLD
    - CHA
    - Sarcoidosis
    - Malignancy

  - o *Hard*
    - *Malignancy*
  - o *Soft*
    - NASH
    - Cysts in the liver
    - Heart failure
    - Tricuspid Regurgitation

- **Edge**
  - o *Sharp*
    - CLD
    - Sarcoidosis
    - Malignancy

- CHA
  - *Rounded*
    - NASH
    - Heart failure
    - Sarcoidosis
    - PRV
- **Tenderness**
  - Infection
  - Tricuspid regurgitation
  - Heart Failure
25. **Find The Upper Border Of Liver With Heavy Percussion On The Right Side Mid Clavicular Line From Up Downwards and Measure How Many Cm From Costal Margin**
26. **Add Both Measurements; That's The Liver Span** (N=10-12cm)
27. **Feel The Liver Surface By Rubbing With The Palmar Side Of Fingers for**
- **Consistency**
- **Surface**
  - Nodular
    - Cirrhosis
    - Metastasis
  - Smooth
- **Pulsations** → Tricuspid Regurgitation
- **Tendernss**
28. **Do Abdomino-jugular Reflux For 15 Sec.**
29. **Palpate For The Spleen From Rt. Iliac Fossa Diagonally Towards The Lt. Hypochondrium**
30. **If You Can't Find The Spleen Ask the Patient to Roll on His Right Side** and Support The Lt. Costal Area With Your Left Hand And Feel For The Spleen With Your Right Hand fingers.
31. **Percuss The Traube`s Area for Dullness or Percuss Lt. 9ᵗʰ ICS Anterior Axillary Line On Deep Expiration Then On Deep Inspiration ; If Note Changes From Resonance On Deep Expiration To Dull On Deep Inspiration Then +Ve Castell Sign** = Splenomegaly
32. **If You Find an Enlarged Spleen** Measure How Many Cms Below Costal Margin; Comment On **Edge**, **Consistency**, **Surface** And **Tenderness**
33. **For Massive Ascitis Do Dipping Method For Palpating Organs.**
34. **Palpate For Kidneys And Do Ballotment**
- Anterior Ballotment (Moves Anteriorly)
- Posterior Ballotment (Moves Posteriorly)
- A Kidney Mass Should Be Ant & Post Ballotable
35. **Percuss for Ascites**
- Percuss By Light Percussion From Midline Downward Until You Find Resonance (Below Umbilicus Is The Best)
- Then From Resonance Percuss Parallel To Midline Towards Lt. Side Looking for For Dullness In Flanks
- Then Ask The Patient To Turn On Right Side while your finger is still on the same place of dullness And wait 30 seconds and percuss again See If Dullness becomes Resonant (**Shifting Dullness**)
- Percussion for ascites should be done on both sides.
- For Massive Ascitis Do Fluid Thrill Test
36. **Auscultate** Liver, Spleen, Renal Arteries, Intestinal Sounds, Venous Hum Above Umbilicus.
37. **Examine For Inguinal Hernias**
38. **Examine The Legs for**
- Lower Limb Edema → CLD, RF, NEPHROTIC
- Clubbing
  - CLD
  - FAP
  - Crohns
  - Celiac

- o Bilharzial Polyposis
- Purpura
- Amputations
- Necrobiosis Lipoidica → D.M. →Renal Failure
- Pyoderma Gangrenosa → IBD, RA
- Erythema Nodosum → IBD, Sarcoidosis
- Vitiligo =AIH, PBC (Primary Biliary Cirrhosis)
39. <u>**Thank The Patient**</u>
40. <u>**Cover Him**</u>
41. <u>**Formulate Your Diagnosis:**</u>
- **Diagnosis** (HSM, Renal Transplant)
- **Possible Causes** (Viral Hepatitis, AIH, Chr.Hemolytic Anemia Lympho-Prolefrative, Sarcoidosis, Myelofibrosis)
- **Complications** (Decompensated Chronic Liver Disease, Nephrolithiasis, Choledeco-lithiasis, Cholecystectomy)

Abdominal Case Presentation

This Gentleman Is Lying Comfortable In Bed With Average Built, He Has Signs Of CLD In The Form Of ...../He Has No Stigmata Of CLD , He Has Hepatomegaly ...Cm Span , Sharp Edge , Firm Consistency , Smooth Surface, Non-Tender, Non-Pulsatile With No Bruit Over it, He Has Splenomegaly ...Cm Below Lt. Costal Margin, Sharp Edge , Smooth Surface, Firm Consistency, Non-Tender, No Bruit Over It , No Shifting Dullness/+ve Shifting Dullness

My Diagnosis is ... as evidenced by ....

I Would Like To Complete My Examination By Examining Hernia Orificies, External Genitalia, Doing P/R, Urine Dipstick, Looking At Patient Observation Charts.

Abdominal Examination Common Pitfalls

1-Starting examination directly without the 30 seconds general survey of the patient, as result you will miss very obvious and helpful findings such as temporalis wasting, purpura...etc.

2-Starting superficial palpation without asking the patient if he has any pain in his tummy, and hurting the patient.

3-Superficial palpation of the abdomen without looking to his face, as a result, you will hurt the patient.

4-Forgetting to examine for flapping tremors.

5-Overlooking any palpable masses under your hands during superficial palpation

6-Imagening an enlarged Lt. Lobe of the liver as a palpable spleen (Enlarged spleen equals dullness in Traube`s area)

7-Imagening an enlarged spleen as an enlarged kidney

	Enlarged Spleen	Enlarged Kidney
Extent	Cannot get above mass	Hand can get between mass & Costal Margin
Mobility	Moves downwards & Medially with inspiration	Limited movement downwards on inspiration
Shape	Splenic Notch	No Notch
Percussion	Dull	Resonant
Ballotment	Not Ballotable	Ballotable

8-Imagening an appendectomy scar as a kidney transplant scar

• You will feel a mass under the Scar if it is a transplanted Kidney

9-Omitting examination of inguinal orifices at the end of the examination.

Abdomen Cases

Chronic Liver Disease

Clinical Examination

- Stigmata of Chronic Liver Disease
  - Temporalis wasting
  - Enlarged parotids
  - Clubbing
  - Leukonychia
  - Dupuytren's contracture
  - Palmar erythema
  - Flapping Tremors
  - Multiple spider nevi
  - Fetor hepaticas
- Jaundice
- HSM or Hepatomegaly only or splenomegaly with shrunken liver
- Liver if felt is firm in consistency, sharp edge, could be nodular surface because of cirrhosis.
- ? Ascites
- ? Caput medusa

Look for a cause:

- *Viral hepatitis:* Tattoos, IV drug abuse needle marks.
- *Auto-immune hepatitis*: Steroids use signs, other auto-immune condition e.g. Vitiligo
- *PBC:* Xanthelasma + Scratch Marks +Other auto-immune disorders
- *Haemochromatosis*: Tanning of the skin or medic alert bracelet/Necklace, venesection marks, Arthritis, Signs of D.M (Insulin injection sites , Necrobiosis lipoidica)
- *Wilson:* Kayser flycher ring in eyes
- *Alpha 1 antitrypsin deficiency*: Hyper-inflated chest with wheezing
- *Drugs*: Amiodarone/Methotrexate /INH
- *Alcohol:* Dupuytren's contracture.

Quick Discussion

How Would You Investigate This Case?

1) Investigations To Confirm the Diagnosis
- U/S= cirrhosis of liver, portal hypertension
- Biopsy= bridging necrosis, piece meal necrosis ,fibrosis
- ALT, AST

2) Investigations To Look For A Cause
- Transferin Saturation , Serum Ferritin (Hemochromatosis)
- Urinary copper & Ceruloplasmin (Wilson)
- ANA , LKM , SLA , IgG (AIH)
- Serum Alpha 1 Antitrypsin Levels
- HBsAg, HCV Ab, HCV PCR, HBV PCR
- Serum IGM, and AMA esp M2 (PBC)

3) Investigations For Complications
- Serum albumin, PT (Prolonged PT & Low Albumin, Bilirubin
- Paracentesis For Ascites
- Alpha Feto Protein For Malignancy
- Endoscopy For Esophageal Varices

How would you treat this Patient?

1) Non-pharmacological
- Salt Restriction.
- Water restriction if Serum Na < 120 mmol/L
- Avoid Sedating & Hepatotoxic Drugs
- Alcohol Cessation

2) Pharmacological
- *Treatment of complications:*

o Spironolactone up to 100 mg OD, Furosemide Up to 180 mg/Day for ascites & L.L Oedema Targeting Daily Wt.Loss of ½ Kg if only L.L oedema or 1L if associated Ascites.
o Tapping of ascites with albumin replacement if needed.
o Beta blockers to decrease portal pressure
o Treatment of acute bleeding → Terlipressin, Octreotide, Vit K, Endoscopy, Blood Transfusion.
o Treatment of Encephalopathy → Lactulose, Enema, Rifaximin.
- *Treatment of the cause*
  o Viral hepatitis B
    ▪ peg INF & Anti-viral Medications e.g. Lamivudine, Adefovir, Enticavir
  o Viral hepatitis C
    ▪ Peg INF (Contraindications ; Auto-Immune Thyroid , Decompensation , Depression , B.M Depression , Psychosis , Pregnancy)
    ▪ Ribavirin
    ▪ Novel Anti Hep C Medication e.g. Sofosbuvir, Daclatasvir.
  o Auto immune hepatitis
    ▪ Steroids With Azathioprine
  o PBC
    ▪ Itching = Rifampicin, Naltrexone, Colestyramine , Antihistaminics
    ▪ Cholestasis & Progression Of Disease = Ursodeoxy Cholic Acid
    ▪ Hypercholesterolemia=Statins
  o Wilson
    ▪ D-penicillamine or Trientine
  o Hereditary hemochromatosis
    ▪ Venesection.

3) **Surgical**
- Band ligation for varices
- TIPS for Resistant Ascitis or Esophygeal bleeding
- Liver Transplantion For Cirrhosis (Contraindication= Severe Cardiopulmonary Disease, Alcoholic, End Stage Malignancy)

What Are The Complications Of CLD (Chronic Liver Disease)?

- Hemorrhage
- Esophageal varices
- Portal HTN
- Ascites
- Splenomegaly & Hypersplenisim
- Hepato-pulmonary syndrome
- Hepato-renal syndrome
- Encephalopathy
- SBP (Spontaneous Bacterial Peritonitis)

What Is Hepatorenal Syndrome?

Decreased liver ability to break down Vaso-active substances → Renal arteries vasoconstriction → Oliguria

What Do You Know About Decompensated CLD?

- Ascites
- Encephalopathy
- Astrexis

What Are The Hepatic Findings Of Alcohol Consumption?

- Acute hepatitis, hepatic steatosis, Cirrhosis, HCC (the liver is nodular)

What Are The Causes Of Nodular Enlarged Liver?

- Cirrhosis, Metastasis (carcinoid, malignancy), Hydatid cysts, Pyogenic abscess, Riedle Lobe

What Are The Degrees Of Hepatic Encephalopathy?

O=normal

1=disturbed sleep rhythm + Anxiety +Euphoria

2=Lethargy + Disorientation + Abnormal behavior + Apathy

3=Stupor + Confusion but respond to stimuli

4=Coma

How Do You Asses Child Pugh Classification?

	1	2	3
Bilirubin	<35	35-50	>50
Albumin	>35	28-35	<28
PT	<4	4-6	>6
Ascitis	Absent	Mild	Resistant
Encephalopathy	Absent	Mild	Severe

<7=A , 7-9 =B ,>9=C

If the patient has Ascitis its B or C

What Are The Different Causes Of Ascites ?

By SAAG → if > 1.1 =Transudate, if <1.1 Exudate

1-Chylous

2-Transudates: SAAG >1.1

- Nephrotic, CHF , Bud Chiari , RF (Renal Failure),
- Hypo-albuminemia, CLD
- Hypothyroidism , Meig`s Syndrome

3-Exudates: SAAG <1.1

- Bacterial peritonitis , T.B peritonitis , Malignant
- Pancreatitis

The commonest cause for Ascites with no stigmata of CLD is Malignancy

What Are The Indications For Liver Transplantation in Acute Hepatitis?

Kings College Hospital Criteria

1-*Paracetamol Induced Acute Liver Failure*

- PH<7.3, Garde III, IV encephalopathy, Creatinine > 300 , INR>6.5

2-*Non-Paracetamol Induced Acute Liver Failure*

- INR>6.5 , or INR>3.5 + Age <10 or >40 + Bilirubin >300

What Are The Causes & Effects Of Hemochromatosis?

- Restrictive cardiomyopathy, D.M., Arthropathy, hepatocellular carcinoma
- Autosomal recessive
- HFE gene on chromosome 6

HSM With No Stigmata Of CLD

Clinical Examination

- No Stigmata of Chronic liver disease
- Hepatomegaly
- Splenomegaly

Look For a Cause

- *Chronic hemolytic Anemia (CHA):* Muddy complexion , chipmunk facies
- *Bilharziasis:* Common Only In Some Countries In Which Bilharziasis Is Endemic e.g. Egypt
- *Lymphoprolefrative Disorder:* Generalized Lymphadenopathy.
- *Sacrcoidosis:* Cushingnoid features, Parotid enlargement, Lupus Pernio, Lung biopsy scars, Erythema nodosum (E.N.), Might Have Lung Fibrosis Signs, ? Cervical L.Ns.
- *Myeloprolefrative*:
  o CML
  o Myelofibrosis
  o PRV
- *Myelofibrosis:* Old age + Purpra + Eccymosis+ Massive Splenomegaly
- *PRV (Polycythemia Rubra Vera):* Facial Plethora, Conjunctival Injection
- *Amyloidosis*: Large Tongue (Indentation At Sides) + Carpal Tunnel Scar + Peripheral Neuropathy + ? Cause of Amyloidosis e.g. RA, Bronchiectasis
- *Gaucher`s disease*
- *Glycogen storage disease*
- *Early CLD*
- *Brucellosis:* Examine this farmers abdomen, ? L.Ns
- *Budd Chiari syndrome*: Tender Liver, ? Ascites
- *Congestive heart failure*: Raised JVP, L.L oedema, Tricuspid Regurgitation, Prominent V waves, Enlarged tender liver which is pulsatile , +ve Abdomino-jugular reflux
- *Leishmaniasis* :Common in certain countries

Quick Discussion

How would you investigate this case?

1) Investigations to Confirm The diagnosis

- U/S Scan
- CT Abdomen

2) Investigations for the Cause

- AML→ FBC, Blast cells
- ALL → Blast cells
- CML→ Philadelphia Chromosome (9,22 Translocation) <u>Treatment</u>: Imatinib
- CLL → Increased Lymphocytes, Immunophenotyping
- Chronic Hemolytic Anaemia → Low Hb, Increased Indirect Bilirubin & Retics, Dec. Haptoglobin , Hemopexin
- Thalassemia Hb Electrophoresis → Hb A2 , Hb F, Microcytic Anemia
- Sickle Cell Anemia →Hb Electrophoresis Hb SS, Hb SC.
- Spherocytosis → Osmotic Fragility Test
- PRV → Increased Red Blood Cell Mass , JAK2 Mutation
- Lymphoma → L.N Biopsy , CT For Staging
- Essential Thrombocytosis → Inc. Megakaryocytes In B.M
- Myelofibrosis → Tear Drop In Peripheral Blood, B.M Aspirate Dry Tap
- Gaucher`s Disease →Beta Glucosidase Activity In Leucocytes
- Glycogen Storage → Muscle, Liver Biopsy
- Bilharzia → Ova In Stool Or Rectal Biopsy
- Amyloidosis → Rectal Biopsy & Congo Red Stain
- Sarcoidosis → Serum ACE & Calcium , Chest X Ray
- Echo for TR, CHF

How Will You Treat This Patient?

- PRV → Hyroxyurea, Venesection.
- Lymphoma →Chemotherapy & Radiotherapy
- Bilharzia → Praziquantel
- Spherocytosis → Splenectomy
- Hemolytic Anemia → Blood Transfusion
- Surgical Removal Of Spleen If Massive Or Hypersplenism With Giving Lifelong Penicillins & Pneumococcal, Meningiococcal, Influenza Vaccines

N.B: Sickle Cell Anemia =No Splenomegaly

What Is Felty`S Syndrome?

RA + Splenomegaly + Neurtopenia (Signs Of Infection).

Hepatomegaly With No Stigmata Of CLD

Clinical Examination

- No Stigmata of CLD
- Liver Span >12cm
- No Ascites
- No Splenomegaly

Look for a Cause:

- *Viral Hepatitis*: SIRS, Tender Hepatomegaly
- *NASH:* Soft non tender
- *Chr. Haemolytic anemia* esp. sickle cell anemia: Afro-Caribean, Jaundice, ? infarcts, ? Amputations)
- *ADPKD:* Enlarged Ballotable Kidneys/Nephrectomy, Signs of Renal Replacement therapy, Tender Liver
- *Carcinoid syndrome*: Nodular liver, Facial Flushing & Telangectasia, Wheezing
- *Malignancy (Nodular Liver)*
- *CHF (congestive heart failure)*
- *Constrictive pericarditis*
- *Hydatid cyst*

Quick Discussion

What are the Causes of Tender Hepatomegaly ?

- o Acute Viral hepatitis
- o Budd-Chiari syndrome
- o Congestive cardiac failure
- o Malignancy
- o Tricuspid regurgitation (pulsatile)
- o Polycystic Liver

What Do You Know About Carcinoid Syndrome?

- Tumor Of Entero-Chromaphin Cells causing Hepatic Metastasis
- **Symtpoms:**
  - o Abdominal Pain, Wt. Loss, Flushing, Diarrhea,
  - o Hypotension, Tachycardia, Wheezing, Tricuspid Stenosis.
- **Investigations**
  - o Increased Urine 5HIAA, CT Scan To Localize Tumor
- **Treatment:**
  - o Somatostation, Cyproheptadine
  - o Surgical Debulking
  - o Radiotherapy, Chemotherapy

Splenomegaly With No Stigmata Of CLD

Clinical Examination

- No Stigmata of Chronic Liver Disease
- Splenomegaly

Look for a Cause:

- _Bilharziasis_
- _Myelofibrosis_: Massive Splenomegaly, Ecchymosis
- _CML_
- _Infective endocarditis_: Stigmata of IEC
- _RA_ (Felty`s syndrome): RA Hands
- _Splenic Abscess_
- _Splenic vein thrombosis_
- _Malaria_
- _Leshmania_
- _Pernicious Anemia_ (signs of autoimmune disease + Anemia + Neurological deficits)

Thalassemia

Clinical Examination

- Thalassemia facies
  - Prominent Zygoma
  - Widely Spaced Teeth
  - Muddy complexion
    - Jaundice
    - Pallor
    - 2ry Haemochromatosis
- HSM/Hepatomegaly
- ? splenectomy scar
- ? Laparoscopic cholecystectomy scar
- No stigmata of chronic liver disease
- Stigmata of Chronic Liver if HCV infected from repeated blood transfusion

Quick Discussion

What Is The Mode Of Inheritance Of Thalassemia Major?

- Autosomal Recessive

What Are The Complications Of Thalassemia?

1) Complications Of The Disease
- Skeletal deformities
- Severe Anemia
- Heart failure
- Gall stones

2) Complications Of Blood Transfusion
- Infections (HBV, HCV, HIV)
- 2ry hemochromatosis
  - Cardiomyopathy
  - Diabetes mellitus (pancreas)
  - Diabetes insipidus (pituitary)=Polyuria
  - Liver cirrhosis

3) Complications of Treatment (Iron chelators)
- Desferoxamine (parentral)→ Corneal deposits, SNHL (Sensory-neural hearing loss), Renal failure
- Deferrapron, Deferrazorax (Oral) → Arthropathy, Agranulocytodsis

What Type Of Hb Is Found In Thalassemia?

- HbA2, Hb F

What Is The Treatment Of Thalassemia?

1) Non –pharmacological: Education
2) Pharmacological:
- Regular blood transfusion → keep Hb.>10
- Iron chelating medications
- Desferoxamine /Deferraprone , Deferrazorax (Oral)

3) Surgical:
- Splenectomy
- B.M transplantation is the definitive Treatment

What Are The Indications For Splenectomy?

- Hyper-splenism
- Pressure symptoms

What Are The Causes Of Haemolytic Anemia?

- **Chronic:**
  - Spherocytosis (AD)

- o Thalassemia (AR) ,
- o Sickle cell (XL-R)
- **<u>Acquired:</u>**
  - o Autoimmune
    - Cold Antibodies (Mycoplasma , EBV)
    - Warm Antibodies (Lymphoma, Leukemia , SLE))
  - o Micro-angiopathic (DIC, TTP, HUS)
  - o Prosthetic valves

Crohn`s disease

Clinical Examination

- Underweight if active
- Clubbing
- ? Pallor
- Lip hyperplasia
- Oral ulcers
- Multiple abdominal scars (Bowel resection)
- Might have Right Subcostal scar / Laparoscopy scars for cholecystectomy (Gall Stones)
- Right iliac fossa mass
- ? Ileostomy ? Colostomy
- Erythema nodosum
- Pyoderma gangrenosum

Quick Discussion

What Are The Investigations?

- *Colonoscopy* reveals: Strictures, Masses, Hyperaemic mucosa & For Biopsy→ Granuloma.
- *Fecal Calprotectin*
- *ESR, CBC, Crp*
- ASCA (Anti S Cerevisiae Ab).

What Are The Treatments For Crohn`s?

1) Acute Attack: To Induce Remission
- Steroids
- Cytotoxic medications e.g. Azathioprine, Cyclosporine
- Biological therapy e.g. Infliximab, Adalimumab
- Metronidazole 1-2 m for peri-anal disease
- Enteral Nutrition
- 5-ASA Treatment

2) Between Attacks: To Maintain Remission
- Azathioprine
- 5-ASA
- Smoking Cessation

3) Indications for Surgery
- Persistent Symptoms Despite High Dose Steroids
- Toxic Megacolon
- Strictures
- Intractable Fistula
- Perforation Or Cancer

PEG tube

Clinical Examination

- Tube inserted in the epigastric region for feeding
- Be familiar with its shape

Always look for a cause

- Stroke (Hemiplegia Signs)
- CP (cerebral palsy)
- Head injury
- Brain tumors
- MS (Multiple sclerosis)
- MND
- Parkinson's disease (Static Tremors, Bradykinesia, Rigidity)
- Head & Neck cancer → there is a risk of seeding from standard pre-oral pull through technique of NG tube.

Quick Discussion

What Are The Complications Of Peg Tube Insertion?

- Hemorrhage
- Perforation
- Peritonitis
- Pneumonia
- Occlusion
- Displacement
- Death

Nephrotic Syndrome

Clinical Examination

- Leuconychia
- Bilateral L.L edema
- Puffiness around eyes
- Xanthelasma
- No Organomegaly
- ? Signs of Pleural effusion

Quick Discussion

What Is Nephrotic Syndrome?

It is a clinical syndrome characterized by:

- Nephrotic range proteinuria (> 3-3.5 gm > 24 hrs)
- Hypo-albuminaemia
- Hypercholesterolaemia
- Oedema

What Are The Causes Of Nephrotic Syndrome?

1) **Primary:** Idiopathic
2) **Secondary**
- *Minimal Change G.N*: Lymphoma, NSAIDS
- *FSGN*: HIV,Heroin, Sickle Cell
- *Membranous:* HBV, SLE, Gold, Neoplasia, Aceis
- *Mesansgiocapillary*: (SLE, Cryoglobulinemia)
- *Amyloidosis*
- *D.M*
- *IgA Nephropathy* with nephrotic range proteinuria

What Are The Investigations For nephrotic Syndrome?

1) **Investigations to confirm the diagnosis**
- Urine analysis for: Proteins, Casts, Active urinary sidements
- 24 Hr. Urinary protein → > 3gm
- PCR > 300 mg/mmol
- Cholesterol
- U&Es: Creatinine is usually normal unless complicated (AKI, associated nephritis)
2) **Investigations for the cause**
- Renal biopsy
- Fundoscopy looking for Diabetic changes to confirm Diabetes as a cause
- ANA, ANCA, C3, C4
- Serology (HBV, HCV, HIV)
- Rectal Biopsy for Amyloidosis
- PLA2R (Phospholipase A2 Receptor Antibody): Diagnosis of primary membranous nephropathy
3) **Investigation for complications**
- U/S KUB
- CXR for effusion
- Doppler for L.Ls for DVT
- Doppler of renal veins to R/O Renal Vein thrombosis
- Investigations for complications of the cause; e.g. Echo for amyloidosis

What Are The Complications Of Nephrotic Syndrome?

- Renal vein thrombosis (protein C & S deficiency)→ Sudden loin pain and hematuria, AKI.
- Atheroma & IHD
- Malnutrition
- Recurrent Infections (Loss of Immunoglobulins in urine)
- DVT (Hypercoagulable state)

What Are The Treatments For Nephrotic Syndrome?

1) Non-Pharmacological

- low salt diet, Water Restriction
- TEDS stocking to prevent DVT

2) Pharmacological

- Diuretics
- Statins
- Anticoagulation
- Treatment of the cause (2ry Causes)
- Idiopathic Nephrotic syndrome
    Steroids
    Cytotoxic medications.

ADPKD

Clinical Examination

- Patient Might Be Using a walking aid (Rupture of Berry Aneurysm)
- Flushed face with Conjunctival injection (Polycythemia)
- Bilaterally enlarged Ballotable kidneys
- Enlarged Cystic Tender liver
- ? Nephrectomy Scar

Look For Signs & Complications Of CKD/ESRD

- o Half & Half Nail
- o Fluid overload
- o Scratch Marks
- o Uremic Fetor
- o Parathyroidectomy scar

Look for Signs Of Renal Replacement Therapy

- o A-V shunts or
- o Dialysis catheter (Chest, Neck, Abdomen)
- o Transplanted kidney With Immuno-suppression signs

Quick Discussion

What Are The Causes Of Renal Cysts?

- ADPKD, ARPKD
- Von Hippel Lindu & Tuberous Sclerosis
- Simple Cyst

What Are The Causes Of Enlarged Kidney?

- Cystic Renal Diseases
- Renal Mass
- Hydronephrosis
- Infiltration (Amyloidosis, Metabolic Storage Diseases)

What Are The Complications Of ADPKD?

- ESRD
- Rupture of Berry`s aneurysm → SAH → Neurological deficit
- Recurrent urinary infections & Recurrent abdominal pain
- 2ry polycythemia → Hyper-Coagulable State
- HTN
- MVP (Mitral Valve Prolapse)
- Recurrent Kideny Stones (Uric Acid/Oxalate)

What Are The Cause Of ADPKD?

- Autosomal Dominant
  - o PKD1 on chromosome 16
  - o PKD2 on chromosome 4

What Are The Indication for Nephrectomy in ADPKD?

- Peristent Pain
- Recurrent Pyelonephritis
- Rescurrent Stone formation
- To Obtain Extra Rooom for Renal Transplantation If Massively Enlarged.

Renal Transplant

Clinical Examination

- Right iliac fossa scar / Lt.iliac fossa scar
- Rt.iliac fossa mass / Lt.iliac fossa mass (Transplant) Desrcibe:
  - Size
  - Site
  - Shape
  - Surface
  - Tenderness (Non-tender unless complicated)
  - Attachement to the surroundings
  - Percussion Note (Usually Dull)

Look For Signs Of Previous Renal Replacement Therapy

- Scars on Neck for central lines.
- Scars on Chest for Permcath dialysis
- Scars of PD on abdomen (Tenchkoff`s Catheter)
- A-V Fistula
  - Functioning (Bruit /Thrill) or Non functioning
  - Recently used or not

Look For Signs of Graft Dysfunction

- Raised JVP
- Uraemic Odor
- L.L Oedema
- Fine Crackles at the Lung Bases
- Signs of Ongoing Other Renal Replacement therapy Modalities
  - Current Central Lines
  - Fresh Puncture sites on a fucntiong A-V Fistula
  - Tenchkoff`s Cather in situ

Look For Signs & Complications of Immunosuppression

  - Cushingnoid features (Rounded plethoric face, Truncal obesity and Striae rubra, The Scars appear red, Thinning of skin , Petichie and Echymosis)
  - Gum hypertrophy → Cyclosporine
  - Fine Tremors → Tacrolimus
  - Skin lesions → SCC, BCC
  - Lympho-adenopathy

Look for Signs of the Causes & Complications of Renal Failure

- Nephrectomy scars
- B/L Enlarged Kidneys Which Are Ballotable + Enlarged Tender Cystic Liver (ADPKD)
- Neck scar for parathyroidectomy
- Hearing Aid (Alport`s)
- Diabetic Dermopathy, Cahrcoat Joint, Walking aid, Necrobiosis Lipoidica (D.M)
- Facial Lipo-atrophy → Messangio-capillary G.N

Quick Discussion

What Are The Main Causes of ESRD?

- Diabetes Mellitus
- HTN
- Inhereted Disease e.g. ADPKD, Alport`s
- Chronic G.N. (Glomerulopnephritis)
- Obstructive Neuropathy
- Vasculitis

What Are The Common Immuno-suppressants Used in Renal Transplant?

- *Steroids*
- *Calcineurin inhibitors*

- o Tacrolimus (Prograf)
- o Cyclosporin (Sandimmune)
- *mTOR Inhibitors*
  - o Sirolimus (Rapamune)
  - o Everolimus (Certican)
- *Antiproliferative Agents*
  - o Azathioprine
  - o Mycophenolate Mofetil (Cellcept)
  - o Mycofenolic acid (Myfortic)

What Are The Causes Of Tenderness Over The Graft?

- Graft Rejection
- Graft Infection

What Are The Complications of Renal Replacement Therapy?

1) **Complications Of Hemodialysis**
- Cardiovascular complications e.g. Ischaemic heart disease, Heart failure, Arrhythmias
- Vascular access Problems/Failure
- Hypotension
- Life Style Intolerance

2) **Complications Of Peritoneal Dialysis**
- Peritonitis
- Tube Related Problems
- Peritoneal Membrane Dysfunction
- EPS (Encapsulating Peritoneal Sclerosis)

3) **Complications Of Renal Transplantation**
- *Cardiovascular Complications*
- *Graft Rejection*
- *Immuno-Suppressants Complications*
  - o Recurrent Infections
  - o Malignancy
  - o Specific Complications for Cytotoxic medications
    - Steroids : D.M, Osteoprosis
    - CNIs: Hyperkalaemia, Hypertrichiosis, Post Transplant D.M., Graft Fibrosis
    - mTORs: Delayed wound healing, Hypercholesterolaemia
    - Antiprolefratives: Anaemia, Bone Marrow depression

How Would You Like To Investigate This Case?

Laboratory tests

- FBC
  - o Raised WBCs → Infection
  - o Low WBCs → CMV infection
  - o Anaemia → MMF
- U&Es
- Fasting blood sugar → Tacrolimus induced diabetes
- Tacrolimus/Cyclosprine levels
- VBG

Tests for Opportunistic Infections

- CMV PCR
- Polyoma Virua (BK) PCR
- PCP BAL

Imaging

- Renal U/S
- Renal Biopsy if suspected rejection /Unexplained Rise in U&Es
- CXR: if Fluid overload /Infection suspected.

What Are The Causes Of Masses In Lt. Iliac Fossa?

- Transplanted kidney

- Carcinoma of colon
- Neoplasia Lt. Ovary
- Fecal Mass

What Are The Causes Of Epigastric Mass?

- Carcinoma of Stomach (Virchow`s)
- Carcinoma of Pancreas (Courvoisier sign; enlarged gall bladder)
- Lymphoma
- Left Lobe Of The Liver
- Abdominal Aortic Aneurysm

What Are The Causes Of Masses In Rt. Illiac Fossa?

- Illeocecal T.B
- Carcinoma caecum
- Lymphoma
- Appendicular abscess
- Neoplasia of ovary
- Ileal carcinoid
- Pelvic kidney
- Transplanted kidney
- Crohns disease

Why In Alport`s Syndrome Kidney Transplantation May Be A Problem?

Because is Alport`s Syndrome, Patients lack collagen IV, So they develop anti-glomerular B.M antibodies after transplantation → Good pasture syndrome

What Is The Main Cause Of Mortality In ESRD?

Cardio-vascular diseases

Summary of HSM

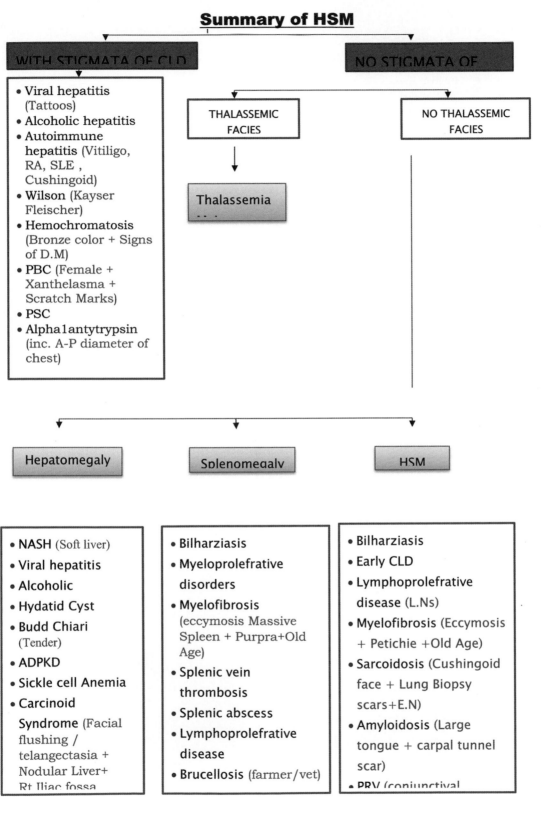

WITH STIGMATA OF CLD

- Viral hepatitis (Tattoos)
- Alcoholic hepatitis
- Autoimmune hepatitis (Vitiligo, RA, SLE , Cushingoid)
- Wilson (Kayser Fleischer)
- Hemochromatosis (Bronze color + Signs of D.M)
- PBC (Female + Xanthelasma + Scratch Marks)
- PSC
- Alpha1antytrypsin (inc. A-P diameter of chest)

NO STIGMATA OF

THALASSEMIC FACIES

Thalassemia

NO THALASSEMIC FACIES

Hepatomegaly

- **NASH** (Soft liver)
- Viral hepatitis
- Alcoholic
- Hydatid Cyst
- Budd Chiari (Tender)
- ADPKD
- Sickle cell Anemia
- Carcinoid Syndrome (Facial flushing / telangectasia + Nodular Liver+ Rt Iliac fossa

Splenomegaly

- Bilharziasis
- Myeloprolefrative disorders
- Myelofibrosis (eccymosis Massive Spleen + Purpra+Old Age)
- Splenic vein thrombosis
- Splenic abscess
- Lymphoprolefrative disease
- **Brucellosis** (farmer/vet)

HSM

- Bilharziasis
- Early CLD
- Lymphoprolefrative disease (L.Ns)
- Myelofibrosis (Eccymosis + Petichie +Old Age)
- Sarcoidosis (Cushingoid face + Lung Biopsy scars+E.N)
- Amyloidosis (Large tongue + carpal tunnel scar)
- PRV (conjunctival

STATION II

History Taking Skills

Introduction To Station II

Before You Start The Station You Have 5 Minutes To Read The Instructions; Read Them Well, Understand The Information Given, And Understand Your Task.

You Will Be Given A Pencil And A Paper; You Can Right Some Notes For Yourself Before You Get Into The Room:

- Your Role (SHO/Registrar Of …Clinic).
- The Patients Name.
- Differential Diagnoses.
- Important History That You Can Miss.
- And Highlights In The Information Given To You.
- The History Taking Scheme Outlined Below.

Station II Is An Easy Station To Pass And An Easy Station To Fail, So Be Prepared Well.

History Taking Is The Core Of Station V As Well.

The Key To Master This Station Is The Ability To Plot Sensible Differentials After Proper Analysis Of The Major Complaint.

While Carrying On With The Station And With Proper Analysis Of Your Major Complaint, New Complaints Will Arise And Accordingly You May Shorten Your List Of Differentials.

During Your Consultation You Should:

- Listen Attentively
- Satisfy The Patient By Explaining What's Wrong, And What You Can Do To Help
- Support And Empathy The Patient
- If You Are Going To Take Notes, Ask Your Patient First Or Let Them Know
- Explore The Problem With Open Questions
- Then Narrow Your Differentials By Asking Closed Targeted Questions.

General Scheme

The following Scheme should give you a broad idea and a Scheme that you should follow during your history taking scenario.

1. **Greeting**
2. **Introduce** yourself clearly and explain your role e.g: "Good morning I am Dr.... SHO of the general medical clinic".
3. Double   check the **Identity Of The Patient**; Name, Age , DOB
4. Establish a **Rapport** (break down the ice)
5. Explain **The Aim Of The Appointment** e.g.: "I received a letter from your GP stating that you have problems with your breathing, is that right"?
6. **Analysis Of The Complaint** with Open questions e.g.: "Can you tell me more about that?" This should be followed by further questions to analyze the complaint; each symptom analysis will be discussed later.

The complaint could be in the form of pain or not.

- If pain remember *SOCRATES* (site, onset, course, radiation, associated symptoms, exacerbating factors, severity),
- If not pain then remember *OCDAE* (onset, course, duration, associated symptoms, exacerbating factors)

7. Ask about **Symptoms Relating To The Main Complaint**; *To R/O Differential Diagnosis,* Symptoms of the **Same System**, symptoms of **Related Systems**.
8. **System enquiry**:

Cardiology Symptoms

- Chest pain **(Cardiac or non-cardiac)**
- Racing heart **(Palpitations)**
- Shortness of breath **(Dyspnea)**
- **Left side heart failure symptoms** (Shortness of breath on lying flat (orthopnea), waking up from sleep short of breath needing to sit up (paroxysmal nocturnal dyspnea))
- **Low Cardiac output symptoms** (dizziness , headaches , leg cramps , Black outs or funny turns)
- **Right side heart failure symptoms** (pain in tummy (right hypochondrium), swollen legs)

Chest Symptoms

- Chest pain
- Shortness of breath
- Coughing
- Phlegm production **(Sputum production)**
  - What Color is it?
  - How frequent?
  - Amount?
- Coughing blood **(Hemoptysis)**
- Noisy chest **(wheezing)**
- Sore throat **(URTI)**
- Runny nose
- Snoring **(Upper airway obstruction/OSA)**

Gastrointestinal Symptoms:

- Tummy pain **(Abdominal pain)**
- Feeling sick **(nausea)**
- Heart burn **(Reflux)**
- Difficulty swallowing **(Dysphagia)**
- Painful swallowing **(Odynophagia)**
- Vomiting **(Throwing up)**

- How frequent do you open your bowels **(General question about bowel habits)**
- Lose motions **(Diarrhea)**
- Is it easy to flush it down **(Steatorrhea)**
- Vomiting of blood **(Hematemesis)**
- Bleeding with back passage **(Hematochezia)**
- Pain with the back passage
- Passing black Tarry Offensive motions **(Melena)**
- Swollen tummy **(Distended abdomen)**
- Yellowish discoloration of the eye white **(Jaundice)**
- Change in color of motions; Paller Or Darker.

Neurological Symptoms

- Headaches , neck stiffness **(Meningeal irritation)**
- Dizziness
- Weakness of arms or legs
- Abnormal sensation in hands or feet like pins & needles.
- Handshakes **(Tremors)**
- Abnormal movements of arms or legs
- Gait disturbances / unsteadiness on your feet **(Ataxia)**
- Fits, seizures
- Speech abnormalities
- Visual disturbance
- Double vision
- Hearing problems
- Memory problems
- Confusion
- Autonomic Dysfuntion
  o Urinary Retention / Incontinence
  o Constipation
  o Impotence

Endocrinology Symptoms

- Intolerance to hot or cold weather
- Shoes size does it still fit, ring size does it still fit
- Weight gain/loss
- Bowel motions
- Abnormal pigmentations on your skin
- Any problems with sexual drive/intercourse
- Drinking more water than usual/passing more urine (water works) than usual
- Eating more than usual

Rheumatological Symptoms

- Joint pains; Analyze Joint Pains Using mnemonic "**PND + 3S**"
  o *Pain* **(SOCRATES)**
  o *Number:* No. Of Joint affected
  o *Deformity:* present or absent
  o *Stiffness:* Present or absent, if present for how long & when
  o *Swelling*
  o *Symmetry*
- Skin rash, Bruising, Acne
- Oral sores
- Morning stiffness of joints
- Skin tightness
- Muscle pains

- Muscle weakness

Genito-Urinary

- Hesitancy, straining , poor flow , dribbling and sense of incomplete evacuation **(Males)**
- Passing less/more urine than usual **(Polyuria/Oliguria)**
- Burning pains with your water works **(Dysuria)**
- Change in color or smell of your water works
- Abnormal discharge from private areas
- What about your periods? Regular? Any problems? Problems with amounts or timings? When did you first start to have periods? Using any methods of contraception? Are you using the pill? **(Females)**

General Symptoms

- Rise in body temperature
- Tiredness
- Lumps or Bumps
- Weight loss/Gain
- Bluish discoloration of the lips
- Pallor
- Hair Loss, Excessive Hair Growth
- Eye Symptoms

Psychiatry:

- What about your mood?
- If severely depressed ask about suicidal attempts; not in all cases
- Unusual thoughts, Thoat broadcast, Thought insertion.
- Hallucinations "Do You See Things That People Can not See?, Do You Hear Voices people Can not Hear"
- Delusions.

9. Past medical history:

- Ask the patient does he have any past medical or surgical history?
- Ask the patient specifically about:
    o T.B, D.M , HTN, heart disease , lung diseases
    o Blood transfusion
    o Previous hospital admissions
    o Diseases of endemic areas if a traveler
    o Previous surgeries and whether they were eventful or uneventful?

10.   Drug history:

- Any regular medications?
- Any over the counter medications/Remedies?
- Female patients ask about the Pill? (oral contraceptive pills)
- Any use of recreational drugs?
- Any allergies to ....?

(medications/ latex/ Anything else/ pets/ When Moving houses, ...etc)?

11.   Family history

- Any similar conditions in the family?
- Any diseases running in family?
- How are the parents and siblings; any diseases? And cause of death if appropriate?
- Are the parents relatives?

12.   Social history

- *Occupation*; what do you do for living?
- *Residence*; where do you live? Is it a house, flat, bungalow?
    o See if there is impact of residence on the symptoms?

- *Impact of symptoms on daily life?*
- *Impact of daily life on symptoms*
- *Financial issues? any problems?*
- *Do you drive?*
- *Do you smoke?* If yes, How many cigarettes/packs daily?? For how long?
- *Do you drink alcohol?* If yes, how frequent??

> If the patient drinks alcohol heavily, you need to ask about the (C A G E) questionnaire. This easy-to-use patient questionnaire is a screening test for problematic drinking and potential alcohol problems
>
> **C**: Have you ever felt you should **C**ut down on your drinking?
>
> **A**: Have people **A**nnoyed you by criticizing your drinking?
>
> **G**: Have you ever felt bad or **G**uilty about your drinking?
>
> **E**: Have you ever had a drink first thing in the morning to steady your nerves or to get rid of a hangover (**E**ye opener)?
>
> Two "yes" responses indicate that the possibility of alcoholism should be investigated further. In that situation, it would be nice to offer help as referring to (Alcohol cessation clinic/ Rehabilitation for alcoholism).

13. Sexual history

Ask about sexual history in details if you feel that this would help you reach your diagnosis: HIV, STDs ...etc.

Must ask in a very polite and conservative way. "I would like to ask you some private questions about your sexual life if you don't mind. Is that OK?"

Ask about: **"4Ps"**

- **P**artner? (Single Vs Multiple)
- **P**references? (Homosexual/Bisexual/Heterosexual)
- **P**rotection? (Using Condoms)
- **P**roblems during Sexual Intercourse.

14. Travel history

Has the patient travelled abroad recently?

15. The main concern

Ask the patient specifically about his concerns and *manage it.*

"So What Are Your Concerns?"

16. Surprise

Here you should write down *Symptoms appearing during taking the history*, which will narrow your Differential diagnosis

Each symptom should be analyzed in details just as analyzing the major symptom.

17. Differential diagnosis

Before entering the station you may have a long list of differentials.

While taking history some of the differentials will be excluded and *the list will be shortened*, **it is important to re-arrange your list starting with the most probable diagnosis according to the symptoms you gathered from your patient**, Then the close differentials to this diagnosis.

During your conversation with the examiner, try to justify your diagnosis (what is with, and what is against) and why you did exclude other differentials.

18. Plan

You need to *re-assure the patient* and *explain honestly* what you are thinking about. You should *sort out a plan* in order to reach your diagnosis and *ensure patient safety.*

This plan may include;

- Bloods
- Scans
- Senior Opinion
- Referral To Other Specialties
- Admission If Necessary Or
- Sorting Future Appointments In Clinics.
- Driving Advice
- Specialist Nurse Referral
- Specialist Team referral
- Support Groups referral
- Written Information

The following scheme is a draft for you to use in the exam in order not to miss any item and keep important points in front of your eyes, please memorize it well.

GENERAL SCHEME

A: Analysis of complaint (HPI)
S: System enquiry
P: Past history
F: Family history
A: Allergies
S: Social history
S: Sexual history
T: Travel history

CONCERN

SURPRISE

Here you should write down
Symptoms appearing during
taking The history, which will
narrow your Differential
diagnosis

ANALYSIS OF THE COMPLAINT

Pain	Not
S: Site	**O:** Onset
O: Onset	**C:** Course
C: Course	**D:** Duration
R: Radiation	**A:** Associations
A: Associations	**E:** Exacerbations
T: Timing	
E: Exacerbating & relieving Factors	
S: Severity	

DIFFERENTIAL DIAGNOSIS

Here you should write down your
differential diagnosis for the
leading symptoms given you in
the scenario before entering the
station.

SYSTEM ENQUIRY

Genito-Urinary	Psychiatry	General Symptoms

PLAN

- Blood
- Scans
- Admission
- Referrals
- Next appointments/Follow up
- Notification if needed
- Driving advice
- Social advice (Smoking, alcohol, etc...)

Case Scenarios

Headache

Differential Diagnosis

Serious Causes	Common Causes	Other Causes
• Subarachnoid Hemorrhage	• Migraine	• Brain Abscess, HIV
• Meningitis	• Tension Headache	• Smoking Cessation
• Carotid Or Vertebral Artery Dissection	• Autonomic Cephalgias (Cluster Headache)	• Carbon Monoxide Poisoning
• Cerebral Venous Thrombosis	• Exertional	• Alcohol withdrawal
• Pituitary Apoplexy	• Medication Overuse Headache	
• GCA	• Trigeminal neuralgia	
• Intracerebral Hemorrhage	• Benign Intracranial HTN	
• Brain tumors:1ry or 2ry	• Metabolic Causes (Dehydration, Hyponatraemia)	
	• Uncontrolled HTN	
	• Errors of Refraction	
	• Referred Pain: Tooth, Ear, Sinuses, Eyes, Face, Neck	

Analysis Of Complaint

- Initially double check **What Is Meant By Headache**?
  - Headache is pain of the head vault.
  - It is different than facial pain or neck pain, but patients may name all (headache).
- Headache is pain, so **Follow SOCRATES.**
  - Where Exactly In Your Head?
  - How Did It Start; Suddenly Or Gradually?
  - How Long?
  - Is It Getting Better Or Worse?
  - Could You Describe The Pain?? Is It Throbbing, Band Like, Boring Pain??
  - Is It Radiating Any Where Else?
  - Do You Have It All The Time/Attacks? When Mostly? (Tension At Night, Increased ICP In Morning)
  - What Makes It Better? What Makes It Worse?
  - How Would You Give It On A Scale From 0-10? Is It The Worst Headache In Your Life?

Questions To R/O Differential Diagnosis

Encephalitis / Meningitis

- Have You Noticed Any Fevers? Skin Rash? Stiffness Of Your Neck?
- Any Contact With Sick Children?

- Change In Behavior? Consciousness?

PMR/GCA

- Is It On The Temporal Side Of the Head?
- Any Pain & Stiffness in Your Shoulders?
- Head Pain, Jaw Cramps/Claudication While Eating?
- Any Visual Problems?

Sub/Extra Dural Hematomas

- Did You Hit Your Head?
- Are you on Any Blood Thinners?
- Change In Behavior? Consciousness?
- Any Associated weakness?
- Do You Drink Alcohol? *(Chronic Subdural)*

Sub-Arachnoid Hemorrhage

- The Worst headache Ever?
- Neck Stiffness?
- Are you Taking Any Blood Thinners?
- *PMH* of Kidney problems?
- *FH*: Of Bleed In the Brain?

Increased ICP

- Does It Occur In The Early Morning?
- Do You Through Up?
- Any Blurring Of Vision?
- Any Weakness in Arms or Legs?
- Any Fits?

Pituitary Tumors

- Signs of Increased ICP: See Before
- **Acromegaly**:
  o What About Your Shoe And Ring Size, Do They Fit?
  o Can You See The Sides Of The Road?
- **Prolactinoma:**
  o Any Breast Discharge?
  o Decreased sexual desire?
- **Pituitary Apoplexy**
  o Any Sudden Severe Bleeding?
  o Associated Endocrine Symptoms?

Cerebral Sinus Thrombosis

- Any PMH of Having Clots in Your Legs or Lungs?
- Double Vision?
- Any Medication Causing your Blood to be Thicker, e.g. HRT, OCPs.
- Are You Pregnant? (For female patients)
- Acute Onset, Thunder Clap Headache.

Benign Intracranial Hypertension

- Have You Gained Weight Recently?
- Do You Have Double Vision?
- Are You Taking Steroids, Vit. A, Tetracyclines, OCPs?
- All tests Done are Normal?

Tension Headache

- Is It Band Like Over Your Head, Occurs At The End Of The Day?
- Have You Been Stressed Recently?
- What About Your Mood?

Migraine

- Is It Unilateral?

- Is It Preceded By Any Unusual Sensations, Taste In Your Mouth?
- Any Weakness?
- Any Blurry Vision? (Aura)
- Eased by sitting in Dark Quiet Room?

Cluster Headache

- Is It Around the Eyes?
- Occurring in Clusters?
- Any Watering Of Your Eyes? Redness?
- Runny Nose, Nose Blockage?
- Does It Occur Several Times In The Day?
- Does It Occur At The Same Time Each Year?

Trigeminal Neuralgia

- Any Pain In Your Face, Triggered By Chewing, Washing Face?

Carbon Monoxide Poisoning

- Does It Get Better When You Are Away From Home?
- Other Family Members having The Same Symptoms?
- Do You Have Any Fuel Burning Devices (Furnaces, Gas Heaters, Gas Boilers, Gas Working Stoves, Gas Generators, and Power Tools?

Medications Induced headache

- Nitrates?
- Sildenafil?
- Long standing Analgesics (Opioids & Non-Opioids) Use?

Hypertension

PMH of HTN or New Diagnosis?

Quick Discussion

How Would You Investigate This Case?

- **CT Head With or Without Contrast / MRI Brain for:**
  - o Brain Tumors
  - o Bleeds
  - o SAH
  - o Meningitis/Encephalitis
- **Lumbar Puncture**
  - o SAH→ Xanthochromia
  - o Meningitis→ raised proteins, Raised WBCs, Glucose abnormality according to the cause
  - o Idiopathic Intracranial HTN → Raised opening pressure & therapeutic
- **Temporal Artery Biopsy** → GCA
- **Pituitary Function tests** → Pituitary Tumors/Apoplexy
- **VBG** → CO Poisoning

How Would You Treat This Case With Headache?

- Analgesia
- Admit to hospital If Alarming Symptoms
- Treat The Cause
  - o *Migraine* → Analgesia Sumatriptan, Prevention with Betablocker & TCA
  - o *Cluster Headache* → high Flow Oxygn , Analgesia , prophylaxis with CCBs
  - o *Brain Tumor* → Neurosurgical R/V
  - o *Pituitary Apolpexy* → Endocrine/Neuro-surgical R/V
  - o *Meningitis* → Antibiotics + Admission to hospital
  - o *Blood Pressure Control*
  - o *Trigeminal Neuralgia* → Carbamazepine

Chest Pain

Differential Diagnosis

Cardiac Causes:

- Ischemic Heart Disease
  - ACS
    - Unstable angina
    - NSTEMI
    - STEMI
    - Stable Angina
- Myocarditis
- Pericarditis
- Dissecting Aortic Aneurysm
- Pulmonary Embolism
- Aortic Stenosis
- Arrhythmias
- Mitral Valve Prolapse

Non-Cardiac

- **Respiratory**
  - Pleurisy
    - Chest Infection
    - Collagen disorders e.g. SLE, RA
    - Poly-serositis e.g. FMF
  - Pneumothorax
  - Pleural Effusion
  - Asthma
- **Chest Wall**
  - Trauma
  - Myositis
  - Tietze`s syndrome (Costochondtritis)
  - Rib Fractures
- **Eosophygeal**
  - Rupture esophagus (Boerhove`s)
  - GORD
  - Diffuse esophageal spasm
- **General**
  - Sildenafil
  - Cocaine
  - Anemia
  - Fibromyalgia

o Herpes Zoster

Analysis Of Complaint

Follow SOCRATES.

- *Where Exactly* In Your Chest?
  - o Ask The Patient To Point out where he feels the pain with his hand
    - If The Patient Can Localize the pain with 1 finger→ it is non-cardiac
    - If the Patient Localizes the pain with a fist→ Possibly cardiac
- How Did It Start; *Suddenly Or Gradually*?
  - o Cardiac Ischemic pain is usually sudden, acute or subacute.
- *How Long*?
  - o Chest pain more than 30 minutes in duration is less likely ischemic
- Is It *Getting Better Or Worse*?
- Could You *Describe The Pain*?? Is It Stabbing Like, Heaviness Like, Burning Like, Tearing Like?
  - o Heaviness →Cardiac Ischemia
  - o Stabbing → Pleurisy, Pneumothorax, PE, Pleural effusion
  - o Burning → GORD ?? Cardiac
  - o Tearing Pain Radiating to the Back→ Aortic Dissection
- *Is It Radiati*ng Any Where Else?
  - o Cardiac Ischemic Pain radiates to the Jaw, Lt. Arm or epigastrium
  - o GORD → Radiates to The Throat
  - o Aortic dissection→Radiates to the back
- *Do You Have It All The Time*/Attacks? When Mostly?
  - o Ischemic cardiac Pain occurs with exertion unless Unstable angina develops it becomes more frequent and not related to exertion.
  - o Myocardial Infarction Pain is Not relieved by GTN or rest.
  - o Aortic Dissection Pain is very severe.
  - o Pericarditis chest pain improve by leaning forwards and NSAIDs and worsens by Laying flat.
  - o GORD is worse by fatty meals and Laying Flat, Improved by sitting Up.
- *What Makes It Better? What Makes It Worse?*
  - o Typical Cardiac Ischemic Chest Pain → Worse after exertion & heavy Meals, Relieved by rest
  - o Pleuritic Pain Worse on Inspiration.
- *How Would You Give It On A Scale From 0-10?*
- *Associated Symptoms?*

Cardiac Ischemic Pain	N & V, Sweating, Pallor, SOB ,Palpitations And Dizziness, Or Symptoms Of CCF
Respiratory Tract Infection	Cough, Sputum, Fever, Hemoptysis
PE	SOB, Palpitations, Non Productive Cough, Hemoptysis, Low Grade Fever, Calf Muscle Pain Or Swelling
Lung Malignancy	Productive Cough, Hemoptysis, Weight Loss, Loss Of Appetite
Pericarditis	Flu Like Symptoms
Peptic Ulcer	N & V, Hematemesis, Melena
GORD	Acid Taste In Mouth, Dysphagia If Esophageal Strictures, Water brash.
Musculoskeletal	Back And Joint Pain
Aortic Stenosis	Syncope, Exertional SOB, Chest pain

Past Medical History:

- HTN, DM, High Cholesterol, Smoking → **Ischemic Heart Disease**
- Menopause → **Ischemic Heart Disease**
- Previous DVT, Recurrent Miscarriages → **PE**
- Pneumothorax → **Recurrence In 15-40%**
- Asthma/COPD → **Pneumonia, Pleurisy, Pneumothorax**
- Marfan syndrome/ Ehlers Danlos / Pseudoxanthoma → **MVP**

Drug History:

- Cocaine→ **Chest Pain, ACS, Aortic Dissection.**
- COC, HRT → **DVT** and **PE**
- Sildenafil causes **Chest Pain**

Family History:

- Ischemic heart disease
- Thrombophilia → **PE**

Social History

- Smoking → **CVS risks, GORD**
- Alcohol → **Peptic ulcer, Atrial Fibrillation**
- Occupational:
  - Heavy lifting → **Musculoskeletal Chest Pain** & **Aggravates Cardiac Ischemia**
- Sexual Intercourse → **Potentiate Cardiac Ischemia**
- Long Halt Flights → **PE**

Quick Discussion

How Would You Investigate This Case?

- ECG
- Cardiac Troponins
- D-Dimers→ PE, Dissection
- CTPA → PE
- CXR → Effusion, Infection, Pneumothorax
- CT Aortogram → Aortic Dissection
- ECHO → Aortic stenosis, MVP, Missed Infarction
- Esophageal manometry → Diffuse esophageal spasm

How Would You Treat This Case With Headache?

- Analgesia
- Admit to hospital If Serious Cause Suspected
- Treatment of the cause
  - *ACS protocol* → ACS
  - *Anticoagulation* → PE
  - *PPI & Life Style modification* → GORD
  - *CCBs or Nitrates* → Diffuse esophageal spasm
  - *Aspiration or chest drain* → Pneumothorax
  - *NSAIDs* → Pleurisy
  - *Antibiotics* → Pneumonia
  - *Control B.P and call Vascular* → Aortic dissection

Hypertension

Differential Diagnosis

Essential Hypertension

- Positive family history
- Middle aged people

Secondary Hypertension

- **Renal Causes**
  o Renal Artery Stenosis
  o ADPKD
  o RCC
- **Endocrinal Causes**
  o Cushing Syndrome
  o Conn`s disease
  o Thyrotoxicosis
  o Pheochromocytoma
  o Acromegaly
  o PCO
- **Haematological**
  o PRV
- **Vasculitis**
  o Polyarteritis nodosa
  o SLE
- **Coarctation of the Aorta**
- **Drugs** (Steroids, MAOI, COC, Cocaine, Amphetamines, NSAIDs)
- **Pregnancy Induced**
- **Pre-Eclampsia**
- **White Coat HTN**
- **Metabolic Syndrome**

Analysis Of The Complaint

Symptoms:

- Headache
- Blurring of vision
- Nose Bleeds

Complications:

- Coronary Artery Disease
  o Chest Pains on exertion
  o SOB on exertion
  o Any heart attacks

- Peripheral Vascular Disease
  - Leg Cramps on Walking
- Cerebrovascular Disease
  - Any Strokes
- Retinal Disease
- Renal Disease

Personal history:

Age:

- If Young Age Suspect 2ry Causes
- If Old Could Be 1ry Or 2ry (So Always Ask For 2ry Causes)

Job:

- Stress Is A Contributing Factor.

Sex

- Polyarteritis Nodosa is Common in Males
- SLE is more Common in Women

History Of Presenting Illness (R/O Differential Diagnosis)

Hyperthyroidism

- Do you tend to feel the Hot weather more than usual?
- Excessive sweating?
- Lose motions?
- Palpitations?
- Irritability?
- Weight loss despite an increased appetite?
- Any neck swelling?

Acromegaly:

- What about your Ring & Shoe Size? Do they fit?
- Excessive sweating?
- Ask about S/S of MEN I?

Cushing's Syndrome

- Weight gain more in The Face, Tummy & around the neck & Back?
- Striae on your Tummy?
- Weakness of shoulders & Hips?
- High Blood sugar

Pheochromocytoma

- Headaches & excessive sweating in attacks, Post Exertional?
- Weight Loss?
- S/S of MEN II?
- Renal Cell Carcinoma
- Blood on Passing urine?
- Pain in Loins?

SLE

- Mouth sores?
- Butter Fly rash on nose?
- Sensitivity to light?
- Raised ESR on Blood tests.

Drug History:

Steroids, OCPs, MAOIs, NSAIDs, Nasal Sprays (Ephedrine Or Pseudoephedrine), Cyclosporine, Cocaine And MDMA, Anabolic Steroids.

Family History:

Essential HTN runs in families

Social History:

- Any Possibility You Are Pregnant?
- Detailed Alcohol and Tobacco history

Quick Discussion

What Investigations You Would Like To Do?

- Examine fundus
- ECG
- ECHO
- _Urinary Catecholamines_ → Pheochromocytoma
- _Urinary 24 hours Cortisol_ → Cushing`s disease
- _Dexamethasone suppression test_ → Cushing`s disease
- _Renin/Aldosterone ratio_ → Conn`s disease
- _ANA_ → SLE
- _Doppler U/S of Renal Arteries_ → Renal artery stenosis

What Treatment You Would Like To Offer?

- ACEIs if < 55 years old
- CCBs, Diuretics > 55 years old
- Treat the reversible causes
- Treatment of complications

Breathlessness

Differential Diagnosis

Cardiac (heart failure)	1. **Systolic Dysfunction** (Ischemia, Cardiomyopathy, Myocarditis, Aortic Stenosis) 2. **Diastolic Dysfunction** (Left V. Hypertrophy, Constrictive Pericarditis, Pericardial Effusion) 3. **Arrhythmias** 4. **Structural Cardiac Lesion** (Valvular, VSD, HOCM) 5. **Iatrogenic** (Excessive IV Infusion, NSAIDS, Steroids) 6. **Increase Demand** (Anemia, Pregnancy, Fever, Thyrotoxicosis, AV Fistula, Paget's Disease
Respiratory	1. **Airways** (Tumor, Foreign Body, Obstructive Lung Diseases → Asthma/Occupational Asthma/COPD) 2. **Parenchyma** (Pulmonary Fibrosis, Alveolitis ,Sarcoidosis, TB, Pneumonia ,Tumors) 3. **Circulation** (PE, Vasculitis, PH) 4. **Pleural** (Pneumothorax ,Effusion) 5. **Chest Wall Deformities** 6. **Neuromuscular** (Myasthenia Gravis, Guillain Barre, Neuropathies, Muscular Dystrophies)
Others	1. **Anemia** 2. **Metabolic acidosis** (Renal Failure) 3. **Obesity** 4. **Psychogenic** 5. **Carcinoid Syndrome**

Analysis Of The Complaint:

Grade or severity

- Dyspnea with effort may be normal.
- It becomes a symptom if it occurs with exercise levels below those expected for the patient age and degree of previous fitness

Onset, Duration and progression

- Occurred **suddenly and progressed rapidly over minutes**
  - PE
  - Pneumothorax
  - Acute LV Failure
  - Asthma
  - Inhaled Foreign Body
- Occurred **gradually and progressed rapidly over hours or days**
  - Pneumonia

- o Asthma
- o COPD
- Occurred **gradually and progressed gradually over weeks, months or years**
  - o Anemia
  - o Effusion
  - o COPD
  - o Pulmonary Fibrosis
  - o Tb
  - o Neuromuscular Disorders
  - o CCF

Variability, Aggravating /Relieving Factors

- Worse When lying flat (**Orthopnea**)
  - o LV failure
  - o Respiratory muscle weakness
  - o However orthopnea could be present with any sever lung disease
- Wakes the patient from sleep (**Paroxysmal Nocturnal Dyspnea**)
  - o LVF
  - o COPD (Nocturnal Hypoxia)
- Dyspnea on **waking up** that is relieve with coughing is typical of
  - o COPD
  - o Asthma
- **Exercise induced asthma**
- Dyspnea **That Improves On Weekends** is typical of:
  - o Occupational Asthma
  - o Extrinsic Allergic Alveolitis

Severity

- Limitations to physical activity (NYHA)
- How far the patient can walk before stopping to rest because of dyspnea (not leg pain)
- Inquire about hobbies the patient used to do and whether dyspnea has stopped him or not

Associated symptoms?

Wheeze and cough	Asthma, COPD, Occupational Astma, Cardiac Asthma, Carcinoid syndrome, Anaphylaxis
Central chest pain	MI, Massive PE
Pleuritic chest pain	Pneumonia, Pneumothorax, PE, Rib fracture
No chest pain	PE, pneumothorax, metabolic acidosis, hypovolemia, LV failure, Anemia, Panic Attacks
Palpitations, Syncope, Presyncope	Arrhythmia, AS, HOCM
Oedema	RVF (LVF, Massive PE, Core-Pulmonale)
Fevers with purulent Productive cough	Pneumonia
Haemoptysis	Lung CA, PE, LVF, Mitral stenosis

Past Medical History:

- Enquire About CVS Risks, Previous Tests Or Echo
- Previous Cardiac
- Pulmonary Disease

Drug History

- Inhalers

- Steroids
- NSAIDs

Family History:

Ischemic heart disease, Pulmonary HTN

Social History

- Smoking: (Ask about active or passive smoking)
  - Risk for MI
  - COPD
  - Worsening Asthma
- Alcohol: Risk for dilated cardiomyopathy
- Detailed occupational history
  - Occupational Asthma (Isocyanates...etc)
  - Asbestosis Exposure
  - Extrinsic Allergic Alveolitis
    - Farmers
    - Malt workers
    - Coal Miners
    - Bird Keepers
- Habits like bird raising; psittacosis

Quick Discussion

What Investigations You would like to do?

- *Asthma/ COPD* → PFTs, ABGs, CXR
- *LVF* → Echo
- *PE* → CTPA
- *Pneumothorax* → CXR, CT chest
- *EAA* → HRCT
- *Pneumonia* → CXR, Blood tests

How Will you treat this patient?

- Asthma → Inhalers, Steroids
- COPD → Inhalers, Steroids
- LVF→ Diuretics, ACEIs, BBs
- PE→ Anticoagulants
- Pneumothorax→ Drainage
- EAA & Lung Fibrosis → Steroids

Palpitations

Analysis Of The Complaint

Age of onset:

Young patients with a history of palpitations in childhood or adolescence

- SVTs
- Congenital long QT Syndrome
- HOCM
- Congenital Heart disease

Nature Of Palpitations:

"what do the palpitations feel like?"

- Racing heart → Tachyarrhythmia
- Heart misses a beat, then pounding or jumping → Ventricular or Atrial extrasystoles
- Pounding in the neck or everything stopped for a moment →AV dissociation or bradycardia.

Rate And Rhythm:

- Fast or slow?
- Regular or irregular? (Ask them to tap the rhythm)

Time Course, Onset An Frequency:

- How Long Have You Had The Palpitations?
- How Often?
- How Long Episodes Last?
- Do They Start Gradually Or Suddenly?

Precipitants:

- Exercise, Coffee, Tea, Coca, Stress, Alcohol, Emotion, Cocaine, Amphetamine, Recent Illness → Tachyarrhythmias
- Sudden Standing up → Postural Hypotension
- Exercise → Exercise induced tachycardia ? VF
- Medications induces e.g. Salbutamol Nebs
- Chest pain → ACS
- Alcohol → AF

Termination:

- SVTs can be terminated by Valsalva & other Vagal Maneuvers
- Ectopic beats can be terminated by exercise

Associated symptoms:

- Dyspnea (With Most Arrhythmias)
- Syncope Or Presyncope (Hemodynamic Instability)
- Chest Pain, Nausea, Sweating (Ischemia)

- Exertional Dyspnea, Orthopnea, Ankle Swelling, Reduced Exercise Tolerance (HF)

Past History:

- Endocrinal diseases: Hyperthyroidism, Pheochromocytoma, hypoglycemia
- Cardiac disease
- Cerebrovascular Accidents (complication to AF)
- Psychiatric illness (anxiety)
- Asthma (Beta agonists)

Family History:

HOCM and long QT syndrome are inherited

Drug History:

- Beta agonists
- Theophylline
- Thyroxine
- MAOI
- Amphetamines
- Cocaine
- Drugs Causing Electrolytes Imbalance e.g. Diuretics
- Drugs that cause long QT $
  - Amiodarone
  - Macrolides e.g. Erythromycin
  - Antihistamines
  - Anti-malarials
  - Antipsychotics
  - SSRIs
- **Social History:**
  - Alcohol, Caffeine, Smoking, Stressful Job.
  - Driving; should inform DVLA and stop driving if any LOC.

Quick Discussion

What Investigations You Would Like To Do?

- *ECG* → To determine the Type of arrhythmia
- *ECHO* → Look for Structural heart disease
- *CXR* → Look for Cardiomegaly, Lung disease
- *Electrophysiological studies*
- *Myocardial Perfusion Scan* → Look for Ischemic Heart Disease
- *Serum Electrolytes*
- *TFTs*

How Would You Treat Him?

- Treat The cause
- Stop Offending drugs
- Correct electrolytes imbalance
- Beta-blockers for exercise induced VT
- Beta blockers for AF
- Cardiology R/V

Cough

Differential Diagnosis

Acute	Chronic
URTI : • Common Cold ,Influenza • Sinusitis • Whooping Cough • Allergic Rhinitis e.g.Hay Fever **LRTI:** • Acute Bronchitis • Pneumonia • Flare-Ups Of Chronic Conditions Such As COPD, Asthma, Bronchiectasis, Fibrosis • Inhale Foreign Body **Cardiac** • Left Ventricular Failure **Others** • Granulomatosis Polyangiitis • Churg Strauss	**Environmental** • Cigarette Smoke, Cigar And Pipe • Dusts, Pollens, Pet Dander, Industrial Chemicals And Low Environmental Humidity. **Lung Conditions** • Asthma, COPD • ABPA • Cancer • Sarcoidosis • Lung Fibrosis (See Respiratory) • Bronchiectasis (see Respiratory) **URTI** • Chronic Sinusitis • Chronic Postnasal Drip • Infections Of The Throat **Drugs** • ACE Inhibitor • Cancer **GIT** • GERD **Cardiac** Left ventricular failure

Analysis Of The Complaint

Onset And Duration:

- **Acute**: less than 3 weeks
- **Subacute:** 3-8 weeks
- **Chronic:** more than 8 weeks

Age Of Onset:

Chronic cough in childhood: mostly asthma

Frequency, Pattern, Progression:

- **Frequency:** Daily, intermittent or seasonal
- **Pattern:**
  o Cough worse in the morning: Chronic bronchitis/Asthma
  o Nocturnal cough: Asthma, GERD, or LV failure

- **Progression:** consider lung cancer in a smoker with a change in nature of cough

Precipitating Factors:

- Food or drink → **GORD** or **Aspiration**
- Posture; worse on bending forward or lying flat → **GORD**
- Irritants → **Rhinitis** or **Asthma**
- Cold weather, Exercise → **Asthma**

Associated Symptoms:

- Weight loss and anorexia → Think about **Lung CA**
- Fever and night sweats → **T.B., Vasculitis**
- Erythematous tender papules on shins (Erythema Nodosum) and eye symptoms suggest → **Sarcoidosis**
- Purpuric rash, Mononeuritis Multiplex with Asthma or Rhinitis suggests → **Chrug Strauss**
- Urinary incontinence → **Stress incontinence** as complication
- Syncope → Cough Syncope due to excessive coughing
- Chest pain → Either due to **Tear in the Chest wall muscles** or secondary to the **Cause e.g. Pleurisy**
- Other Associated symptoms as described in the following table:

Sputum Production	Determine quantity ,character ,and color
	• Clear →**Chronic Bronchitis**
	• Yellow or green → **Acute Infection**
	• Rusty brown + foul smell and taste → **Bronchiectasis**
	• Frothy pink → **LV failure** (lung congestion)
	On the other hand **Dry cough** may be with viral illness, GORD ,Interstitial Lung Disease
Haemoptysis	Blood tinged → **Infection** and **LVF**
	Frank →**Lung cancer** and **T.B, PE, Bronchiectasis, Granulomatosis Polynagiitis, Good Pasture`s syndrome**
Chest pain	Pleuritic→ **Acute Infection** and **PE**
	Tightness→ **Asthma** and **COPD**
	Cardiac origin→ **LVF** 2ry to MI
	Musculoskeletal → 2ry to severe coughing
Dyspnoea	Sudden onset→ **Asthma, PE, Acute pulmonary edema or foreign body**
	Subacute → **Pneumonia, Aspiration, COPD, Asthma**
	Gradually progressive → **COPD, LV failure**
	Orthopnea and PND → **LV failure**
Wheezes	**Asthma, COPD, Cardiac failure, Churg strauss $, Carcinoid syndrome**
Hoarseness	Vocal cord paralysis due to : Laryngitis ,Laryngeal Malignancy, **Bronchogenic Carcinoma** (invading recurrent laryngeal N)
Nasal symptoms	Rhinorrhea or Nasal discharge → Rhinitis, URTI, Churg Strauss
	Throat clearing an sensation of dripping at the back of throat → **Post Nasal Drip**
GIT symptoms	Retrosternal pain, burning pain dyspepsia, vomiting → **GORD**

Past History:

- *History of Atopy* → Asthma, Hay Fever
- *History of Respiratory Illness* → Childhood Asthma, Recurrent Chest Infections, COPD, Previous T.B., Sinusitis
- *History of acid related GIT disorders like peptic ulcer*

Family History:

- Atopy
- Lung cancer
- PE or Hypercoagulable state
- Congenital heart disease
- Ischemic heart disease

Drug History:

- ACE Inhibitors → Dry Cough
- NSAIDs, BBs → Triggers Asthma
- Nitrates, CCBs, Theophyllines, Bisphosphonates → trigger GORD
- Nitrofurantoin, Methotrexate, Amiodarone, Busulphan → Pulmonary Fibrosis

Social History:

- Occupational history to determine any triggers to cough as:
  - Solvents
  - Fumes
  - Vapours
  - Animals And Dust
  - Occupational Asthma
    - Isocyanates → Painters
    - Wheat → Bakers
    - Avian Proteins
    - Tobacco
  - Extrinisic Allergic Alveolitis
    - Birds Droppings → Bird Fancier
    - Cheese workers
    - Malt workers
    - Farmers
- Have the patient been exposed to asbestos?
- Smoking : COPD, lung cancer ,laryngeal cancer
- Travel abroad where T.B is endemic

Quick Discussion

What Investigations You Would Like to do for this case?

- CXR
- HRCT for pulmonary fibrosis
- ECHO for heart failure
- Blood tests looking for raised inflammatory markers
- p-ANCA for Churg Strauss
- C-ANCA for Granulomatosis Polyangiitis
- Aspergillus percepitants
- CTPA for PE
- PFTs for COPD
- PEFR with reversibility for Asthma
- Sputum MC&S & for Acid Fast Bacilli

How Would You Treat This Case?

- Support ABCDE
- Treat Acute exacerbations of asthma & COPD with Nebs & Steroids & Antibiotics if needed
- Clexane for PE
- Inhalers for Asthma / COPD
- Avoidance of the cause
- Stop smoking
- Antibiotics for T.B.
- Plasma Exchange & Immuno-suppressants for Wegner`s & Churg Strauss

Wheezes

Wheezes are high pitched whistling sound produced by air passing through narrow airways. Typically wheezes are limited to expiration, If it occurs in inspiration that means severe airway obstruction Or Stridor.

Wheezes that causes night wakening is typical of asthma, while wheezes after wakening in the morning is typical of COPD

Wheezes	Stridors
Expiratory	Inspiratory
Whistling or musical sound: • High pitched →small airways • Low pitched →large airways	Loud high pitched
Due to obstruction of small airways	Due to partial obstruction of large airways (necessitate intervention)

Analysis Of The Complaint

Details of symptoms:

"What do you mean by wheeze?" As patients may use the term to Describe Rhonchi, Cough Or Dyspnea

Progression Of Symptoms:

Asthma: usually intermittent with exacerbation caused by obvious precipitant symptoms are reversible with bronchodilators

Onset:

Acute ± Clear Precipitant	Subacute	Chronic
• Anaphylaxis • Acute Exacerbation Of Asthma Or COPD • PE • Aspiration • Foreign Body • Acute LVF	• Respiratory Tract Infections • PE • LV Failure	• Asthma • COPD • Lung cancer • Carcinoid syndrome • Churg Strauss

Associated symptoms:

Respiratory	**Cough :** • Chronic non-productive cough troublesome at night occurring together with wheezes is suggestive of asthma • Chronic cough for > 3 months for > 2 years in the morning is suggestive of COPD **Dyspnea:** Common with most causes **Chest tightness:** Asthma or COPD **Chest Pain:** Infection, PE **Hemoptysis:** PE or Lung cancer If PE is suspected ask about its symptoms and risk factors **Change in voice:** Bronchogenic carcinoma ,laryngeal disease **Constitutional symptoms** : Infection or Malignancy
Cardiac	Heart Failure Symptoms
Others	Symptoms of **Anaphylaxis** (Urticarial rash, Tongue Swelling, Angioedema, N.V) Symptoms of **Churg strauss** $ (Rhinitis, Asthma, Rash, Mononeuritis Multiplex) Symptoms of **Carcinoid $** (Diarrhea, Flushing, weight loss) Symptoms of **GORD**

Precipitants:

"Have you noticed anything that triggers the symptoms?"

• **Asthma:** Smoking, Pollen, House dust, Mold, Cold air, Exercise, Emotional stress
• **Anaphylaxis**: Ingestion of nuts, Wasp or Bee sting, Medications

Past History:
• **Atopy**
  o Eczema
  o Anaphylaxis
• **Asthma**
  o What is Your PEFR?
  o Have you been admitted to hospital because of your asthma
  o What treatment are you on?
• **Cardiac disease**
• **GORD**
• **COPD**
  o How Far Can you Walk Before Feeling SOB?
  o Are you on Home Oxygen?
  o Are you on Home Nebulizers?
  o Are you on Home BIPAP?
• **Previous Anaesthesia**, Endotracheal intubation?

Drug History:
• Induce Broncho-constriction: NSAID, Aspirin, BBs
• Inhaled Cocaine can exacerbate asthma
• OCPs, HRT → PE

Social History:
• **Detailed Occupational History**:
  o Occupational Asthma
  o Extrinisic Allergic Alveolitis
  o Asbestos

- **Smoking History** :
  - Asthma
  - COPD
  - Bronchogenic And Laryngeal Carcinoma

Family History:
- Atopy
- DVT

Quick Discussion → See before

Hemoptysis

It is important to determine whether the blood has been coughed up (Respiratory Tract), Vomited (GIT) ,or has suddenly appeared in the mouth without coughing (Nasopharyngeal)

Differential Diagnosis

Tumors	Bronchogenic Carcinoma, Metastases, Kaposi's Sarcoma, Bronchial Carcinoid
Infection	T.B., Bronchiectasis, Abscess, Mycetoma, Cystic Fibrosis
Vascular	PE, A-V Malformation
Vasculitis	Wegner's, Good pasture's
Trauma	Inhaled Foreign Body, Chest Trauma, Iatrogenic
Cardiac	Mitral Valve Disease, Acute LV Failure
Haematological	Hereditary Hemorrhagic Telangiectasia(HHT), Anticoagulation

Analysis Of The Complaint

Age of onset:

- Consider lung cancer, Bronchiectasis, PE, Infections, LVF in a patient over 50 years old.
- Infections, PE and HHT should be considered in younger patients

Amount:

How many teaspoons or cups /24 hours? More than 200 ml carries a bad prognosis

Duration and Frequency:

- **Intermittently for years:** Bronchiectasis
- **Daily** (for a week or more): lung Cancer, TB, lung abscess, Vasculitis
- **Single episode:** need immediate action if they are very large or associated with symptoms like pleuritic chest pain suggesting PE

Appearance:

- *Streaking of clear sputum or blood clots* for more than a week → suggestive of Lung Cancer, but can also occur in Chronic Bronchitis and Bronchiectasis
- *With purulent sputum* → is suggestive of Infective Cause (e.g. Bronchiectasis, Pneumonia)
- *Diffuse staining of sputum with blood* (Pink Frothy)→ Acute Pulmonary Edema
- *Large amounts of pure blood* → Bronchiectasis, TB. Lung cancer, PE, Lung Abscess, Mycetoma , Granulomatosis Polyangiitis

Associated Symptoms:

- Cough and sputum
- Dyspnea
- Pleuritic Chest pain
- Fever, rigors, night sweats
- Hoarseness of voice, and dysphagia

- Weight loss and anorexia
- Rash, arthralgia ,and myalgia
- Bleeding
- Leg pain ,swelling ,and erythema
- GIT symptoms (differentiate hemoptysis from hematemesis)

Past History:

- DVT or any thrombus
- Bleeding disorders
- Recurrent chest infections (bronchiectasis or cystic fibrosis)
- Childhood rheumatic fever (Mitral Stenosis)
- Malignancy (Metastases or PE)
- AV malformation in cerebral or GIT(HHT)
- Chronic liver disease (coagulopathy or hematemesis mistaken for hemoptysis)
- Immunosuppression (opportunistic lung infections, and reactivation of TB

Family History:

- Lung malignancy
- TB
- HHT
- Bleeding disorders and thrombophilia
- Factor V Layden → PE

Drug History:

- Anticoagulants and anti-platelets
- OCPs, HRT → PE
- Cocaine: pulmonary hemorrhage and infarction

Social History:

- Smoking (Single most important risk factor for lung cancer)
- Occupational history: Asbestos
- Travelling abroad to areas endemic for TB
- Pregnancy → Increased risk for PE

Quick Discussion → See before

Ankle Swelling

Differential Diagnosis

Unilateral	Bilateral (systemic)
• DVT	• Heart failure
• Venous insuffiency	• Hypo-proteinemia
o Varicose Veins	o Nephrotic Syndrome
o Post-phlebetic Limb	o Liver Cirrhosis
• Cellulitis	o Kwashiorkor
• Immobility	o Malabsorption Syndromes
o Hemiplegia	• Hypothyroidism
o Arthritis	• Chronic venous insufficiency
• Hematoma	• IVC obstruction
	• Lymphatic obstruction by pelvic Tumor or Filariasis
	• Thiamine deficiency
	• Milroy's disease (unexplained lymphedema appearing in puberty, more common in females)
	• Immobility
	• Drugs (Amlodipine)

Analysis Of The Complaint:

Onset And Duration:

• Acute onset (< 72 hours) is strongly suggestive of DVT

Symmetry:

Symmetrical or asymmetrical

Extent:

• How far in legs does the swelling extend?
• Is there any swelling in scrotum or penis?
• Is there abdominal swelling?
• Is it confined to joints?

Pattern:

• Pitting or non-pitting?
• Does pressing on the swelling leave finger marks?
• Lymphoedema and hypothyroidism are non-pitting

Aggravating factors:

• Venous insufficiency: swelling worse at the end of the day
• Drugs (CCBs)
• Trauma, animal bites or stings

Relieving factors:

- Venous insufficiency: Relieved by leg elevation or compression stockings
- Ask if diuretics have been used and if it reduced the swelling

Others:

- Oozing or not?
- Skin discoloration?
  - Brown hemosiderin over the medial aspect of ankle suggests venous insufficiency
- Trophic changes to skin? Previous ulcers
- History of trauma or injuries

Associated Features:

- Painful or painless: Pain is with DVT, Cellulitis, Lymphedema is painless. Others cause low grade aching
- Ask about symptoms of causes
- Ask about risk factors of DVT
  - Hypercoagulable states
  - Prolonged immobility
  - Long Flights
  - Malignancy
- Itching common with venous insufficiency
- Red, Painful, Hot with fevers & Shakes Suggestive of Cellulitis

Past History:

- Cardio-Vascular:
  - Risk factors of Cardiac ischemia and if controlled or not
  - Any Previous ECHOs
  - PCI or CABG?
  - Valvular Heart disease
- Respiratory:
  - Any chronic respiratory disease or symptoms?
- Thyroid disease
- Renal disease
- Chronic liver disease
- Previous surgery or irradiation: lymphedema
- Previous DVT or varicose veins ;venous insufficiency
- Any hematological disease

Family History

- DVT or PE
- Hypercoagulable states:
- Factor V Leyden
- Homocysteinuria
- Protein C & S Deficiency
- Cardiac disease (Ischemic, Dilated cardiomyopathy, HOCM)

Social History

- Smoking (CVS risk factors)
- Alcohol (dilated cardiomyopathy, chronic liver disease)
- Travelling long distances →DVT
- Pregnancy → DVT

Drug History:

- **DVT Risk**
  - OCPs
  - Tranexemic acid
  - HRT

- **Fluid Retention**
  - CCBs
  - steroids
  - Hydralazine
  - Minoxidil
  - Methyldopa
  - Thiazolinediones
  - MAOI
  - NSAIDs
- Nephrotoxic medications can aggravate Renal Failure
- Fenfluramine causing Pulmonary HTN

Quick Discussion

What Investigations You Want To Do For This Patient?

- DVT
- Raised D-dimers
- Doppler U/S legs
- ECHO for heart failure & Pumonary HTN
- Cellulitis → Raised inflammatory markers
- LFTs & serum albumin
- Abdomen/Pelvis CT Scan if Pelvic tumor suspected
- TFTs if Hypothyroidism

How Would You Treat This Patient?

- Anti-Coagulants for DVT
- Diuretics for Heart failure
- Hold off the offending medication
- Treat the Cause

Diarrhea

Differential Diagnosis

Acute	Chronic

• **Infective GE:**
 o Staphylococcus Toxin
 o Bacillus cereus
 o Salmonella
 o E-coli
 o Shigella
 o Campylobacter
 o Giaridiasis
 o Amoebiasis
 • **Drugs**
 o Antibiotics
   ▪ Direct effect
   ▪ CDIF
 o Laxatives
 o PPIs
 o Metoclopramide
 o Eryhthromycin
	• **Infection:**
	 o Parasitic infestation HIV(Cryptosporidium)
	 • **Malabsorption Syndrome:** *(Intestinal, pancreatic, biliary)*
	 o Inflammatory bowel disease
	 o Post bowel resection
	 • **Neurological:**
	 o Irritable bowel $
	 o Autonomic neuropathy
	   ▪ Diabetes Mellitus
	   ▪ Parkinson Plus
	 • **Tumors:** → Colorectal cancer
	 • **Drugs:**
	 o Laxative abuse
	 o Antibiotics
	 o Cytotoxics
	 • **Endocrinal disease:**
	 o Hyperthyroidism
	 o Pheocromocytoma
	 o Carcinoid Syndrome
	 o Zollinger Ellison Syndrome
	 o VIPOMA
	 • **Mechanical:**
	 o Fecal impaction (Over Flow Diarrhoea)

Analysis Of The Complaint

- Onset, Course, Duration
- Amount
- Frequency
- Does The patient wake up from his sleep to Open his Bowels
  - If Yes → Organic Cause
  - If No → No Organic Cause **(Irritable Bowel Syndrome)**

Associated Symptoms:

- Bloating, Abdominal Pain, Constipation, Hematemesis, Melena
- Fever → **Infective Causes**
- Blood? Mucous? → **Dysentery/Colitis**
- Pale, Hard to flush? Offensive? → **Malabsorption**
- Weight Loss → **Malabsorption, Malignancy**
- Heat Intolerance, Sweating, Palpations, Irritability → **Hyperthyroidism**
- Flushing, Bronchospasm, Lower Limb Edema (TR) → **Carcinoid Syndrome**
- Clubbing → **Inflammatory Bowel Diseases, Whipple's, Coeliac Disease**
- Erythema Nodosum (Painful Red Rash on Shins) → **Inflammatory Bowel Disease**
- Pyoderma Gangrenosa (Violaceous Ulcer on Legs)→ **Inflammatory Bowel Disease**

- Lymph Nodes → **Whipple's Disease**
- Itchy Rash over elbows or buttocks (Dermatitis Herpitiform) → **Coeliac Disease**

Past History:

- Peptic ulcer (Zollinger's Ellison syndrome, Vagotomy)
- DM
  - o Coeliac Disease
  - o Autonomic Neuropathy
- Surgeries (Vagotomy, Blind loop, Bowel resection, Pancreatic surgery)
- Hypertriglyceridemia → **Chronic Pancreatitis**
- Scleroderma → **Small bowel Bacterial Overgrowth**
- Parkinson`s disease → **Autonomic neuropathy**
- Hyperthyroidism

Drug History

- Laxatives
- Antibiotics
- Cytotoxic
- PPIs → **Bacterial Overgrowth, CDIF**
- Metoclopramide
- Erythromycin

Family History

- Coeliac disease
- Medullary carcinoma or MEN → **VIPOMA**
- Inflammatory bowel disease
- Familial hypertriglyceridemia → **Chronic Pancreatitis**

Social History

- Crohn`s disease is more common in smoker
- Alcohol is related to Chronic pancreatitis
- Travel History → Increase suspicion of infectious origin

Quick Discussion

What Investigations Would You Like To Do For The Patient?

- *Stool Cultures, MC & S*
- *Carcinoid syndrome* → 5-HIAA in Urine
- *Coeliac Disease*
  - o Tissue transglutaminase
  - o Anti-Gliadin antibodies
  - o Endoscopy with jejunal Biopsy
- *Inflammatory Bowel disease*
  - o Fecal Calprotectin
  - o Colonoscopy & Biospy
- *Thyroid Function tests*
- *Chronic pancreatitis*
  - o Fecal elastase
  - o Fecal fat
  - o ERCP
  - o Investigations for D.M
- *Malabsorption* → Fecal Fat

How Would You Treat This Patient?

- *Treat The Cause*
- *Stop the offending medication*

- *Supportive treatment* with replacement of fluids & electrolytes
- *Coeliac disease*
  - Gluten free diet
- *Inflammatory bowel disease*
  - Mesalazine
  - Steroids
  - Azathioprine
- *Hyperthyroidism* → Carbimazole
- *Bacterial overgrowth* → antibiotics
- *Infectious diarrhea* → antibiotics
- *CDIF* → Antibiotics

Vomiting

Differential Diagnosis

- **GIT Causes:**
  - PUD, Gastritis
  - Food poisoning ,GE
  - Liver failure, HCC
  - Gastric Cancer
- **Kidney:**
  - Renal Failure
- **Neurological Causes**
  - Raised intracranial pressure
  - Migraine
  - Gastroparesis
  - Labyrinthitis
- **Psychiatric Causes:**
  - Anorexia
  - bulimia
- **Endocrinal Causes**:
  - Addison's disease
  - Panhypopituitarism
  - DKA
- **Medications**
  - Chemotherapy
  - Opiates
  - Theophylline toxicity
  - Digoxin toxicity
- **Cyclic vomiting Syndrome**
- **Pregnancy**

Analysis Of The Complaint

You should differentiate between vomiting & regurgitation; Vomiting its forceful contraction of the stomach to expel food out, whilst regurgitation is passive regurgitation of the food due to local obstruction or stenosis associated with Dysphagia.

Onset, Course, Duration

- Acute Onset Suggests Infections or Gastritis.

Associated Symptoms

- Abdominal pains → **GE, Gastritis**
- Weight loss, early satiety → **CA Stomach**
- Epigastric mass, L.Ns → **CA Stomach**
- Tanning of the skin, generalized weakness → **Addison`s disease**
- Dizziness on standing up, Palpitations → **Dehydration signs**
- Fevers → **Infectious cause**
- Jaundice → **Hepato-Biliary cause**
- Known Diabetic, weight loss, Polyuria, Dizziness , Dehydration, not taking insulin → **DKA**

- Headaches, blurring of vision, vomiting → **Raised Intracranial pressure**

Past Medical History

- CA on chemotherapy → Chemotherapy related
- D.M → Gastroparesis, DKA
- PUD → Gastritis or PUD
- CKD
- Psychiatric disorders
- AF on Digoxin
- COPD on Aminophylline

Drug History

- Chemotherapy
- Opiates
- Theophylline toxicity
- Digoxin Toxicity

Family History

- FH of Gastric CA

Social History

- Alcohol → Gastritis, Gastric CA
- Smoking → Gastritis & Gastric CA
- Pregnancy

Quick Discussion

How Would You Investigate This Case?

- U & Es for dehydration & AKI
- FBC, Crp for signs of infection
- Endoscopy with Biopsy for gastric CA
- CT head for increased intracranial pressure
- Digoxin Level
- Aminophylline Levels
- Short Synacthen test for Addison's disease
- Gastric Motility Studies for Gastroparesis
- VBG, Serum Ketones, Blood sugar for DKA

How Would You Treat This Case?

- Supportive treatment for dehydration and IV fluids
- Anti-emetics
- Treatment of the cause
- Addison's disease → Dexamethasone
- Gastric CA → Upper GIT MDM
- Digoxin Toxicity → Stop & FAB Fragments
- Aminophylline toxicity → Dialysis
- DKA → Insulin, fluids, heparin
- Gastroparesis → Metoclopramide, Erythromycin

Dysphagia

Differential Diagnosis

Congenital	Esophageal Atresia	
Acquired	**In the lumen:** Foreign body **In the wall:** • Stricture *(GORD, Candidiasis, Caustic)* • Achalasia • Carcinoma • Plummer Vinson $ • Scleroderma • Irradiation • Chagas' disease • Diffuse esophageal Spasm **Others:** • Anxiety (Globus hystericus) • Drugs: NSAIDs, bisphosphonates	**Outside the wall:** • Pharyngeal pouch • Mediastinal tumors *(Bronchial carcinoma, Lymphoma)* • Enlarge left atrium (Mitral Stenosis) • Aortic aneurysm **Neuromuscular disorders:** • Bulbar and pseudobulbar palsy • Guillian Barre Syndrome • Myasthenia Gravis • Stroke • Motor Neuron disease • Parkinsonism • Multiple sclerosis • Advanced Dementia

Analysis Of The Complaint:

Onset, Course, Duration

• **Acute Onset**
  o Food Bolus obstructing the esophagus
  o Guillian Barre syndrome
  o Bulbar, Pseudobulbar Palsy
• **Chronic**
  o Achalasia
  o Tumors

More To Solids or Liquids?

• Achalasia is more to Liquids initially
• Esophageal Cancer is more to solids initially

Is There Any Pain During Swallowing? (Odynophagia)

• Esophagitis (CMV –EBV-Candidiasis)

Associated Symptoms:

• *Achalasia:* Heart Burn, Chest Pain, Halitosis, Nocturnal Cough, Regurgitation Of Food.
• *Carcinoma:* Weight Loss, Anorexia, History Of GORD, Smoking, Alcohol.

- ***Plummer Vinson S***: Postmenopausal Women, Iron Deficiency Anemia, Esophageal Webs, Koilonychia, Glossitis
- ***Scleroderma***: Calcinosis, Raynaud's, Sclerodactyly, Telangiectasia, Pulmonary HTN
- ***Guillian Barre***: Recent Viral illness, Ascending weakness

Past Medical History

- Scleroderma
- Strokes
- Dementia
- Parkinsonism
- MND
- Multiple sclerosis
- Lung CA

Drug History

- Bisphosphonates

Social History

Smoking, Alcohol → Cancers

Quick Discussion

What Investigations You Want To Do For This Patient?

- Barium Swallow
- CXR
- Endoscopy
- CT CAP
- Swallowing Studies

How Would You Treat This Patient?

- Treat the Cause
- IV fluids temporary
- PEG Tube for Advanced non reversible diseases
- NG Tube temporary

Jaundice

Differential Diagnosis:

Prehepatic	Hepatic	Cholestatic

Congenital:
• Gilbert's disease
• Crigler-Najjar
Hemolysis:
• **Congenital:**
  o Hereditary Spherocytosis
  o Sickle cell anemia
  o GP6D deficiency
  o Thalassemia
• **Acquired:**
• Incompatible blood transfusion
• Malaria
• Autoimmune hemolytic anemia
• Hypersplenism
• Metallic Heart Valves
• TTP
• HUS
• DIC
	Acute:
	• Viral hepatitis (A, B, C, CMV, EBV)
	• Leptospirosis
	• Autoimmune Hepatitis
	• Paracetamol overdose
	• Halothane
	• Toxins
	• Statins
	• Metastasis
	Chronic:
	• Chronic viral hepatitis
	• Chronic autoimmune hepatitis
	• Alcoholic hepatitis
	• Cirrhosis
	• Haemochromatosis
	• Wilson's disease
	• Alpha 1 antitrypsin deficiency
	• T.B.
	• Histoplasmosis
	• Syphilis
	Others:
	• HCC
	• Budd Chiari $
		Intrahepatic:
		• 1ry biliary cirrhosis
		• Pregnancy
		• Chlorpromazine
		• Co-amoxiclav
		Extrahepatic:
		In the Lumen:
		• Gallstones
		• Parasites (schistosomiasis)
		In the Wall:
		• Congenital biliary atresia
		• Cholangiocarcinoma
		• Sclerosing cholangitis
		Outside the wall:
		• Carcinoma or LN compressing the CBD
		• Cancer head of pancreas.

Analysis Of The Complaint

OCDAE

Associated symptoms:

• Malaise, Weight loss → **Carcinoma**
• Dark urine ,pale stools, itching → **Cholestasis picture**
• No pale stool & Slightly darker Urine → **Hepatic Jaundice**
• Anemia symptoms → **Hemolysis**
• Joint pain, skin discoloration, Impotence, D.M. → **Hemochromatosis**
• Psychiatric/Neurological Problem → Wilson`s Disease
• Auto-immune disorders (Vitiligo, Thyroid disease) → **Auto-immune Hepatitis/ PBC**
• Abdominal pain preceding jaundice → Biliary colick followed by impaction of stone, Alcoholic hepatitis infective hepatitis, drug induced
• Hematemesis → **Cirrhosis Of The Liver**

Past History

- Ulcerative Colitis → **Sclerosing Cholangitis**
- Auto-immune disorders → **PBC, Auto-immune hepatitis**
- Blood transfusion → **Viral Hepatitis**
- DVT, PE → **Bud Chiari Syndrome**
- Underlying Malignancy → **Metastasis, Bud Chiari Syndrome**
- COPD in Young age → **Alpha 1 antitrypsin deficiency**
- MEN I S/S → **Panceratic Cancer**

Drug History

- Augmentin
- Macrolides
- Statins
- Anti-Tuberculous medications
- Anti-Epileptic medications
- Cimetidine
- Estrogen

Family History

- Hypercoagulable states → **Budd Chiari Syndrome**

Social History

- Travel → **Malaria, Viral Hepatitis**
- IV Drug Abuse → **Viral hepatitis**
- High risk jobs (Nurses) → **Viral Hepatitis**
- Pregnancy

Quick Discussion:

What Investigations You Would Do For This Patient?

- FBC
- Split Bilirubin
- Reticulocytic count, Haptoglobin, Haemopexin → Hemolysis
- CT Abdomen for CA Pancereas
- ECRP / MRCP for Biliary stones
- See Station I Abdomen

How Would You Treat This Patient?

- Stop Offending drug
- Treat the cause
- ERCP & Sphincterotomy with stone extraction for Biliary stones
- Oncology for CA Pancereas
- See Station I Abdomen

Constipation

Congenital	Hirschsprung's disease
Acquired	• Lack Of Fibers In Diet • Irritable Bowel syndrome • Intestinal Obstruction • Colonic Cancer • **Painful Anal Conditions** (Fissure, Abscess, Hemorrhoids) • **Ileus** (Hypokalemia, Recent Surgeries, Immobility (Parkinsonism, Stroke) • **Endocrinal**: Hypothyroidism, Diabetic Neuropathy, Hyperparathyroidism (High Calcium) • **Hypercalcemia**: Sarcoidosis, Metastatic CA, Hyperparathyroidism • **Drugs**: Codeine, Morphine, Atropine, TCA • Depression

Analysis Of The Complaint:

• Has constipation been lifelong or it's of recent onset?
  o Recent Change in Bowel Habits in old age showed alert you about Carcinoma
• Do you mean by constipation hard stool or decreased frequency?
• Are You Passing Wind? Or its absolute constipation?
• How often do You Open Your Bowels each week?
• Has the shape of the stool changed? Pellet-like?
• Full dietary history
• Diverticular disease is a complication so ask for it (Painful Tummy, Fevers, Bleeding P/R)

Associated Symptoms:

• Intolerance to Cold, Lethargy, Weight gain → **Hypothyroidism**
• Polyuria, Polydipsia, Abdominal pains , Depression → **Hypercalcemia**
• Vomiting → **Intestinal Obstruction, Ileus**
• Tenesmus (Mucus)→ **Important In Acute Constipation Of Infective Origin**
• Painful defecation → **Painful Anal Conditions**
• MEN I or MEN II → **Hypercalcemia**

Past History

• Parkinsonism, Stroke
• Hypothyroidism
• Prolonged immobility
• Sarcoidosis → Hyperkalaemia

Drug History

• Buprenorphine Patch
• Codeine
• Morphine
• Atropine
• TCA

Family History

Colorectal cancer

Quick Discussion

How Would You Manage This Patient?

- P/R
- AXR to R/O Obstruction
- Laxatives
- Enema
- Stop the offending drug
- Investigations for the cause
- Treatment of the cause

Abdominal Pain

GP Letter

Medical SHO On Call

Dear Dr

Re: P.J. (DOB: 12/01/1957)

I would be grateful if you kindly review this 59 years Old lady who is complaining of abdominal pain for the last few days, I advised her to go immediately to the hospital if the pain doesn't settle down.

Kind regards

Differential Diagnosis

Abdominal Quadrants

Right		Left
Gall Bladder Liver	Gastritis, Pancreatitis, Cardiac Causes	Spleen
Renal	Mesenteric ischemia , Irritable bowel $, Inflammatory bowel	Renal
Appendicitis Terminal ileum Ovarian	Gynecology Urology	Constipation Ovarian

+Porphyria   +Lead poisoning

+Familial Mediterranean fever   +Vasculitis (PAN)

+Adrenal insufficiency   +Sickle cell disease

Analysis Of The Complaint

SOCRATES + Relation To Food, Defecation + Timing

- Ask The patient to point out on his body where exactly he feels this pain.
- **Pancreatic Pain:**
  o Epigastric
  o Radiates To The Back
  o Precipitated By Eating, Relieved By Leaning Forward
  o Associated with vomiting
  o Diabetes if Chronic
- **Biliary Pain:**
  o Right Sided (Right Hypochondrium)
  o Precipitated By Eating
  o Associated With Nausea
  o Positive Murphy`s sign if Acute Cholecystitis
  o May be Associated with Jaundice
- **Peptic Ulcer Disease**
  o Epigastric
  o Colicky/ Burning
  o Radiating to the back
  o Related to food either eating or Fasting.
- **Colonic Pain:**
  o Lower Pain
  o Colicky
  o Partially Relieved By Defecation
- **Cardiac Pain:**
  o Epigastric
  o Precipitated by exertion or heavy meals
  o Might be radiating to jaw and arms
  o Associated With Dyspnea
  o Chest Pain

- **Renal Pain**
  - Colicky / Dull Aching
  - Radiating to Groins
  - Might be Associated with urinary symptoms

Alarm Symptoms:

A anemia

L loss of weight

A anorexia

R recent onset of progressive symptoms

M melena or hematemesis

S swallowing difficulty

Past History

- D.M, HTN → Ischemic colitis, IHD
- AF → Ischemic colitis
- Biliary stones → Biliary Colic, Cholangitis, and Cholecystitis
- ADPKD → Renal Stones, Infections
- FMF
- Vasculitis → Ischemic colitis
- Sickle cell disease

Drug History

- Sudden withdrawal of steroids → Addison's
- Opiates → Constipation
- NSAIDs → PUD

Family History

- FMF
- Cancers
- Social History
- Travel History → Infectious cause
- Alcohol → Pancreatitis, Gastritis, PUD
- Smoking → IHD, Ischemic colitis
- Partners → Pelvic Inflammatory Disease
- Occupation → Lead Poisoning

Quick Discussion

How Would You Manage This Patient?

- CT Abdomen → Pancreatitis, Intestinal Obstruction, Cancers
- AXR → Intestinal Obstruction
- Serum Amylase → Pancreatitis
- Endoscopy for PUD
- U/S for Renal & Hepatic Causes
- CT KUB for renal causes
- Treat The Cause
- Analgesia

Dyspepsia

Is Indigestion

Chronic Recurrent Upper Abdominal Pain + Feeling Full Early ±Bloating ± Bleching ± Heartburn

Differential Diagnosis

1. GORD
2. Gastritis
3. Peptic ulcer
4. Malignancy
5. Pancreatitis
6. Cholecystitis
7. Cardiac pain
8. Drugs

Hematuria

Differential Diagnosis

Diagnoses in < 45 years	Diagnoses in > 45 years	Diagnoses to consider in any age
Pulmonary renal Syndrome • Good pasture's • Granulomatosis Polyangiitis • Microscopic polyangiitis **GNs:** • IgA nephropathy • Post streptococcal GN • Alport`s syndrome **Other Vasculitidis:** • PAN • HSP **CT diseases:** • Systemic sclerosis • Lupus nephritis **Congenital** • ADPKD • ARPKD	**Malignancy:** In Kidney ,bladder , or prostate **Benign:** Benign prostatic hypertrophy **Infection:** Prostatitis	**Renal stones** **Infections:** • UTI • Pyelonephritis • IEC • TB • Cystitis **Drugs:** • Anticoagulants • Thrombolysis • Cyclophosphamide **Others:** • Bleeding tendency • Catheterization • Radio/chemotherapy

Analysis Of The Complaint

OCDAE

Associated symptoms

• Hemoptysis → **Good Pasture`s, Granulomatosis Polyangiitis**
• Dysuria, Fevers, Frequency, urgency → **UTI**
• Loin Pains, Fevers → **Pyelonephritis**
• Loin Pains → **Stones**
• Renal Colick → **Stones**
• Sore throat → **IgA Nephropathy**
• Dermatitis Herpitiform → **IgA Nephropathy**
• Hesitancy, Poor stream, Dribbling at the end, sense of incomplete evacuation → **Prostatism**

Past History

• Celiac disease → **IgA Nephropathy**
• ADPKD
• Recent Catheterization

- SLE
- SAH → **ADPKD**
- Acromegaly → Renal Stones
- Hypercalcemia (MENI/MENII/Sarcoidosis) → **Renal stones**

Drug History

- Anticoagulants
- Cyclophosphamide

Family History

- RCC
- ADPKD
- Stones

Social History

Menstruation → Could it be menstrual blood

Quick Discussion

How Would You Manage this patient?

- CTKUB for renal stones
- Urine dip
- Urine MC & S
- U/S KUB
- Group and save blood
- ABCDE
- Renal/Urology R/V

Polyuria

Differential Diagnosis

Osmotic	1ry Polydypsia	Inability To Concentrate Urine	
		Cranial DI	**Nephrogenic DI**
• DM	• Psychogenic	• *Idiopathic*	• *Familial*
• Uremia	• Habitual	• *Post*: Surgical, Radiation, Trauma	• $\uparrow Ca2+ , \downarrow K+$
• Diuretics		• *Tumors*	• *Drugs:* Lithium, Tetracyclines, Amphotrecin
		• *Vascular*: Apoplexy, Aneurysm	• *Tubulointerstitial diseases:*
		• *Infiltration*: Sarcoidosis , Histocytosis	o Sickle cell anemia
		• *Infection:* TB, Meningitis	o Obstruction
		• *DIDMOAD*	o Pyelonephhritis

Analysis Of The Complaint

OCDAE

Associated symptoms

• Weight Loss, Polyphagia → **Diabetes Mellitus**

• Lupus Pernio rash, E.N. → **Sarcoidosis**

• S/S MEN I & II → **Nephrogenic DI**

• Drinking A lot of Fluids daily → **Psychogenic Polydypsia**

Past medical history

• CKD

• Meningitis

Drug history

• Diuretics

• Lithium

Quick Discussion

How Would You Manage This Patient?

• Basic blood tests

• Water deprivation test with desmopressin replacement

• Serum Calcium

• Investigations for the cause if present

• Fasting Blood Sugar

• HbA1C

• Desmopressin for Cranial DI

• Thiazides diuretic for Nephrogenic DI

Calcium Disorders

Differential Diagnosis

Causes of Hypercalcemia	Causes of Hypocalcemia

• Hyperparathyroidism
  ○ 1ry
  ○ Tertiary
  ○ part of MEN
• ↑ Vit D
• Bone tumors
• Multiple Myeloma
• **Drugs:** Thiazies, Lithium
• Sarcoidosis
• Milk alkali syndrome
• Dehydration alone
• Familial hypocalciuric hypercalcemia
• Metastatic CA to the bones
	• ↓ Albumin
	• Vit D ↓ *(Liver, renal or malabsorption)*
	• Hypoparathyroidism
	• Acute pancreatitis
	• ↓ Mg2+ *(Resistance to PTH)*
	• Acute ↑ PO4+
	  ○ Renal failure
	  ○ Rhabdomyolysis
	  ○ Tumor lysis Syndrome
	• **Drugs:** Cisplatin, bisphosponates
	• AD hypercalciuric hypocalcemia

Analysis Of The Complaint

OCDAE

Symptoms Of The Cause

Symptoms Of Hypercalcemia

• Constipation
• Abdominal pains
• PUD
• Bony Pains
• Renal Stones & Hematuria
• Depression

Symptoms Of Hypocalcemia

• Tingling around the mouth & finger tips
• Tetany
• Palpitations

Past History

• Parathyroid disorders
• S/S MEN I, II → **Hypercalcemia**
• S/S Polyglandular deficiency → **Hypocalcaemia**
• Cancers

Drug History

• Lithium
• Thiazides
• Bisphosphonates

Quick Discussion

What Investigations You Want to do?

Hypercalcemia

- PTH levels
- If PTH high → Primary hyperpathyroidism
- If PTH Low → Malignancy
- Sestamibi Scan for Parathyroid glands
- ACE levels for Sarcoidosis
- Admit if Ca > 3

Hypocalcemia

- Vit D Levels
- Serum Mg
- U & Es

How Would You Treat This Patient?

Hypercalcemia

- IV Fluids
- Bisphosphonates if severe & Malignancy related
- Cinacalcet for primary hyperparathyroidism not fit for surgery
- Treat the cause
- Surgery for Primary & Tertiary hyperparathyroidism

Hypocalcemia

- IV Calcium Gluconate
- Oral Calcium supplements
- Treat the cause

Renal Impairment

Differential diagnosis

Prerenal	Renal	Postrenal
Volume depletion • Diarrhea • Bleeding • Vomiting • Diuretics • Poor intake	**1ry GN :** Nephritic or nephrotic **2ry GN:** SLE ,RA ,MC TD, HUS ,TTP, DIC, Cryoglobulinemia, Malignancy, Good pasture, Granulomatosis Polyangiitis, Easinophilic polyangiitis **Alport`s syndrome** **DM** **Amyloidosis** **Vascular:** Vasculitis, HTN Nephrosclerosis, Renal Vein Thrombosis **Tubulointerstitial** **Congenital disorders:** ADPKD, VHL ,Tuberous Sclerosis **IV Contrast** **Drugs:** Gentamicin PPIs Penicillins	Obstruction *(ask about pain)*

Analysis Of The Complaint

OCDAE

Symptoms of Uremia:

SOB, Itching, Mouth odour, lethargy, Nausea, Vomiting

Symptoms of Overload:

SOB, L.L. Edema

Urinary Symptoms:

Hematuria, Frequency, Urgency, Oliguria, Polyuria, Dysuria, Proteinuria *(puffy eyelids, LL swelling, Frothy Urine)*

Symptoms/ History of The Causes

DM /HTN/ Stones /Reflux /APKD /VHL/Tuberous Sclerosis /Analgesics /dehydration

Quick Discussion

How Would You Manage This Patient?

• U & Es
• FBC , Crp

- Urine Dip
- Urine MC&S
- U/S KUB
- Urinary Na
- Stop offending drugs
- IV Fluids if pre-renal
- Monitor Urine output closely
- Dialysis if
- Pericarditis
- Resistant Hyperkalaemia
- Resistant acidosis
- Fluid overload resistant to treatment

Dizziness

Patients may use terms as dizziness, vertigo or feeling light headed

Differential Diagnosis

Peripheral	Central
• Perilymphatic fistula	**Cerebellar And Brainstem Dysfunction:**
• BPPV	• Multiple sclerosis
• Meniere's disease	• Cerebellopontine angle tumors
• Ototoxicty (SNHL)	• Basal meningitis
• Migraine	• Vertebrobasilar ischemia or hemorrhage
• Arrhythmia	• Drugs
• Labyrinthine dysfunction:	• Migraine
○ Labyrinthitis	• Alcohol
○ Vestibular neuritis	• Postural Hypotension
○ CV disease that leads to labyrinthine	• Cervical Ribs
hemorrhage or ischemia	• Subclavian Steel Syndrome
○ Trauma (Petrous temporal bone)	• Normal pressure Hydrcephalus
• Acoustic Neuroma	**Cerebrum:**
	• Temporal lobe epilepsy
	Hereditary:
	• Arnold-Chiari malformation
	• Forereach's ataxia
	• Spinocerebellar ataxia
	• Ataxia Telangectasia
	• Hypoglycemia

Analysis of The Complaint

1st make sure what does the patient means exactly

- Vertigo: The room spinning around the patient
- Syncope: LOC
- Lightheadedness/ Dizziness not feeling alright

Age Of Onset:

- Vestibular Dysfunction, Stroke, Cardiac Causes → More With Old Age
- Pre-syncope → More Common in younger Ages

Onset:

- Acute vertigo is mostly due to cerebro-vascular disease or peripheral vestibular dysfunction
- Insidious onset is mostly due to central vestibular dysfunction

Duration:

- Dizziness lasting less than a minute→ Presyncope or BPPV
- Lasting minutes to few hours→ Labyrinthitis, vestibular Neuritis, TIAs, Migraine
- Prolonged vertigo→ Stroke, Multiple sclerosis
- Persistent vertigo lasting months is mostly psychogenic as the CNS adapts to the defect
- Recurrent vertigo →BPPV or Meniere's

Description Of Symptoms:

- Associated features *preceding, during* and *after* the event
- Open questions followed by close Q. to differentiate vertigo, syncope and presyncope
  - "DO you experience light headedness as if you are about to faint?"
  - "DO you lose consciousness?"
  - "DO you feel the room is spinning around you or you yourself are spinning?"

Precipitants:

- Sudden head and neck movements → Vestibular dysfunction , vertebra-basilar ischemia, BPPV
- Coughing, sneezing, and straining→ perilymphatic fistula
- Viral illness → Layrinthitis or vestibular Neuritis
- Trauma→ carotid or vertebral artery dissection
- Standing Up Suddenly → Postural Hypotension

Exclude Precipitants Of Syncope/ Presyncope:

- Standing from sitting → Orthostatic hypotension
- Prolonged standing, large meal, hot environment → Vasovagal
- Prolonged fasting → Hypoglycemia
- Cough, Micturation, Defecation →Situational syncope

Relieving Factors:

- Sitting down relieves presyncope
- Limiting head movements improves BPPV, Labyrinthitis, Vestibular neuritis
- Fixation on a distant object improves peripheral vestibular dysfunction

Associate Symptoms:

Nausea & Vomiting	Vestibular dysfunction
Sensoy neural hearing symptoms	• Tinnitus, Deafness, Ear Fullness → Meniere's disease or Acoustic Neuroma
Neurological symptoms	• Headache, N/V , Seizures, Blurred Vision →**Space Occupying Lesion Or Migraine** • Diplopia, Dysarthria, Dysphagia ,Limb Weakness ,Sensory Disturbance, Loss Of Consciousness → **Brainstem Symptoms** • Tremors ,Ataxia ,Gait An Balance Disturbance → **Cerebellar** • Facial Sensory Loss And Weakness+ Hearing Loss →**Cerebellopontine Angle Tumors**
Cardiac symptoms	Palpitations before the feeling → **Postural Hypotension / Tachyarrhythmia**
Psychiatric symptoms	Anxiety, panic attacks

Past History:

- Cardiac diseases
- Neurological diseases (Epilepsy, MS, Migraine)
- Vascular risk factors (DM, HTN, Hyperlipiemia ,previous vascular events)
- Head injuries
- Malignancy (paraneoplastic Syndrome that affect cerebellum)

Drug History:

- Phenytoin, Carbamazepine → Cerebellar Syndrome
- Antihypertensive → Orthostatic hypotension
- Aminoglycosies, NSAIDs, Furosemide, Cisplatinum → Ototoxicity
- Insulin, Oral hypoglycemic medications → hypoglycemia and presyncope

Social History:

- Alcohol: chronic excessive consumption can cause cerebellar ydrome

Syncope – Presyncope

Patients Use Various Terms as Collapse, Funny Turns, Dizziness, Passing Out, Faints, Fits So It's Important to Determine What Does the Patient Mean Exactly

Differential Diagnosis

Cardiac	• **Arrhythmias** :
	  o Sinus bradycardia, sick sinus syndrome
	  o Heart block, sustained ventricular tachycardia
	  o Prolonged QT syndrome
	• **Aortic stenosis**
	• **HOCM**
	• **MI**
	• **Carotid sinus hypersensitivity**

Neurological	• **Epilepsy**
	• **Autonomic failure**
	  o DM/Parkinson's/Multisystem atrophy
	• **Neurally mediated syncope** :
	  o Vasovagal /situational (Cough, Micturation, Defecation)
	• **Vertebrobasilar ischemia**

Metabolic	• **Hypoglycemia**
Others	• **Orthostatic Hypotension** o Drugs, Hemorrhage, Dehydration, Hypoadrenalism, D.M., Parkinson`s • **Hyperventilation $** • **Anemia**

Analysis of The Complaint

OCDAE

Frequency

Symptoms Preceding The Event:

Prodromal symptoms:

"How did you feel just before the collapse?"

- Nausea, abdominal pain, flushing, light headedness, blurred vision → **Neurally mediated**
- Aura (strange sensation) → **Seizures**
- Focal neurological symptoms → **Cerebrovascular disease** or if seizures occurs after → **2ry generalization of a partial seizure**
- Sudden onset headache and neck stiffness → **Subarachnoid hemorrhage**
- Headache, Neck Stiffness, Fever and Rash → **Meningitis**
- Chest Pain, Dyspnea, Palpitations → **Cardiac cause** (however a sudden loss of consciousness without warning with rapid recovery mostly represents **Arrhythmia**)

Precipitants:

"What were you doing just before the collapse, anything triggered it?"

- Exercise: is **Cardiac** until prove otherwise
- Flashes of light/Sleep deprivation /hunger /recent illness /illicit drugs /alcohol and its withdrawal: **Seizure**
- On Standing or change in posture: **Orthostatic Hypotension** and **Autonomic Dysfunction**
- Hot weather /prolonged standing /large meals: **Vasovagal**
- Micturation /defecation /coughing /sneezing: **Situational**
- Neck movements /shaving /tight collar: **Carotid hypersensitivity**
- Raising the arm: **Subclavian steel**
- Prolonged fasting: **Hypoglycemia**
- Anxiety, Fear: **Hyperventilation**

Events during the attack:

- "Did You Lose Consciousness? Did You Hit Your Head Or Injure Yourself?"

- "Do You Remember Falling To The Ground? Can You Remember What Happened?"
- "Collateral History: Color Of The Patient, Seizure Activity"
  - Looking Pale + LOC for few seconds or minutes → **Cardiac, Neurally mediated**
  - Fits with Biting of tongue & urinary Incontinence → **Seizures**
  - If a patient has LOC he can have some shakes without being a fit without tongue biting of urinary incontinence due to cereberal hypoxia

Symptoms after the attack:

- Time to recovery? Rapid in Cardiogenic and vasovagal , prolonged after seizures
- Any confusion, headache ,limb weakness (Post ictal)
- Injury: from tonic clonic seizures or from the fall
- Number or previous attacks

Drug History:

- Insulin and Sulphonylurea → Hypoglycemia
- Antihypertensives → Hypotension
- BBs → Bradycardia

Seizures

Differential Diagnosis

- **Primary /Unprovoked**
- **Secondary /Provoked:**
  - **Infection:** Acute meningitis, Post meningitis, Encephalitis, Cerebral malaria, Abscess, TB
  - **Neoplastic** :1ry or 2ry
  - **Vascular**: Stroke and post-stroke, A-V malformation, Cerebral venous thrombosis
  - **Trauma:** Head injury, Birth injury (cerebral palsy)
  - **Metabolic:** ↓ glucose , ↓Na+, ↓Ca2+, Uremia, Porphyria
  - **Drugs:** sub therapeutic levels of antiepileptic, Lithium, TCA, Recreational drugs, alcohol and benzodiazepines
  - **Syndrome associated with seizures** :Tuberous sclerosis, Sturge-Weber, Down Syndrome

Analysis Of The Complaint

Differentiate True Seizures From Conditions That Mimic Seizures.

  - These are: Syncope, TIA, migraine, panic attacks, breath holing attacks & hyperventilation

A Collateral History Is Important, Ask about:

- If this is the first time? or the patient is known to have epilepsy
- Age of onset
- Total number of events
- Duration of each episode
- Time interval between each episode
- Pattern of symptoms of each episode

Symptoms Preceding The Event:

- **Prodromal** :usually present with syncope and not seizures
- **Precipitants**
- **Aura:**
  - Auras can be motor, sensory, autonomic, or cognitive
  - "Did you experience any strange smells, tastes, or other sensation before you lost consciousness?"

Associated Symptoms For Etiology look for symptoms of:

- Meningitis
- Cerebrovascular disease
- Raised ICP
- Recent ear or URT infection
- Head injury

Events During The Attack:

- Impairment of consciousness (in generalized and complex partial ,but not in simple partial)
- If yes, then a collateral history must be obtained

Symptoms After The Attack:

- Limb weakness (Todd's paresis)
- Confusion and headache
- Disturbed LOC
- Injury
- Time to full recovery

Weakness of Arms or Legs

- Diseases of nervous system
- Diseases of neuromuscular junction
- Muscle disorders

Analysis Of The Complaint

History Aims:

- Differentiate true muscle weakness from motor impairment of systemic illness
- Localize the lesion
- Determine the cause

Establishing True Weakness:

Patients could mean tiredness, malaise, rigidity, and incoordination

Distribution:

Which areas are affected and if symmetrical or asymmetrical

- Asymmetrical weakness → CNS or P.N. (Peripheral neuropathy)
- Symmetrical → Muscle disease or P.N. (Peripheral neuropathy)

Onset:

- Acute → Vascular event
- Subacute → Inflammatory, infectious, traumatic
- Chronic → Neoplastic, Degenerative, Metabolic

Duration, Progression, Recovery:

- TIA < 24 hours or stroke
- Stroke > 24 hours
- Multiple sclerosis, there will be periods of recovery

Functional Impairment:

"What activities can you no longer do because of the weakness?"

Climbing stairs, writing, standing from sitting position, combing hair

Associated Neurological Symptoms:

Dysphasia	Cortical sign
Facial weakness and sensory loss	Crossed or Uncrossed Hemiplegia, MS
Sensory disturbance	Depends on the site of the lesion
Visual disturbance (Amaurosis Fugax)	Thromboembolism or vertebrobasilar ischemia
Bulbar symptoms (Dysphagia, Dysarthria, Dysphonia, Diplopia, Vertigo, Vomiting, Hearing Impairment)	Brainstem involvement
Gait disturbance	Depends on the site of the lesion
Cerebellar symptoms (Dysathria, Ataxia, Tremors, Incoorination)	Cerebellar affection commonly MS
Sphincter disturbance	Distal spinal cord disease
Headaches	↑ ICP
Seizures	Todd's paralysis

Associated Non-Neurological Symptoms:

Fever	Infective or inflammatory
Neck pain	Carotid dissection, Vertebral Artery Dissection or subarachnoid hemorrhage
Back pain	+ LL weakness + sphincter disturbance is an emergency → Cauda Equina lesion
Constitutional symptoms	Systemic illness ,malignancy

Muscle Weakness

Differential Diagnosis

UMNL	LMNL	Neuromuscular junction	Muscle
Brain and Brainstem: Stroke MS Space occupying lesion Seizures (Todd's paralysis)	**Peripheral neuropathy:** Polyneuropat - ies Mononeurop a-thies Mononeuritis multiplex	Mysthania Gravis Drugs induced MG Lambert Eaton Syndrome Botulism Organophosph -ate toxicity	**Hereditary:** Muscular dystrophy (Duchenne, becker, fascioscapulohumeral) Myotonic dystrophy Hypo/Hyper kalaemic periodic paralysis
Spinal cord: Trauma ,tumors Myelitis (MS) ,infections Hematoma ,A-V malformation			**Acquired:** Polymyositis/ Dermatomyositis Inclusion body myositis Electrolyte imbalance Endocrine disease (cushing,Addison,hypothyroidism) Infections(Viral ,Toxoplasmosis, trichinosis, cysticercosis) Drug induced myopathy Rhabdomyolysis
Anterior horn cell: Motor neurone disease Polio Lead poisoning			

Analysis Of The Complaint:

Differentiate functional weakness which is due to pain, depression, or chronic illness from true weakness

Age Of Onset:

Hereditary myopathies and Some peripheral neuropathies present in childhood

Onset ,Course, Duration:

- **Acute weakness rapidly progressive** → Guillian Barre Syndrome, Stroke, Botulism, Organophosphate, Lead, Transverse myelitis, Myasthenia Gravis crisis
- **Chronic weakness with slow progression** → Space occupying lesion ,Myasthenia Gravis
- **Episodic weakness** (sudden onset and full resolution) → hypo/hyper periodic paralysis

Distribution:

- Generalized weakness
- Localized weakness
- Distal symmetrical weakness
- Proximal symmetrical weakness

Pattern:

- Ascending weakness: Guillain Barre $ and spinal cord disorders
- Descending Weakness: Organophosphate, lead, Botulism, Miller fisher syndrome

Precipitating and relieving factors:

- Exercise and meals rich in carbs and Na+ →hypokalaemic paralysis
- Diet rich in K+→ hyperkalaemic paralysis
- Exercise → aggravates MG and improves Lambert Eaton $

Associated symptoms:

- Muscle cramps and stiffness
- Dyspnea
- Bulbar symptoms → Stroke, MS, MND
- Neurological symptoms :Visual disturbance ,diplopia ,Ptosis ,speech disturbance, Parasthesia, seizures, back pain, gait disturbance , sphincter disturbance
- Thyroid disease: hypo/hyper
- Cushing's syndrome: proximal myopathy

- Addison's disease: Generalized weakness
- Rash: dermatomyositis
- Constitutional symptoms
- Depressive symptoms
- Respiratory symptoms → Dermatomyositis, Polymyositis

Functional Status:

- Patients finding difficulty in climbing stairs, combing hair, standing up from seated position may have a proximal myopathy
- Patients finding all types of daily activities difficult may be having functional weakness

Gait Disturbances

Differential diagnosis

Neurological	Non-Neurological

• Frontal lobe diseases
  o *Dementia*
  o *Normal pressure hydrocephalus*
• Cerebellar ataxia
• Parkinsonism
• Spasticity (UMNL)
• Flaccidity *(P.N./myopathy)*
• Sensory ataxia
	• Musculoskeltal
	• Arthritis
	• Claudication
	• Postural hypotension
	• Alcohol
	• Drugs
	  o Benzodiazepines
	  o Antidepressants
	  o Antipsychotics

Analysis Of The Complaint

OCD AE capacity + Nature of Gait

Alarming Symptoms

- Acute onset
- Sphincter disturbance
- Sensory Level
- Systemic symptoms

Nature of Gait:

- **Spastic gait (Scissoring):** *"Do you have to drag both feet? Does your foot cross over when walking?"*

  o Ms,

  o Friedrich`S Ataxia,

  o Sub Acute Combined Degeneration

  o Anterior Spinal Artery Occlusion (Dissociated Sensory Loss)

- **Hemiparetic gait:** "Do you drag 1 leg at the side to walk?"
  o Stroke

- **High Steppage gait:** "Do you have to lift your feet high up?"
  o Peripheral neuropathy

- **Ataxic gait:**
  o Cerebellar (Drunken gait): *"Do you have troubles maintaining your balance? Do you fall at one side?"*

    ▪ Cerebellar disease

  o Sensory: *"Do You have to look to your feet while walking? Do You feel unsteady when closing your eyes?"*

    ▪ Tabes Dorsalis

- **Parkinsonian gait (Shuffling /Festinant):** *"Do your feet shuffle along the ground? Do you have difficulty starting to walk?"*

- **Waddling gait:** *"Do you feel as if you are waddling from side to side?"*

  o **Duchene muscle dystrophy**

  o **Becker`s muscle dystrophy**

- **Antalgic gait**: painful gait

- **Choreic gait**

Serious Causes That Must Be Excluded:

- Spinal cord compression
- Stroke
- Spinal cord ischemia
- Guillain barre
- Normal pressure hydrocephalus

Acute Confusion (Delirium)

Delirium: sudden onset and fluctuating ↓ in cognitive function and consciousness. It is reversible

Dementia: progressive and irreversible ↓ in cognitive function without any ↓ in consciousness

In all ages	> 65 years	< 65 years
• **Electrolyte imbalance**: ↑ Ca2+, Low Na, High Na • Hypercapnia • Infection • **Metabolic**: liver, kidney, Thyroid, Glucose ↓ or ↑ • Brain tumors • MI • PE • Alcohol intoxication & withdrawal • Drugs: Anticholinergic, Opiates, Dopamine agonists, Steroids	• Polypharmacy • Stroke /Subdural hematoma • UTI, Respiratory infections • Acute urinary retention • Fecal impaction • Dehydration	• Recreational drug use and withdrawal • Meningitis • Encephalitis • HIV

Diagnosis Of Delirium Requires 1 And 2 + 3 Or 4:

1. Acute Onset And Fluctuating:

Is this a dramatic change in behavior from baseline? Does the abnormal behavior comes and go during the day?

2. Inattention:

Does he/she have difficulty focusing? Is he/she easily distracted?

3. Disorganized Thinking:

Do you have difficulty following their conversation?

4. Altered Level Of Consciousness:

Does he/she have episodes of drowsiness or agitation?

Dementia

Differential Diagnosis:

1ry causes	2ry causes
Neurodegenerative conditions	**Metabolic:**
• Alzheimer's	• Vit B12, Folic acid, thiamine ↓
• Parkinson plus syndromes:	• Thyroid ↓
o Progressive supranuclear palsy	• Cushing`s syndrome
o Corticobasal degeneration	• Wilson's disease
o Dementia with Lewy bodies	**Vascular:**
o Frontotemporal dementia	• Stroke
• CJD	• Subdural hematoma
• Huntington's disease	• Antiphospholipid $
	Neoplastic:
Others:	• 1ry or 2ry
• Vascular dementia	**Inflammatory:**
• Normal pressure hydrocephalus	• SLE
	Drugs And Toxins:
	• Anticholinergics
	• Alcohol (Korsakoffs $)
	• Heavy metal exposure
	Infection:
	• Syphilis
	• AIDS dementia

Analysis Of The Complaint

OCD AE

Characteristics

- **Memory loss:** for short or long-term events
- **Attention and concentration** : lost early in Lewy dementia
- **Orientation:** Loss of special awareness in Alzehiemer`s disease
- **Aphasia**: *"use wrong words for familiar objects? Difficulty understanding written information, use same word to answer different questions?"*
- **Apraxia:** *"difficulty dressing or washing?"*
- **Fluctuation:** there are good & bad times in Alzehiemer`s disease

Fevers

Analysis Of The Complaint

OCD

Characteristics:

Continuous: Typhoid, pneumonia, Brucellosis, UTI, T.B, LRTI.

Remittent:

- The temperature remains above normal throughout the day and fluctuates more than 2 degree Celsius in 24 hours
- IEC, Typhoid

Intermittent:

- The temperature is present only for some hours in a day and remains to normal for the remaining hours.
- Malaria ,Kala azar ,sepsis

Relapsing (undulant)

- Brucellosis

Associated Symptoms → System inquiry

If Returning Travelers

- Date of travel and duration of stay
- Nature of area and accommodation
- Means of transportations
- Activities :
  o Sexual contact (Protected/Unprotected)
  o Animal contact
  o Insects exposure
  o Needles and Blood exposure
  o Hospital admission
  o Food and drink
  o water sports and lakes
  o Use of IV Recreation Drugs
- Vaccination
- Malarial prophylaxis
- Symptoms Onset in Relation to the Travel History (Incubation Period)
- Any symptoms arose besides Fevers
- Common causes
  o Gastro-enteritis
  o Infective diarrhea
  o Malaria
  o Legionella Pneumonia
  o Viral Penumonitis

Occupation

- Sewage Workers → Leptospirosis
- Farmers → Brucellosis

Differential Diagnosis

- Infections including T.B, HIV seroconversion
- Malignancy
- Vascular: Acute MI, PE , Pontine hemorrhage
- Trauma : massive crush injury
- Collagen disorders
- Endocrine: Thyrotoxicosis and Addison's
- Neuroleptic malignant syndrome, Seretonin syndrome

Systemic Lupus Erythematosis

GP Letter

Rheumatology Clinic

Dear Dr

Re: P.J. (DOB: 12/01/1985)

I would be grateful if you kindly review this 31 years Old lady who was complaining of lethargy, painful hand joints & Photosensitivity, I am thinking she might be having SLE..

Kind Regards,

Criteria For Diagnosis:

1. Malar rash
2. Discoid rash
3. Photosensitivity
4. Oral ulcers
5. Renal
6. CNS :fits ,dementia ,depression ,weakness, pins/needles ,Transverse myelitis
7. Serositis
8. Arthritis
9. Blood: ↓RBCs ,↓PLTs, ↓WBC (lymphopenia)
10. ANA
11. Anti-DNA, Antiphospholipid

Quick Discussion

What Are The Causes Of Photosensitivity?

- SLE
- Porphyria Cutanea Tarda
- Erythropoietic Porphyria
- Pemphigoid
- Pemphigus
- Drugs
  - Thiazides
  - NSAIDS
  - Sulphonamides
  - Tetracyclines
  - Ciprofloxacin
  - Antihistamines
  - OCPs

How Would You Investigate This Patient?

- U& Es
- FBC
- Clotting
- ESR
- CrP
- ANA
- Anti DsDNA
- Renal Biopsy if needed

How Would You Treat This Patient?

- Steroids
- NSIADS
- Anti-Malarials
- DMARDS

<u>SLE Nephritis Treatment:</u>

- **Type 1, Type 2**:
  - o No treatment except for antiproteinuric (ACE or CCBs)
- **Type 3, Type 4**:
  - o Steroids + Cyclophosphamide → If falied Mycophenolate Mofetil
- **Type 5:**
  - o Less steroids + Cyclophosphamide → If failed Mycophenolate mofetil
- **Type 6:**
  - o Renal replacement therapy

N.B: Recurrence of lupus nephritis in transplanted kidney is 5 %

Weight Loss

Differential Diagnosis

Intentional

Non-Intentional:

Paradox (Normal Appetite)	Not Paradox (Poor Appetite)

• Uncontrolled DM
• Hyperthyroidism
• Pheocromocytoma
• Malabsorption syndrome
	• Chronic infections
	  o TB, HIV, Brucella
	• Chronic diseases:
	  o Liver, kidney, heart, respiratory
	• Inflammatory disorders:
	  o SLE, RA
	• Malignancy
	• Depression or anorexia nervosa
	• GIT diseases causing vomiting, dysphagia or abdominal pain

Analysis Of The Complaint

How Much Weight Over How Much Period Of Time?

Significant weight loss is loss of **4.5 kg** or >**5%** of the usual body weight over a period of 6 - 12 months.

Alarm Symptoms?

• **GIT:** **D**ysphagia, **D**iarrhea, **E**arly satiety, **A**bdominal pain, **M**elaena / hematochezia + Change in bowel habit
• **Constitutional symptoms:** Fever, Night sweats, Fatigue

Gastro-Intestinal Symptoms

Renal Symptoms

Respiratory Symptoms to R/O Cancers of Lung, T.B.

Endocrine Symptoms to exclude DM, Hyperthyroidism, Addison

Psychiatric History to R/O Depression

Questions To R/O Different Causes

Weight Gain

Differential Diagnosis

Intentional

Unintentional

Endocrinal	Fluid retention	Drugs	Others
• Hypothyroidism • Cushing • Insulinoma • PCO • Hypothalamic (Trauma, tumor, inflammation, surgery)	• Congestive HF • Nephrotic or CKD • Liver cirrhosis • Meig's syndrome	• NSAIDs • Steroids • Anabolic steroids • OCPs • Antipsychotics • Antidepressants • Antiepileptics • Insulin & sulphonylurea & Glitazones	• Pregnancy • Abdominal /Pelvic mass • Obesity • Nicotine withdrawal • Prader-Willi syndrome

Analysis Of The Complaint

How Much In How Much Period Of Time?

Where Exactly?

- **Cushing**: Truncal, Interscapular, Face
- **Hypothyroidism:** Facial Puffness, Leg Oedema (Non-Pitting)

Questions For The Complications Of Obesity:

CVS, DM, GORD, Gallstones, OSA, Malignancy

Ask About Symptoms to R/O Different Causes:

Drug History

- NSAIDs
- Steroids
- Anabolic steroids
- OCPs
- Antipsychotics
- Antidepressants
- Antiepileptics
- Insulin
- Sulphonylurea
- Glitazones

Neck Lump

Differential Diagnosis:

Cervical L.N.s

- Swelling on the sides of the neck, Multiple, Tender or non-tender
  - **Hematological Causes:**
    - Lymphoma
    - CLL
    - ALL
  - **Infections:**
    - HIV
    - EBV
    - CMV
    - T.B.
    - Toxoplasmosis
    - Brucellosis
  - **Infiltration**
    - Sarcoidosis
    - Amyloidosis
    - Metastasis From Near By Tumour
  - **Collagen Disorders**
    - Felty`s syndrome
    - SLE
    - RA
    - SJogran
  - **Drugs**
    - Phenytoin
    - Atenolol
    - Allopurinol
    - Cephalosporin antibiotics
    - Brucellosis

Thyroid disease

- Swelling In The Centre Of The Neck Moves With Swallowing, Might Be Tender
  - **With Hyperthyroidism :**
    - Graves's disease (Eye Signs & Nail changes)
    - Multinodular Goiter
    - Subacute Thyroiditis Solitary Nodule
    - Adenoma

  - **With Hypothyroidism :**
    - Hashimoto's Thyroiditis
  - **With No Hormonal Change:**
    - Thyroid Cancer Alone or as part of MEN 2

Others:

  - **Congenital:**
    - Branchial (One on lateral side of the neck)
    - Thyroglossal Cyst (Central Small Moves With Swallowing)
    - Dermoid Cyst
  - **Vascular:**
    - Carotid Artery Aneurysm

o Carotid Body Tumor (Chemodectoma)

o **Neoplastic**

o **Cervical rib**

Salivary gland disease:

- Inflammation or Tumor
- Parotid gland swollen in
    o Sarcoidosis
    o SJogran
    o Pleomorphic adenoma
    o Cancer
    o Stones
    o Mumps

Analysis Of The Complaint

OCD AE

Lump Characteristics

- *Site*
    o *L.Ns are on sides of the neck and submental, submandibular*
    o *Ask about L.Ns in Groin & Axilla*
    o *Thyroid is central and moves with swallowing*
- *Size*
- *Shape*
    o *Butterfly is thyroid*
    o *Rounded could be L.Ns*
- *Number*
    o *L.Ns are multiple*
- *Consistency*
    o *Firm L.N.s could be due to infection or malignancy*
- *Mobility*
    o *L.Ns are freely mobile*
- *Tenderness*
    o *L.N.s if Tender → Infection*
    o *Thyroid if tender → Thyroiditis*

Ask About Symptoms to R/O Different Causes:

Diabetes Mellitus

Background of DM:

- **Type and estimated duration**
  - Long Duration is associated with Micro & Macrovascular complications
- **Control:**
  - **Symptoms of hyperglycemia**
    - Weight loss
    - Polyuria
    - polyphagia
  - **Symptoms and Frequencies of hypoglycemia**
  - **Recent home glucose monitoring or HbA1C**
  - **Admissions with DKA or HONK**
  - **Current treatment**
  - **Diet and exercise**
- **Occupation & Driving If The Patient Is On Insulin**
  - HGV drivers are banned if they are on insulin

Complications of DM:

- **Macrovascular :**
  - Coronary Artery Disease
  - Cerebrovascular Accident
  - Peripheral Vascular Disease
- **Microvascular:**
  - Retinal
  - Renal
  - Neuropathy
  - Autonomic Neuropathy
  - Foot Disease
- **HTN**
- **Hyperlipidaemia**

HIV + ve Patient

Specific History:

- When Were You Diagnosed? How?
- How Did you Catch It?
- What Was your Last CD4 Count?
- Any Contact With People With Long Standing Chest Infection? (T.B)
- Do you Have Any Resistance or Sensitivity to Any Medication?
- What Medications Are U Taking Now?
  - **Abcavir** Causes Fever, Rash , Diarrhea , Abdominal Pain
  - **Efaverinz** Causes Fever, Rash Inc. Liver Enzymes
  - **Zidovudine:** Headaches , Diarrhea , Abdominal Pain
  - **Lamivudine:** Headaches , Loss Of Appetite
  - **Neverapine:** Headaches , Allergy, Liver Toxicity , Diarrhea

Systemic Review

Sexual History

Social History

Causes Of Abdominal Pain In HIV Patients

- Infections :Cryptosporodium (Flourescent microscopy with auramine stain or Abs)
- Dedanosine pancereatitis
- Peritonitis
- Kaposi Sarcoma

Joint Pain

Differential Diagnosis

Mono/oligoarthritis	Polyarthritis
• Trauma	• RA
• Septic arthritis	• SLE
• Crystals arthritis	• Viral infection
• Sero –ve arthritis	• Vasculitis
• Osteoarthritis	• Sero –ve arthritis
• Lyme disease	• Osteoarthritis
• Malignancy	• Sarcoidosis
	• Malignancy
	• Parvovirus B 19
	• Hemochromatosis

Unilateral	Bilateral (Sym/Assym)
• Trauma	• SLE
• Septic arthritis	• RA
• Crystal arthritis	• Sero –ve arthritis
o Gout	o Enteropathic Arthrtitis
o Pseudogout	▪ Inflammatory Bowel Disease
• Sero –ve arthritis	▪ Whipple`s disease
• Osteoarthritis	o Reiter Syndrome
• Haemoarthrosis	o Psoriatic arthropathy
• Gonococcal arthritis	o Ankylosing Spondylitis
• Osteomyelitis	o HLAB27 +ve, RF -ve
• Osteosarcoma	• Osteoarthritis
• Rheumatic fever	• Sarcoidosis
• RA	• Malignancy
	• Parvovirus B 19
	• Hemochromatosis

Analysis Of The Complaint

SOCRATES + 3 D + 3 S

- **Distribution**
  - o 1 or many Joints?
  - o Large Or Small Joints?
- **Deformity**
  - o RA
  - o Psoriatic Arthropathy
  - o Gout

- **Duration**
  - ○ Acute vs Chronic arthritis
- **Systemic Symptoms** = symptoms of collagen diseases
  - ○ Rash, Hair Loss, Fevers, Painful Eyes, Muscle Pain, Recent GIT Or Urogenital Infections
- **Symmetrical or Asymmetrical**
  - ○ RA is B/L Symmetrical
- **Stiffness**
  - ○ RA Stiffness > 1 hour
  - ○ OA / Psoriasis < 1 hour

Questions To R/O Different Causes

Back Pain

GP Letter

Rheumatology Clinic

Dear Dr

Re: P.J. (DOB: 12/01/1946)

I would be grateful if you kindly review this 70 years Old lady who is complaining of back pain for the last 3 months, the pain is not improving despite voltarol gel and paracetamol, I requested an x-ray of his back still A/W to be done, Presented today to my clinic with severe pain with weakness in his R leg.

Kind regards,

Differential Diagnosis:

Mechanical	Inflammatory	Developmental	Neoplastic
• Osteo-arthritis (Spondylosis) • Paraspinal Muscles spasm • Disc Prolapse • Fracture vertebrae (Osteoporosis) • Spinal Canal Stenosis	• Sero-negative arthropathy e.g. Ankylosing spondylitis • Discitis • Osteomyelitis • Brucellosis • T.B. • Spinal abscess	• Scoliosis • Spondylolisthesis • Spina Bifida • Leg Length Discrepancy	• Multiple myeloma • Metastasis • Bony Tumor

Visceral Causes	Others
• Gastritis • Pancreatitis • Renal Colic / Pyelonephritis • Aortic dissection	• Retroperitoneal fibrosis • Meningitis • SAH • Transverse myelitis • Multiple sclerosis

Analysis Of The Complaint

SOCRATES

- Seronegative Arthropathies are worse in the morning with morning stiffness but improve with movement
- Mechanical pain is worse on movement and relived by rest

Neurological symptoms

- Weakness
- Paresthesia
- Sphincter Control
- Saddle Anesthesia
- Gait disturbance

Alarm Symptoms (Red Flags)

- History of malignancy ,↓ immunity, HIV
- Age> 50
- Fever, night sweats, Weight loss
- Duration > 1 month

- No response to analgesia
- Night pain
- Thoracic pain (Radicular Pain)
- Neurological Symptoms

Questions to R/O Different Causes

Quick Discussion

What Is Cauda Equina Syndrome?

- Cauda equina syndrome occurs when the nerve roots in the lumbar spine are compressed, disrupting sensation and movement & Pelvic autonomic functions
- This is a neurological emergency

What Is Cord Compression?

- Compression of one or more of the segments of the spinal cord causing paraparesis & Parasthesia below the lesion with sensory level.
- This is a neurological emergency

How Would You Investigate This Case?

- MRI Back if Alarm Signs
- Protein electrophoresis & urine for bence jones proteins for MM
- HLAB27 for seronegative arthropathies
- x-ray back shows sacro-ilitis in seronegative arthropathies & Spondylotic changes in spondylosis (Osteophytes & Loss of joint space)
- X-Ray is diagnostic for spondylolisthesis
- Investigations for the cause

How Would You Manage This Patient?

- Treatment of the cause
- Steroids & Radiotherapy for malignanct causes
- Analgesia

Dry Eyes

Differential Diagnosis

- Sarcoidosis

- Keratoconjuctivitis Sicca → RA

- Sjogren syndrome

- Inflammatory bowel

- Behcet's syndrome

- Facial Nerve Palsy

Analysis Of The Complaint

OCDAE

Visual Problems

- Loss of vison
- Blurring of vision
- Pain in Eyes
- Redness of the eyes

Oral Ulcers

Differential Diagnosis

- Aphthous ulcer
- Traumatic
- Drug induced: Bisphosphonates
- Bechet`s disease
- Reiter`s syndrome
- Inflammatory bowel diseases
- Celiac disease
- Pemphigus valgaris
- SLE
- Infections: Syphilis ,HSV ,Candida
- Malignancy :SCC, BCC

Analysis Of The Complaint

OCDAE

Any Other Sores In The Body

How Did The Sore Look Like In The Beginning

Questions To R/O Different Causes & Complications Of Causes

e.g. DVT & Iritis in a case of Behcet`s disease

Amenorrhea

Differential Diagnosis

1ry Amenorrhea	2ry Amenorrhea
• Turner	• Pregnancy
• Testicular feminization $	• Pituitary failure : trauma, tumor, infection, infiltration, Sheehan syndrome
• Congenital adrenal hyperplasia	• Hyperprolactinemia
• Chronic childhood illness	• PCO
	• Anorexia nervosa /Bulemia

Analysis of The Complaint

OCD AE

Usual Cycle Habit

Milk

• Hyperprolactinemia → Galactorrhea
• Failure of lactation → Sheehan Syndrome

Questions to R/O Different Causes

Hirsutism

Excessive hair growth in unusual sites

Differential Diagnosis

- Racial /familial
- Old age
- Pituitary: Acromegaly, ↑prolactin
- Ovarian: PCO, tumors
- Adrenal: congenital adrenal hyperplasia, Cushing, adrenal tumor
- Porphyria
- Drugs: Minoxidil, Cyclosporin, Danzaole, Phenytoin

Analysis Of The Complaint

OCD AE

Distribution

Virilism

- Clitoromegaly
- Male Baldness
- Deeper Voice

Drugs

Loss of Libido

Differential Diagnosis

	Males	Females
Causes	**Physical:** • Alcoholism • Abuse of recreational rugs • Obesity • ↑ Prolactin • ↓Testosterone • Thyrotoxicosis *(loss of libido + gynecomastia)* • Drugs: antiandrogen, thyroid hormones, anabolic steroids • Any major disease such as DM • Pan-hypopituitarism • Klinfelter`s syndrome **Psychological:** • Depression • Stress	**Physical:** • Alcoholism • Drug abuse • ↑ Prolactin • Drugs: tranquilizers • Any major disease such as DM • After childbirth **Psychological:** • Depression • Stress
History	• Hair distribution • Morning erection • Impotence • Testicular volume (masses or ↓) • Gynecomastia *(never ask for discharge)*	

Summary for Common Conditions

Veteranian (Farmer) + Arthritis+ Sweating + Depression = BRUCELLOSIS

- Undulant fever +Migratory Arthralgia & Myalgia +SPLEENOMEGALY
- Transmitted by close contact with animals secretions , drinking unpasteurized milk
- Transmition between humans by sex
- FBC: Leucopenia + Anemia + +ve Bengal rose reaction
- Blood culture & Detection of antibodies
- TTT: IM streptomycin 1gm for 14 days + Doxycyline 100 mg twice for 45 days

Hyponatremia + Fatigue +Chest symptoms (CA) = SIADH

- Causes: CA lung , Legionella Pneumonia ,Lung abscess , Head injury, Sarcoidosis , Carbamazepine , Morphine, Cholropropamide, SSRI , TCA , hypothyroidism
- Na <134 , Osm <280
- TTT: Cause , Fluid restriction , Demeclocycline , Conivaptan (V1 and V2 receptor antagonist)

Bloody diarrhea + Wt. loss + Abdominal Pain + young age = IBD

- Back Pain, Eye Pain
- INV.: Colonoscopy and biopsy
- TTT: Prednesolone , Mesalazine , Azathioprine , Methotrexate , surgery
- UC can be complicated by **PRIMARY SCLEROSING CHOLANGITIS**
  - Fatigue +obstructive jaundice (pale stool , dark urine) + pruritis
  - ERCP: beading of intrahepatic & extrahepatic bile ducts + P-ANCA
  - TTT: Ursodiol , Rifampicin , Cholestyramine , definitve =liver transplantation
- Crohns Complicated by GALL STONES
- True love and witts criteria for Crohns severity
  - Mild: < 4 motions , ESR is normal , no fever
  - Moderate : > 4 motions < 6 motions
  - Severe : > 6 motions + Fever + ESR > 30

Nephrotic + Hematuria + Loin Pain = RENAL VEIN THROMBOSIS

- CT Angiography
- Membranous G.N then Membrano-prolefrative G.N
- TTT: Anticoagulants, Surgery to remove clot

Pain & Tingling In The Legs At The End Of Day Relieved By Walking + Normal Examination = RESTLESS LEG SYNDROME

- Causes: Fe deficiency, polycythemia, Varicose veins, Thyroid disorders, Uremia, D.M, Antidopaminergic drugs, P.N., Familial (AD)
- INV: NCV, EMG, FBC, TFTs
- TTT: Cause /Dopamine agonist /Gabapentin

Sudden weakness which resolves in 24 h = TIA

- Causes: Athreosclerosis (D.M , HTN , cholesterol), Embolism from Heart, Hypercoagulable state, AF
- Risk of stroke is determined by ABCD2 score:
  - Age >60 =1p
  - Blood pressure >140/90 =1p
  - Clinical: speech but no weakness =1p , weakness =2 p
  - Duration < 1h = 1p , > 1h = 2p
  - Diabetes present =1p
  - 1-3 =mild , 4-5 =moderate , 6-7 high risk
- Hypercoagulable states:
  - Antiphospholipid Syndrome
    - DVT + Recurrent miscarriage + Stroke (recurrent thrombosis); Lupus anticoagulant, anticardiolipin → TTT: Asprin, heparin
  - Pregnancy & OCPs

o PNH (Hematuria + Anemia)

o Behcet`s :oral + genital ulcers + Iritis = pethargy test , TTT:Steroids

o Antithrombin III defiency: AD , Causes heparin resistance →increase the dose of heparin

o Protein C & S deficiency: Nephrotic (Xanthelasma + L.L edema+ Eye puffiness)

o Factor V Leiden :

   ▪ FH of recurrent thrombosis (AD) , the ratio of time for blood to clot

   ▪ Using 2 samples one with APC and other without, genetic testing

o Homocysteinuria

o Nephrotic syndrome

o Myeloproliferative disorders

Headaches by end of day = TENSION HEADACHE

- Band like
- Causes: Stress , Sleep deprevation , Eye strain , Irregular meal times
- TTT: NSAIDs / TCA prevent future attacks

Morning Headache + Obesity /OCP + Blurred vision +Vomiting = IDIOPATHIC INTRACRANIAL HTN

- Causes: OCP, Tetracycline , Vit A , Retinoids, WT.Gain , Steroids
- INV.: CT scan, MRV to R/O Sinus Thrombosis, Lumbar puncture (inc. opening pressure)
- TTT: Repeated lumbar puncture, Acetazolamide Wt.loss

Unilateral Headache (Around eyes) + No Aura + 2 Autonomic symptoms (Ptosis, Miosis, Rhinorrhea, lacrimation, Flushing, Sweating) on same side = CLUSTER HEADACHE

- More common in males
- TTT: Oxygen, Sumatryptan
- Prevention: CCBs, verapamil

Episodes of intense pain in Face for seconds, minutes or hours + triggering area on the Face + Triggered by light touch or air currents = TRIGEMINAL NEURALGIA

- Any division of V nerve (ophthalmic, maxillary or mandibular)
- 10% are bilateral
- Electric , stabbing or burning pain
- Triggered by: Chewing, brushing teeth, Talking, Shaving, Loud noise (concerts)
- Cause: Trauma , CPA tumours , Superior cerebellar artery aneurysm , post herpetic neuralgia , MS , Idiopathic
- TTT: Carbamazepine/Microvascular decompression

Anemia (S/S) + Red urine + Vascular thrombosis (Bud Chiari / DVT/ Mesenteric/ Stroke) = PNH

- INV.: Flow cytometry for CD55 & CD59
- TTT: Heparin / blood transfusion + Ecluzimab = B.M transplantation

Chronic chest infection + pins and needles in hands/proteinuria (Frothy urine) / L.L edema = BRONCHIECTASIS WITH AMYLOIDOSIS

- AMYLOIDOSIS: Abdominal pain , Vomiting , Diarrhea , HSM , P.N , CT$, Macroglossia , Hemoptysis , Cardiomyopathy →CCF, Nephrotic → RF
- INV: CT chest, sputum analysis, Rectal biopsy and staining with congo red for amyloidosis
- TTT: TTT of cause + Melphalan /Cyclophosphamide

ANEMIA + MCV>110 FL = MEGALOBLASTIC ANEMIA

- Dec. Hb., Macrocytosis, Low reticular count
- Platelets may be reduced
- WBC are hypersegmented

- Howell jolly bodies (Pernicious Anemia)
- Pernicious anemia is common with auto-immune conditions (Vitiligo)
- Pernicious anemia is common in the elderly
- <u>INV:</u>Anti-intrinsic factor abs, anti parietal cell Abs
- <u>TTT:</u> Cyanocobolamine every week for 4 weeks then every 3 months
- <u>VIT. B12 DEFIENCY</u>
  - o Pernicious Anemia (Autoimmune)
  - o Ileal resections
  - o Malabsorption $
  - o Gastrectomy
- <u>FOLIC ACID DEFIENCY</u>
  - o Malabsorption & Deficiency of diet
  - o Liver disease & Alcohol
  - o OCPs, Phenytoin, Metformin

Repeated recurrent infections in sinuses, URTIs, LRTIs +Diarrhea (Giardiasis, Cryptosporidium, Helicobacter) = COMMON VARIABLE IMMUNODEFIENCY (Acquired hypogamaglobulinema)

- Recurrent Sino-pulmonary infections +Joint infections + Giardia/ Cryptosporidium / Helicobacter
- <u>INV:</u> low immunoglobulin levels in blood
- <u>TTT:</u> IVIG

Fatigue, Dry eye + Joint Pain+ E.N. =SARCOIDOSIS

- Lupus pernio (Purple rash on nose and cheeks resemble frost bite)
- Cough + SOB + L.Ns
- Bilateral VII Palsy
- Bilateral hilar L.N + E.N = Lofgren syndrome
- Dry eye + Dry mouth = Mikulicz syndrome
- Hypercalcemia signs (Polyuria, PUD, Renal stones, depression , constipation)
- E.N (tender red bumps/rash over shins)
- Other Autoimmune conditions
- <u>INV:</u> CXR , CT Scan , Biopsy , Inc. serum ACE , Hypercalcemia
- <u>TTT:</u> 30-70% no need for TTT
- Chest changes not healing after 2 months Or Uveitis , Neurosarcoidosis , Hypercalcemia → Steroid / Azathioprine

Hypertension in young age + Weight loss = Remember VASCULITIS

- <u>Maltezers Triad</u> (Purpura +Arthritis+ Myositis) + Constitutional S/S (Fever+ Wt.Loss + Night Sweats)
- Nose Bleeds, HTN, G.N, Abdominal pain, Bloody diarrhea, Headaches
- <u>INV:</u> High ESR , biopsy , Angiogram
- <u>TTT:</u> Cyclophosphamide

Bloody diarrhea + Gall stones + fever, Sweating + loss of wt. = IBD (CROHNS) Due to terminal ileitis= Bile salts pool = gall stones

Nose problems (Stuffiness , Crusts , Change in shape) , sinus problems , ear problems (URT problems) +LRT problems (Hemoptysis , SOB) + Elevated creatinine (Hematuria)= GRANULOMATOSIS POLYANGIITIS

- Iritis, scleritis, purpura, Arthritis, Rapidly progressive G.N
- <u>INV:</u> High ESR , C-ANCA , Biopsy
- <u>TTT:</u> Steroid + Cyclophosphamide + Plasma exchange +Rituximab

Repeated Wheezing (shortness of breath) + URT problems + Eosinophilia + Kidney problems (Hematuria, high creatinine) = ESINOPHILIC POLYANGIITIS

- Mononeuropathy (C.Ns)
- Montelukast can cause Churg strauss
- <u>INV:</u> Esinophilia + P-ANCA +Biopsy
- <u>TTT:</u> Steroids + Cyclophosphamide

Dizzy spells + Noisy chest + Flushing + Wt.loss = CARCINOID SYNDROME

- Hypotension + Tricuspid stenosis + Diarrhea + wheezing + hepatomegaly
- Enterochromaphain cells tumour with liver metastasis
- Raised 5HIIA in urine
- <u>TTT:</u> Cyproheptadine & Octereotide

Wt.Loss + Polyuria+ Polydipsia + Infections (UTI, SKIN) = D.M
- Leg Cramps could happen , Diarrhea
- FBS > 7
- RBS or 2 hr Post prandial > 11.1

Inflammatory Diseases & Auto-Immune Gets Worse At Night & Early Morning
- Endogenous Steroids increase By Day and Dec. in evening

Wheezing and shortness of breath which gets better on holidays away of work = OCCUPATIONAL ASTHMA

- Isocyanates (painters of automobile & furniture), Wheat (Bakery workers)
- PEFR, Spirometry AT WORKPLACE , Skin prick test, IgE specific Abs
- Stop job (occupational therapist) + bronchodilators

CHRONIC FATIGUE SYNDROME CRITERIA

- New onset fatigue in 6 months not related to exertion plus:
  - Memory & conc. Problems
  - Headaches
  - Tender L.Ns
  - Sore Throat
  - Myalgia
  - Irritable bowel $

Textile worker + SOB + Cough = BYSSINOSIS

- Similar To occupational Asthma
- From cotton inhalation

Constitutional S/S (fever +Night sweats) + ESR>100 + tooth extraction = INFECTIVE ENDOCARDITIS

- Heart murmur + Inc. Creatinine +Stroke +Gangrene (septic emboli)
- <u>INV:</u> Transesophageal echo (vegetations)+ blood culture (dukes major criteria), RF, Urine Dip
- <u>TTT:</u> IV antibiotics (Hospital Protocol) until C&S
- In people with colon cancer = Streptococus bovis = IV penicillin or IV Ceftriaxone
- <u>Dukes minor criteria:</u> Immunological (Osler , G.N), Embolic manifestations (Roth , splinter Hemorrhage, Jane way), IV drug abuser

Young Age + HTN +Polyuria + Glycosuria + FH of RCC = VON-HIPPEL LINDU

- AD on chromosome 3
- Genetic diagnosis
- CNS tumors (Epilepsy, Headaches) + Retinal hemangiblastoma (loss of vision) + RCC (Flank mass + Hematuria) +Pheocromocytoma + Pancreatic neuro endocrine tumors + pancreatic cyst (Glycosuria +Polyuria) + endolymphatic sac tumors.
- <u>TTT:</u> surgery for tumors, Laser photocoagulation for retina

Fever + Myalgia +Body pains + Rash + Recent visit to Queensland = DENGUE FEVER

- SEROLOGY
- Supportive TTT

Chest pain /Faints + GIT bleeding + Old Age =ANGIODYSPLASIA (HEYDES SYNDROME)

- AS (Aortic stenosis) causes consumption of Von willibrand = Angiodysplasia =bleeding per rectum/hematemesis
- INV: Von Willibrand electrophoresis
- TTT: Desmopressin or Factor VIII/ Aortic valve replacement

Increase cholesterol > 4 mmol = HYPERCOLESTEROLEMIA (hyperlipedemia)

Primary Hyperlipidemia	Secondary Hyperlipidemia
Type I: Hyperchylomicronemia (lipoprotein lipase deficiency) Eruptive xanthoma, colic, retinal vein occlusion, pancreatitis, steatosis, organomegaly	D.M, Alcohol , Hypothyroidism PBC
Type IIa: Familial Hypercholesterolemia Tendon Xanthoma + Xanthelasma + Arcus senilis +Premature CVS events (claudications , Impotence, Infarctions, renal bruits)	Beta blockers, Estrogen, Diuretics
Type IIb: Familial Combined Hyperlipidemia Hypertriglyceridemia + Hypercholesterolemia	Renal Failure Nephrotic
Type III: ABETALIPOPROTIENEMIA Palmar xanthoma+ Retinitis Pigmentosa + Steatorrhea	
Type IV: Familial Hypertriglyceridemia Acute pancreatitis	
Type V: Familial Hyperchylomicronemia + Glucose Intolerance + Hyperuricemia	

Treatment

- Cholesterol =Statins, Ezetemibe, Cholestyramine
- Triglycerides =Fibrates , Omega 3, Ezetemibe, Niacin

Wt.Gain + Cold intolerance + Menorrhagia + Hair loss + Apathy+ Pins & needles in hands (carpal tunnel) + Macrocytic anemia + Hyperlipedemia = HYPOTHYROIDISM

- Hypersomnia + P.N +Resteless Leg Syndrome+Dry skin
- Hashimoto/1ry atrophic / radioactive iodine /Thyroidectomy/Lithium & Amiodarone
- Post partum Thyroiditis ; 30 % will need L.-Thyroxine for life

Young age + HTN + Headaches + Sweats + Polyuria + Glycosuria = PHEOCROMOCYTOMA (Ask about MENII S/S & Neurofibromatosis)

- Tachycardia + Flank pain + Wt. loss
- INV.: 24 hrs urinary catecholamines , metanephrines , Inc. serum chromogranin , CT abdomen
- TTT: Phenoxybenzamine (non-selective alpha blocker) + Labetalol (alpha & beta blocker) + Surgery
- MEN II A is AD RET oncogene (Pheocromocytoma +Medullary carcinoma (thyroid swelling) + hyperparathyroidism = hypercalcemia =constipation , polyuria , PU , psychiatric problems , renal stones (hematuria) , fractures
- MEN II B is AD (Pheocromocytoma +medullary carcinoma + neurofibromas + Marfanoid features)
- Neurofibromatosis I is AD on chromosome 17 (>6 café au lait patches + Optic glioma + >2 Neurofibromas + Axillary freckling + Lisch nodules + epilepsy + pheochromyctoma , CPA (Cerebellopontine angle) $, Jugular foramen $)
- Neurofibromatosis II AD on chromosome 22 Has Acoustic neuroma (Hearing loss + Tinnitus +Vertigo)

History of gall stones/bile duct tumors or intervention + Fever + jaundice + Rt. Quadrant pain = ASCENDING CHOLANGITIS

- Charcot`s triad + shock (hypotension)+ confusion = Raynold`s pentad
- INV.: Inc. ESR , increased ALP , bilirubin , GGT , U/S , MRCP , ERCP , blood culture
- TTT: Usually E.coli→IV fluids → penicillin + gentamycin / ciprofloxacin + metronidazole then ERCP & cholecystectomy
- May be caused by stones, Benign stricture, Malignant stricture, Ascaris

Progressive worsening dyspnea + Antibiotics for recurrent urinary tract infections + Bibasal crackles + Normal FBC, urea & electrolytes = NITROFURANTOIN INDUCED PULMONARY FIBROSIS

- CT , PFTS , CXR
- Drugs causing pulmonary fibrosis :Methotrexate, Belomycin, Busulphan, Nitrofurantoin, Amiodarone

Jaundice + Pain in Rt. Upper quadrant = HEPATITIS (Back pain) or ASCENDING CHOLANGITIS

- In hepatitis fever precedes the jaundice
- In ascending cholangitis fever is with the jaundice

Diarrhea + Wt.Loss + Irregular periods + Sweating + Intolerance to hot weather = THYROTOXICOSIS

- Tremors /L.L swelling/HTN/Palpitations
- Grave`s = Eye signs (Opthalmoplegia , Exopthalmous) + Acropachy+ pretibial Myxdema +Enlarged gland (TSHR stimulating Abs)
- Hashimoto`s = Enlarged gland (Anti thyroglobin , Anti thyroid peroxidise)
- Dequervian = Tender gland
- Amiodarone
- Post-partum Thyroiditis =2-12 m post-partum = hyper then hypo = Antithyroid peroxidise= Resolve in months to years , 30% will neeed L-thyroxine
- INV.: TSH , T3 , T4 , Thyroid Scan , U/S
- TTT: Propranolol , Carbimazole , Propylthiouracil (pregnancy), Surgery , Radioactive iodine

Malabsorption (Pale , Offensive Diarrhea , Floating , Difficult to flush ,Wt.Loss , Vit. deficiencies) + Anemia + Normal colonoscopy = CELIAC DISEASE

- Wt. loss + Mouth ulcers + Itchy Rash (dermatitis herpitiform)
- Associated autoimmune disorders (Hypothyroidism , D.M , Microscopic colitis)
- HLA DQ2 , HLA DQ8
- Always ask about diet
- Vit K defiency (Eccymosis, Petichie , Hematomas)
- B12 , Folic deficiency=Megaloblastic anemia (SOB, palpitation)
- Vit D deficiency (osteomalacia) (Bone pain + Muscle weakness + easy fractures +Hypocalcemia + Inc. ALP)
- IgA nephropathy (Hematuria)
- Inc. IgA , Anti tissue transglutaminase, Anti-Endomysil Abs, Anti gliadin Abs , endoscopy with jejunal biopsy (villous atrophy)
- TTT with Gluten free diet (barely, oats, wheat) .. Rice & maize are ok
- Dapsone for dermatitis herpitiform

Malabsorption + Fever = TROPICAL SPRUE

- TTT: Tetracycline / cotrimoxazole

Malabsorption + Joint pain = WHIPPLE DISEASE

- INV: Biopsy = PAS organism
- TTT: Tetracylcine/cotrimoxazole for 1 year

Resistant celiac not responsive to gluten free diet = INTESTINAL LYMPHOMA (enteropathy associated T Cell Lymphoma)= TTT: CHOP

Diarrhea + Normal colonoscopy + PPIs/NSAIDS over use = MICROSCOPIC COLITIS

- TTT : Antidiarrheal + Mesalazine

Malabsorption (Pale offensive floating, difficult to flush, Vit. Deficiencies, Wt.loss) + History of surgery in bowel (Crohns, Tumors) = SHORT GUT SYNDROME

- < 2 m of small bowel
- May be transient condition for intestinal adaptation
- TTT: Loperamide, Lactase enzyme, PPIs, Vit. injections , Intestinal lengthening surgery, TPN

PPIs/fistulas/diverticula/D.M + Malabsorption + Bloating/Nausea /Vomiting = SMALL BOWEL BACTERIAL OVER GROWTH

- Dec. motility (Scleroderma , Celiac , Bilroth antrectomy (blind loop) , Diverticula)
- Dec. Immunity (Common variable , D.M , Chronic pancreatitis , immunosuppressive medication)
- Inc. small bowel bacterial contamination (Crohns (surgery to remove ileocecal valve) , PPIs)
- Jejunal aspiration = 10^5 bact./ml
- TTT: Norfloxacin /Co-Amoxiclav for 1 week

PPIs Causing Diarrhea

- Microscopic Colitis
- Small bowel Bacterial over growth
- CDIF

Alteration of bowel habits + Chr. Pain (bloating) + No alarm signs (age >50 , Bleeding , Wt. Loss , FH of IBD or colon CA) = IRRITABLE BOWEL SYNDROME

- Usually start after an infection
- Diarrhea predominant or constipation predominant
- Urgency for bowel movement + Sense of incomplete evacuation (tenesmus) + GERD + other psychological related problems (chronic fatigue syndrome, fibromyalgia, Headaches, back aches, depression , anxiety)
- INV. All normal
- TTT: Psychotherapy, laxatives, Antispasmodics, TCA, SSRIs , Lactobacillus

ROME III criteria for IRRITABLE BOWEL SYNDROME

- Recurrent abdominal or discomfort for 3 days/month for 3 months plus:
  - o Relieved by defecation
  - o Altered stool frequency
  - o Altered stool form
  - o Altered stool passage (Urgency/Straining/Tenesmus)
  - o Mucus with stool

Abdominal pain + Fatigue + Tiredness + Jaundice + Itching = PBC

- Auto-Immune more in females
- Xanthelasma + Other Auto-immune disorders (Thyroid , D.M , Vitiligo, RA)
- INV: Inc. IgM , AMA M2, Inc. ALP , Bilirubin , GGT , U/S , ERCP , Biopsy
- TTT: Ursodeoxycholic acid , Rifampicin , cholestyramine , Liver transplantation

Previous URTI + Chest Pain + CCF (Palpitations + SOB + PND+ Orthopnea + Swollen legs) = VIRAL MYOCARDITIS

- Other Causes: Rheumatic fever , Parvo virus B19, Coxackie , Doxorobusin , VASCULITIS
- INV.:ECG , ECHO , CXR
- TTT: TTT of CCF (Nitrates, ACEIs, Diuretics)

CHF signs (Palpitations +SOB+ PND+ Orthopnea + Swollen legs)+ last month pregnancy = PERIPARTUM CARDIOMYOPATHY

- Last month of pregnancy up to 5 months postpartum
- Excessive Wt. Gain in last month of pregnancy
- Dilated cardiomyopathy
- TTT: Diuretics, ACEIs, Nitrates
- Recovery takes few months to years

Mitral stenosis signs (SOB , Cough , Orthopnea , PND) + Palpitations +Wt. Loss + Faints + Murmur = LA MYXOMA

- Fevers + Chest pain
- TTT: Surgery / Mitral valve repair

> 5 Unilateral headache (Pulsating) + Vomiting, Photophobia, Phonophobia + Aura (Vision loss, Sensory , Motor symptoms) = MIGRAINE

- OCP , Pregnancy , Cheese , Tomatoes , Caffeine
- Classic migraine is with Aura
- Common migraine without Aura
- TTT: simple analgesics, sumatryptan, Prevention: BBs , TCA

Old female + Sudden back pain + Radiculopathy (Severe shooting pain in dermatome) = COMPRESSION FRACTURE due to OSTEOPOROSIS

- Could Cause Cauda Equina S/S (Leg pain & weakness (paraparesis) + urinary retention/Incontinence + Saddle Anesthesia +Absent ankle reflex)
- Osteoporosis itself cause no S/S
- Repeated fractures = Stooped posture
- Risks: Alcohol , smoking , under wt. , Cushing , Acromegaly , Anorexia nervosa , hypogonadism , Rheumatoid , Multiple myeloma , Steroids , Glitazones , Anticoagulants, Malabsorptin $
- INV.: DEXA scan : T score < -2.5
- TTT: Bisphosphonates (Alendronate) + Ca + Vit D

Recurrent TIA (Weakness + Normal examination + Resolving) + HTN + Palpitations = AF

- SOB + Orthopnea + PND + Lightheadedness
- Alcohol / HTN / MS/ MR/ Thyrotoxicosis/ pericarditis / Congenital Ht.Ds / Lone AF
- Indication of warfarin CHADSVASC score
- Rhythm control if Acute AF=Amiodarone/DC
- Rate control if Chronic AF=CCBs , BBs , Digoxin

Epigastri pain Resistant to H2 blockers = PEPTIC ULCER DISEASE

- H.Pylori / NSAIDs / Steroids
- Hypercalcemia
- Gastrinoma (Zollinger elisson=Recurrent ulcers+Unusual places) Part of MEN I
- Epigastric pain + Wt.Loss + Vomiting +Hematemsis (coffee ground or frank) + Melena (Black tarry offensive motion)
- Endoscopy with biopsy (exclude malignancy), H.Pylori fecal Ag , Urea Breath Test, H.pylori Abs , Serum Gastrin
- Complications of PUD:
  - o Hematemsis/Melena =Anemia
  - o Perforation
  - o Pyloric obstruction
- TTT: Triple therapy (Clarithromycin/Metronidazole + Amoxicillin+ PPIs) for 14 days

Diarrhea + Recurrent PUD (Epigastric pain + Vomiting + Wt.loss + hematemesis/Melena) + Constitutional S/S (Fever +Night sweats+Wt.Loss) = ZOLLINGER ELLISON

- PUD non responsive to PPIs = Zollinger Ellison or Malignancy

- Ulcers of esophagus , stomach , duodenum , intestine
- Gastrinoma of pancereas
- Part of MEN I (Hypercalcemia +Pit.Tumour+Pacereas Tumour)
- Fasting Serum Gastrin in 3 occasions/Secretin test
- TTT: Octerotide+PPIs /Surgery+ Chemotherapy

Hemoptysis/Cough for years + Inc. Creatinine/Frothy urine/hematuria+ Anemia = GOOD PASTURE`S SYNDROME

- Hemoptysis is late (cough for years with anemia due to pulmonary Hemorrhage before hemoptysis appear)
- Renal failure is late (proteinuria , hematuria are early signs)
- Preceded by viral infection (Influenza)
- Type II hypersensitivity= Crescentic G.N , RPGN
- Anti-glomerular B.M Ab
- TTT: Steroids + Immunosuppression + Plasmapharesis / Renal transplant

Recurrent miscarriage/Pre-eclampsia (proteinuria ,HTN , Edema) + inc. APTT + Thrombocytopenia + Vaso-occlusive S/S = ANTIPHOSPHOLIPID Ab SYNDROME

- Other Autoimmune disorders / SLE
- INV:Anticardiolipin , lupus anticoagulant , inc. APTT , Low platelets

TTT: Asprin , heparin

CA Lung +Severe bone pain (Dull , Constant, Inc. with activity)+Spinal compression +Hypercalcemia S/S (polyuria + polydypsia + PUD+ Depression+ fractures+ Constipation) + Inc. ALP = METASTATIC BONE DISEASE

- CA Breast , Prostate , Lung
- TTT: Bisphosphonates /Radiotherapy /steroids

Recurrent Joint pain & swelling (hemoarthrosis) + Prolonged bleeding after procedures+ FH = HAEMOPHILIA

- XL-R , VIII (A),IX (B)
- INV: Normal bleeding time , platelets , PT , Inc. clotting time , APTT
- TTT: Factor VIII transfusion , Fresh frozen plasma

Easy bruising + Nose bleeds +Bleeding Gums+ Heavy menses + FH = VWBD

- AD
- Normal PT ,Platelets , inc. Bleeding time & APTT
- Measurement of VWB factor
- TTT: Desmopressin

Leg Ulcers + Anemia S/S + Recurrent infection (Autosplenectomy) = SICKLE CELL ANEMIA

- Strokes
- Osteomyelitis+ Slamonella enteritis + DI + Choledocolethiasis
- Vaso-occlusive crisis (Acute chest syndrome , Pain in arms or legs, priapism ,Abdominal pain , Ulcers)
- Acute chest crisis(lung infarction) (Fever, Chest pain , SOB, Pulm.infiltrates)
- Aplastic crisis (Erythema infectiousm parvo virus B19)
- XL-R , Sickling occurs with Dehydration , Acidosis , Infections
- INV.:
  - CBC: Anemia with reticulocytosis , howell jolly bodies
  - Hb electrophoresis
  - Sickling test with Sodium Metabisulphite
  - Genetic councelling
- TTT: blood/penicillin/folic

- o Chest crisis=exchange tranfsuion
- o Vaso-occlusive crisis=Opioids , Oxygen , NSAIDS, IV fluids
- o Bone marrow transplant

Recurrent vaso-occlusive episodes (DVT , PE , Budd chiari , Cerebral sinus thrombosis <inc. Intr.Cr. Pr.>/Stroke) + Mouth ulcers = BEHCET DISEASE

- Oral ulcers +genital ulcers + Uveitis + Vaso-occlusive+ livido reticularis/Erythema nodosum / Pyoderma gangrenosa + Sagittal sinus thrombosis + Hemoptysis + Aseptic meningitis
- Diagnosis : skin lesion +genital lesions + eye lesions + pethargy test
- TTT: high dose steroids+ Infliximab+ Azathioprine+ INF if severe IVIG

Diarrhea With Normal Colonoscopy

- Malabsorption Syndromes
- Microscopic colitis
- Irritable Bowel Syndrome

Common Inherited Cancer Syndrome:

- **HNPCC (Lynch syndrome)**
  - o Colon , Gastric CA/Endometrial CA/Ovarian CA/Pancereatic (biliary)
  - o Keratoacanthomas /Sebaceous adenoma / Skin CA
- **FAP**
  - o APC gene: Autosomal dominant
  - o Gardner syndrome: FAP+Lipomas+osteomas+sebaceous cysts+gatric polyps
  - o Turcot $: FAP+Medulloblastomas (CPA $)
- **Peutz Jeghers**
  - o AD
  - o GIT Hamartomas
- **MEN I , MEN II**
- **Von Hippel Lindu**
- **BRCA I , BRCA II**
- **Breat CA / Ovarian CA / Prostate CA**
- **Leukemia /Lymphoma**

Causes Of Abdominal Pain With Normal Initial Investigations:

- Vasculitis (PAN) =Mesenteric Ischemia
- FMF
- Porphyria
- Addison`s

Working in Hotel/Hospital (A/C) + Cough+ Dyspnea + Hyponatremia + Elevated LFTs + Ataxia + Fever= LEGIONELLA PNEUMONIA

- Reservoirs : A/C , Cooling towers /Nebulizers/Showers/Hot Tubs
- INV: LFTS , KFTs , CXR , CT ,Urinary Ag
- Risks: Immuno compromised/smoking/Chr.Lung Ds
- TTT: Azithromycin / Levofloxacin

Fever + Sorethroat + L.Ns + Wt.Loss + Rash + High Risk Behavior = ACUTE HIV

- <u>INV.:</u> Abs , CD4
- <u>TTT:</u>
  - o HAART (2NRTI + 1 PI/NNRTI) (zidovudine+lamivudine+ neverapine) if
    - CD4<350
    - Coinfection with HBV regardless of CD4
    - HIV Neuropathy regardless of CD4
    - Pregnancy regardless of CD4 count
  - o Cotrimoxazole if CD4 <200

Ataxia + Urinary Incontinence + Dementia (Mental decline= Apathy, forgetfulness, Inattention) =NORMAL PRESSURE HYDROCEPHALUS

- No signs of increased intracranial pressure
- 1ry or 2ry (SAH , Brain infection , tumour , surgery , Trauma)
- INV: CT brain= enlarged ventricles with convoluted atrophy, Lumbar puncture (improvement =success of ventriculoperitoneal shunt)
- TTT: Ventriculoperitoneal shunt

Seizures (Autism , learning disability) + Hematuria + Skin rash = TUBEROUS SCLEROSIS

- Autosomal Dominant
- Commonest brain tumour = Giant Cell astrocytoma
- Renal =Angoimyolipoma , Renal cysts and rarely RCC
- Skin:
  o Adenoma sebaceum (butterfly bumps on nose,cheeks of reddish spots)
  o Shagareen patch (lower back or nape pigmented thick skin)
  o Subungal fibroma (small fleshy tumours under nails)
- INV: renal U/S , CT brain , MRI , fundoscopy , Echo
- TTT: Supportive

Jaundice + Wilson (history of CLD) + Disturbed sleep Rhythm , Agitation,Flapping tremors, personality changes = HEPATIC ENCEPHALOPATHY

- Bleeding /Constipation/high proteins/benzodiazepines/Alcohol /Infections (UTI,Pneumonia) / Hypokalemia (Diuretics)
- Due to GABA mediated inhibition , Build up of Ammonia (metabolic toxins)
- Urgent Admition
- EEG : Triphasic slow Waves
- Enema /Lactulose/Metronidazole/Protien restriction

Old age + Bone pain (Sternum,back) + Frothy urine = MULTIPLE MYELOMA

- High ESR
- Hypercalcemia S/S + Hyperviscosity S/S + Constitutional S/S + Paraprotienemia(P.N) + Amyloidosis(CTS) + Pancytopenia+ Osteoporosis
- Fractures+spinal cord compression+ RF (hypercalcemia, Uricemia, Fanconi, pyelonephritis)
- Cancer of plasma cells
- INV: Protien electrophoresis (polyclonal protein)/B.M examination/X-ray bones
- TTT: steroids/chemotherapy/thalidomide/stem cell transplant

CAUSES OF HYPERVISCOSITY

- PRV
- MM
- Waldenstrom Macroglobulinemia
- Cryoglobulinemia
- Leukemia
- TTT: Plasmapharesis

Enlarged L.Ns + Hypervicosity of bl.(spontaneous bleeding ,visual problems , headaches, vertigo) + P.N + Hepatomegaly = WALDENSTROM MACROGLOBULINEMIA

- Monoclonal gammopathy (IgM)
- B.M sample + flow cytomery +CT+Urine+ESR+KFTS (inc. Creat)
- TTT: if constitutional S/S → Rituximab+Cyclophosphamide+plasmapharesis (hyperviscosity)

Smoking + Old Age+ Cough+ Hemoptysis+ Wt.Loss = BRONCHOGENIC CARCINOMA

- Difficulty swallowing + Clubbing +SOB+Horner (ptosis & myosis)+bone mestastasis
- Caused by Smoking /Asbestosis

- Paraneoplastic
  - SMALL CELL CA
    - SIADH (Hyponatremia , Low serum osmolarity)
    - Inc. pigmentation (ACTH)
    - Ataxia (Anti Hu Abs)
    - Eaton Lambarat $ (Anti voltage gated Ca channels) TTT: Steroids/IVIG
  - NSCC
    - HPOA
    - Hypercalcemia (polyuria , constipation,stones,PUD)
- INV: CXR , CT scan chest , Bronchoscopy with biopsy
- TTT: Lobectomy , pneumonectomy , radiotherapy , chemotherapy (cisplatin,Etoposide)

Old Age > 50 + Pain & stiffness in shoulders + headaches + ESR > 50 + Normal CT = POLYMYALGIA RHEUMATICA

- TTT Steroids
- May cause TEMPORAL ARTERITIS (GIANT CELL ARTERITIS)
  - Headaches + Jaw claudication + Pain in scalp + Loss of vision + very high ESR
  - Causes loss of vision (AAION)
  - Loss of pulsations of temporal artery + tender temporal & Scalp areas
  - Temporal artery biopsy for Giant cells infiltrates
  - High Dose steroids

Young Age (15-40) + Constitutional S/S (Fever, Wt.loss , Night sweat) + Itching + Painless Lumps = HODGKIN LYMPHOMA

- Cancer of lymphoctyes
- Past history of EBV infection/Excessive use of GH
- Pain In L.Ns after Alcohol consumption
- INV: Reed sternburg cells on biopsy/CT & PET Scan for staging
- Stages:
  - STAGE I : Single L.N group
  - STAGE II : 2 or > L.N on the same side of diaphragm
  - STAGE II : Both sides of diaphragm including spleen
  - STAGE IV : extralymphatic spread
  - A: no systemic symptoms
  - B: systemic symptoms
- TTT: Radiotherapy /chemotherapy (Mustin,vincristine,bleomycin,prednisone)

Old Age + Constitutional S/S + Generalized Lumps = NON-HODGKIN LYMPHOMA

- Skin rash (Mycosis fungoids)
- EBV(Burkit),HH8 , HTLV , HIV , H.Pylori ,Autoimmune ds (SLE,RA) , Radiation
- INV: Biopsy/CT
- TTT: chemotherapy/Radiotherapy/B.M trasnplantaion

ESR>100 = T.B, INFECTIVE ENDOCARDITIS , OSTEOMYELITIS, DEEP ABSCESS, GCA , VASCULITIS , METASTAIC CANCERS , WALDENSTROM MACROGLOBULINEMIA

Male +Constitutional S/S + Abdominal pain + Joint pains+ elevated creatinine= POLYARTERITIS NODOSA

- MI + Strokes + HTN + Livedo reticularis +Testicular pain +HBV
- No lung S/S , No purpura (doesn't affect small vessels)
- INV: CBC , ESR , Sural nerve biopsy (rosary beads sign of vessels)
- TTT: Steroids + cyclophosphamide + Rituximab

Previous throat infection/ Impetigo (skin rash ttt with Antibiotics) + Hematuria + Frothy urine + Eye Puffiness =POST STREPTOCOCCAL G.N

- Oliguria + HTN

- DPGN : Type III hypersensitivity
- INV: U&Es/Urine analysis
- TTT: Steroids

D.M + Weakness/Wasting/Pain of thighs/hips/buttocks =DIABETIC AMYOTROPHY

- Proximal diabetic neuropathy
- Due damage to the nerve
- INV: HBA1C , NCV , EMG
- TTT: Control D.M , Physiotherapy , Diet , Gabapentin

Meltzer's Triad (Purpura + Arthritis + Myositis) + Hematuria (IgA nephropathy) +Abdominal pain = HENOCH SCHENOLIEN PURPRA

- Platelets are normal or raised
- History of pharyngitis (Sore throat)
- TTT: Steroids + Azathioprine + IVIG

Meltzer's triad (Purpura + Arthritis + Myositis) + Hyperviscosity S/S (spontaneous bleeding of mucous membranes + blurred vision + headaches + vertigo) = CRYOGLOBULINEMIA

- TYPE I : (Monoclonoal IG) Waldenstrom , Multiple myeloma
- TYPE II : (Monocloncal IG + Circulating ICs)HCV
- TYPE III: (Polycloncal IG + circulating ICs) HCV , SLE
- INV: Cold agglutinins + Cause

Inc. ALP + Normal LFTS+ Proximal weakness + Bone Pains/Fractures = OSTEOMALACIA

- Malabsorption / Dec. intake/RF
- INV: PTH is high , Low Ca , Low P , High ALP
- TTT: Weekly Vit D. 10,000 U IM injection for 6 weeks

Severe pain after eating by 15 mins + Old age + Atherosclerotic manifestations (stroke/cramps/MI) =CHRONIC MESENTERIC ISCHEMIA

- Angiography
- TTT: anticoagulation / Angioplasty / Surgery (endarterectomy)

Malabsoprtion + D.M = CHRONIC PANCEREATITIS/Celiac Disease

- Alcohol, Cystic fibrosis , Idiopathic
- INV.: X-ray→ calcified , CT, Dec. fecal elastase ,secretin stimulation test
- TTT: Replacement (Insulin + Pancereatic enzymes)

URTIs (sinusitis, otitis media) + Chr. Pancereatitis (Malabsorption +D.M)+ Recurrent Chest infection (SOB + Cough+yellow sputum) +Infertility + FH = CYSTIC FIBROSIS

- Salty tasting skin, ABPA, Pseudomonas inf., Borkholderia inf.
- INV: Sweat test Cl > 60 mmol , CFTR gene Ch. 7
- TTT: Replacement therapy + TTT of complications

Dextrocardia + Infertility + recurrent URTIs + Recurrent chest Infections = KARTAGNER SYNDROME

- Immotile cilia syndrome (AR)

Hypoglycemia + HSM + Renomegaly on U/S + Lactic acidosis + Hyperuricemia (Gout) + Infections +bleeding= GLYCOGEN STORAGE DISEASE (VON GIERKES)

- Autosomal recessive
- INV: Liver Biopsy , Glucose-6-phosphatase activity
- TTT: Increase eating starch , glucose/Allopurinol for hyperuricemia

BMI 30 + Waist circumference > 94 cm   + BP >140/90 +FBG >6.1 mmol + Cholesterol > 4 mmol + Triglycerdies > 2 + HDL <1 mmol = METABOLIC SYNDROME

- Due to insulin resistance , Endocrine (PCO , Cushing) , Stress , Sedentary life
- Risks it cause
  - Diabetes
  - Coronary Heart disease
  - Psychosis
  - Rheumatic disease
  - Gout
- TTT: Life style modification , TTT of cause , surgery

Purpra + low platelets + Normal WBC +Abdominal pain+ Normal ESR = IMMUNE THROMBOCYTOPENIC PURPRA

- Increased bleeding (Gums , Menorrhagia)
- INV: inc. bleeding time , low platelets , normal PT , APTT , Clotting
- TTT: Steroids , IVIG, splenectomy

ITP + Autoimmune Hemolytic Anemia = EVAN SYNDROME

Purpura (Thrombocytopenia) + Headache/hallucinations/confusion +Anemia = TTP

- Renal impairement might occur
- Pregnancy , Quinine , Clopideogrel , Cyclosporine , Ticlopedine
- TTT: Plasma exchange / Steroids + immunosupression if recurrence after plasma exchange

Recurrent different neurological deficit+ Uhthoff phenomenon (loss of vision/pins & needles sense with inc. body temp.) = MULTIPLE SCLEROSIS

- Avoid hot bathes and hot showers, exercises (Uhthoff phenomenon)
- Heat inc. demyelination
- May be presented with:
  - Recurrent vertigo
  - Double Vision
  - Pain With Moving Eyes
  - Weakness
  - Unsteadiness
  - Lhermit sign (neck flexion causes pain in back)
- INV: MRI , VEP , CSF
- TTT: Steroids

Anemia + Inc. Creatinine + Low platelets + Recent bloody diarrhea (E-Coli O157:H7) =HUS

- Medical emergency , most will resolve , small % will have Chr. Kidney ds and need replacement therapy
- TTT: Antibiotics , Hemodialysis

Sudden Weakness in foot & Legs + Ascending pattern (diplopia , dysphagia , dec. resp.) = GUILLIAN BARRE SYNDROME

- CAUSES: Campylobacter (diarrhea) , Influenza , CMV (sore throat)
- Blitaeral VII + Areflexia + Motor more than sensory loss
- Low Bl.Pr. + Bladder dysfunction may occur in severe cases but is temporary
- INV: NCV , CSF (inc. protiens)
- TTT: IVIG , Plasmapharesis

Opthalmoplegia + Ataxia + Areflexia = MILLER FISCHER $

- Anti GQ1B Abs

Malabsorption (offensive diarrhea + difficult to flush) + Wt.loss + fatigue + Itchy rash on elbows = CELIAC DISEASE

Low back pain + Dyspnea + Opacities of both upper zones of lungs on CXR = ANKYLOSING SPONDYLITIS

- Anterior uveitis , AR , Achilis tendinitis , Apical fibrosis ,
- HLA B21 , schober test , X-ray showing scaro-iliitis , bamboo spine ,
- <u>TTT:</u> NSAIDS , Sulphasalazine /methotrexate as disease modifying/ physiotherapy

Hypercoagulable state (DVT , PE , BudChiari , Cerebral Sinus Thrombosis) + Hyperviscosity + inc. Hb + Itching with hot bath =PRV

- HSM+Facial Plethora + congested eyes +PUD+ GOUT
- INV.:Inc. Red cell mass + Jak 2 mutation + Thrombocythemia+Dec. ESR
- TTT: Venesection , Hydroxyurea , Bone marrow transplant

Pregnancy + Dyspnea +Anemia + elevated liver enzymes + low platelets = HELLP SYNDROME

- Third timester
- Pregnancy induced HTN or pre-eclampsia
- Exclude fits = Pre-eclampsia
- DIC , Renal failure is a complication
- <u>TTT:</u> Delivery , DIC : Fresh frozen plasma , HTN: labetalol/hydralazine/ Nifidepine

Lymphopenia + Hypothyroidism= DIGEORGE SYNDROME

Lymphopenia + Albinism + peripheral neuropathy= CHEDIACK HEGASHI SYNDROME

Pregnancy + Jaundice + Abdominal Pain + fever = ACUTE FATTY LIVER OF PREGNANCY

- Third trimester +RF +Pancereatitis +Hepatic encephalopathy
- Elevated Liver enzymes
- TTT: Delivery after stabilization (Fluids , Glucose , FFP)

Old Age + Sudden Falls + Bradychardia (<40BPM) = COMPLETE HEART BLOCK

- Causes : Ischemic Ht. Ds , Lyme ds. , Congenital (Anti Ro , la Abs)
- <u>INV:</u> ECG ,ECHO
- <u>TTT:</u> Permanent Pacing

Recurrent Abdominal pain + Recurrent fevers + PH of laparotomy+ Normal tests =FMF

- Serositis (pericarditis, pleurisy , effusions)
- COMPLICATIONS: Amyloidosis & RF
- INHERITANCE : AR
- TTT: Colchicine & NSAIDS

HYPOGLYCAEMIC UNAWARENESS (hypoglycaemia with no alarm Signs)

- Occurs in long standing IDDM who always keep their glucose to normal levels
- Causes:
  - o AUTONOMIC NEUROPATHY
  - o BRAIN DESENSITIZATION TO HYPOGLYCAEMIA (if repeated attacks the brain increases its receptors to glucose)
  - o BETA BLOCKER DRUGS

INCREASED FREQUENCY OF HYPOGLYCAEMIA IN IDDM

- AUTONOMIC NEUROPATHY (Diarrhea , vomiting)
- BETA BLOCKERS
- ADDISON DISEASE (pigmentation + postural hypotension)
- PREGNANCY (Ask about LMP)
- Imbalance between INSULIN & FOOD (irregular eating pattern) & EXCERCISES
- RENAL FAILURE
- INSULINOMA

Old Age +Constitutional S/S +Wt.Loss+inc. ESR >100+ Cough + Pain in chest = TUBERCULOSIS

- Long contact with people with chest infection (Nurse)
- Hemoptysis + osteomyelitis + potts ds of spine + cold abscess in skin + L.Ns
- INV: Sputum analysis with zeil nelson and culture on bactic or lovenstien Jensen
- TTT: admition , isolation , contact tracing , notify local authority
- 2 months Rifmpicin , INH , pyazinamide , ethambutol
- 4 months Rifampicin + INH

Constitutional S/S (Fever +Night sweats + Wt.Loss) = MALIGNANCY /C.T. DISEASE (vasculitis) / INFECTIVE ENDOCARDITIS /T.B / LYMPHOMA

Recurrent Angio-edema (Swelling of the Dermis)+ No Cause= C1 ESTERASE INHIBITOR DEFIENCY

- Inherited as AD or Acquired
- First appears after trauma or dental work
- Abdominal pain and vomiting
- Stridor or suffocation
- No Urticaria
- ACEIs are contraindicated (inc. bradykinin levels)
- INV: Low C1 inhibitor , Low C2 , C4
- TTT: EPI-Pen , Purified C 1 inhibitor, Tranexemic acid

Inc. Intracranial pr. S/S (vomiting , headache , blurred vision) + Amenorrhea =PROLACTINOMA

- Bitemporal hemianopia / Breast discharge
- INV: Inc. Prolactin , MRI , Ca , PTH , G
- TTT: Bromocriptine , Surgery

Pancereatic problem (Glucagonoma :D.M ,polyuria+polydepsia , Insulinoma : Hypoglycemia Gastrinoma : Recurrent PUD , Vipoma : Diarrhea) + Pituitary adenoma(Prolactinoma (Amenorrhea , breast discharge , Acromegaly) + Hyperparathyroidsim (Parathyroidectomy , Recurrent renal stones , HTN) = MEN I

- AD , RET oncogene

Hemodialysis + Painful knee =GOUT

- More in old age / May be +ve FH
- Metabolic syndrome / Glycogen storage ds/ Chemotherapy / Alcohol / Polycythemia / Psoriasis / Thiazides
- X-Ray , Aspirate (Needle like –ve Birefringence on polarized microscopy of Mono sodium urate) , Inc. ESR
- Check KFTS
- TTT = NSIADS , Steroids , Intra-articular steroids /Colchicine
- Prophylaxis by allopurinol after 14 days of attack if:
  - 2 attacks/year or Nephropathy

Sudden Muscle weakness after exercise + Hypokalemia = HYPOKALEMIC PERIODIC PARALYSIS

- AD
- Exercise /High sodium & CHO diet/Excitement /Noise/Infection
- Often misdiagnosed as conversion disorder
- TTT: Acetazolamide , Spironolactone & potassium drinks with exercise

Sickle Cell Anemia (SCA) + Sudden Pain in arms and legs not responding to analgesia= THROMBOTIC SICKLE CRISIS = B.M Infarction

- TTT : Hydration, Analgesia, Blood
- Crisis due to Hypoxia or Infection (UTI =Burning , Polyuria)
- Other Sickle Crisis:

- o Aplastic Crisis
  - Infection with Parvo virus B19
  - Decrease reticulocytes
  - Give blood
- o Hemolytic Crisis
  - If with other hemolytic anemia
- o Acute Chest Syndrome
  - SCA +Lung Infection =sickling=Lung infarction= more Hypoxia , Cough , fever , SEVERE CHEST PAIN
  - Exchange transfusion + Antibiotics

Knee Pain + IV drug Abuser/Sexually active + Constitutional S/S = SEPTIC ARTHRITIS

- Any Blood infection / Near by infection / Sexual partners / IV drug user
- Staph aureus / Gonococcal (Rash on the trunk) / E.Coli (IV drug users)
- Knee x-ray (soft tissue swelling , erosions , subchondral necrosis) , Knee aspiration (Microscopy, Cytology, Gram Stain , Culture, polarizing microscope)
- TTT: IV Flucloxacillin + fusidic Acid
- Exclude Rieter
  - o Conjunctivitis , Uveitis , burning urine/Diarrhea, Back Pain , AR , keratoderma blenorrhagica (rash on feet) , Balanitis
  - o Campylobacter , Chlamydia, Shigella, Salmonella , chlamydia
  - o HLA B27
  - o TTT: NSAID , Steroids , Immuno supressants

Porter (weight lifting) + Chest pain (reflux) + Palpitations (irritation to vagus) + SOB (irritation to diaphragm) + Dysphagia= HIATUS HERNIA

- Obesity /Smoking/Straining/Constipation/Coughing
- Upper GIT endoscopy , Barium swallow with trendlenberg position
- PPIs , Surgery

FH of IHD + Stress /Straining job + HTN + Chest pain = ANGINA PECTORIS must be excluded

- Stress ECG, Dobutamine stress Echo

Recurrent falls with no warning signs (Adam Stock) + Palpitations + Chest pain +Dizziness = SICK SINUS SYNDROME

- Worsens with CCBs , BBs , Digoxin
- Idiopathic fibrosis/Ischemic/Sarcoidosis/Amyloidosis/Chagas/cardiac surgery
- ECG: sinus bradycardia/sinus arrest/AF/Atrial Tachycardia
- TTT: Pacing

Recurrent falls + Old age + No alarming signs = COMPLTE HEART BLOCK

- Idiopathic, Ischemic
- ECG
- TTT: Pacing

Young Age + Syncope during exercise + FH of collapse =HOCM

- Autosomal Dominant
- ECG , ECHO
- TTT: BBs , ICD

Fatigue / Tiredness for 6 months+ Ms / Bone pains + Dec. concentration+ Flu like illness =CHRONIC FATIGUE SYNDROME

- Preceding vial illness
- Irritable bowel $ / Sore throat / Tender L.Ns /SOB/Chest pain/ Headaches
- TTT: CBT , Graded exercise ,SSRI

**Proximal Weakness (Wasting) + Rash on eyes & Fingers + Intact sensations + Arthralgia =
DERMATOMYOSISTIS /MIXED CT.DS.** (Anti RNP)

- Dysphagia / Dyspnea
- Auto-Immune / EBV/ Parvo virus /Malignancy/Breast implants
- Exclude malignancy (GIT)
- Inc. CPK , EMG , Biopsy , Anti Jo-1 , Anti Mi-2
- <u>TTT:</u> Prednisolone, IVIG, Plasmapharesis

Proximal Weakness + Painful Muscles + Intact sensations + No rash = POLYMYOSITIS

- Statins/Malignancy/EBV
- CPK , Biopsy , Anti Jo Abs

Weakness of Hand grip + Weakness Of Thighs = INCLUSION BODY MYOSITIS

- Polymyositis not responding to prednisolone
- Frequent falls
- Dysphagia & foot drop are late
- CPK , EMG ,Biopsy
- <u>TTT:</u> Supportive + Specialized exercise therapy

**Dysphagia + Odynophagia + Homosexual + TTT for oral candidiasis = ESOPHYGEAL
CANDIDIASIS**

- Preceding sore throat (Cold 3 weeks before) = seroconversion
- Testing for HIV , CD4
- Starting HAART (Zidovudine + Lamivudine +Nelfinavir)
- Endoscopy
- <u>TTT:</u> IV Fluconazole

Ascites in Old age + No liver disease = Suspect **MALIGNANT ASCITIS**

**Long history of Asthma (Dyspnea) + Chest pain + New development of L.L edema +FH =
PRIMARY PULMONARY HTN**

- CXR: Prominent pulmonary arteries with clear lung fields
- ECG: Right axis deviation + RVH +strain pattern
- ECHO
- Cardiac catheterization to show inc. Pulmonary Pr. >25 mmhg with CWP <15mmhg
- <u>TTT:</u> Bosentan, Sildenafil, Prostacylins + ANTICOAGULATION

Chest Pain Radiates To Throat, Burning , Worse After Meals = GORD

- Chronic cough worse at night / Lying flat
- 24 hrs ambulatory PH monitoring
- <u>TTT:</u> PPIs

**Recurrent Loss of consciousness/Dizzy spells with SUDDEN TURNING OF HEAD =
CAROTID SINUS HYPERSENSITIVITY**

- Occur with Wearing high collars shirts
- Vasovagal syncope
- <u>TTT:</u> Life style modification / Dual chamber Pacing

Long standing reflux + Dysphagia = BENIGN ESOPHYGEAL STRICTURE , CA ESOPHAGUS

Heparin + Low platelets after 5-14 days =HEPARIN INDUCED THROMBOCYTOPENIA

- HIT + Thrombosis = HEPARIN INDUCED THROMBOCYTOPENIA AND THROMBOSIS
- <u>TTT:</u> Danaproid , Lepirudin, Fondaparinox

Causes Of Zigzag Line Vision

- TIA (Emboli of AF , Carotid Atheroma)
- Macular edema

- Vitrous heamorrhage
- Retinal detachment
- Migraine
- Hypotension
- Hypoglycemia

Surgery in pituitary + Vomiting =ADDISONIAN CRISIS

- Hyperkalemia (Gastro-enteritis causes hypokalemia)
- TTT: IV Fluids & hydrocortisone

Causes Of Howell Jolly Bodies On Blood Film

- Splenectomy
- Sickle cell anemia (Auto splenectomy)
- Celiac disease (Hyposplenism)
- Megaloblastic anemia
- Severe hemolytic anemia

Sjogran (Autoimmune disease) + Elevated Liver enzymes (Rt. Hypochondrial pain + jaundice) = AIH

- Autoimmune disease could be associated all together

WT. gain /Low mood / Depression / Easy bruising /Hirsuitism / Acne = Cushing yndrome

STATION III

Cardiovascular System Examination
Neurological System Examination

Station III Cardiovascular System Examination

1-Wash Your Hands

2-Greet The Patient, Introduce Yourself And Take Permission

3-Position The Patient 45 Degree

4-Expose The Patient Till Mid Abdomen

5-Generally Examine The Patient From The End Of The Bed (take your time) look for:

- **Marfanoid features**=AR (Aortic regurgitation)
  - o Tall with long fingers
  - o Span >height
- **Head & neck:**
  - o *Down syndrome* Face + Short stature → VSD
  - o *Noonan face* + Short Stature → PS (Pulmonary stenosis)
  - o *Turner* = COA (Coarcitation of aorta), AR (Aortic regurgitation), AS (Aortic stenosis)
  - o *Vigorous neck pulsations*=AR (Aortic regurgitation)
  - o *Xanthelasma*
  - o *Cyanosis*
- **Chest:**
  - o Pericordial bulge = Long standing Heart disease
  - o Scars
  - o Pace makers, Defibrillator
  - o Cardiac apex
- **Abdomen**
  - o Distension = Ascites/Hepatomegaly = ? CCF (heart failure)
- **Arms**
  - o Clubbing = Congenital cyanotic Ht.ds / Infective endocarditis
  - o Cyanosis
- **Legs**
  - o Clubbing
  - o Cyanosis
  - o Differential cyanosis =PDA with reversed shunt
  - o Saphenous graft harvest scar=CABG
  - o Diabetic changes (Necrobiosis lipoidica , Dermopathy)

7-Ask The Patient To Spread His Hand And Examine Dorsum For:

- Clubbing → Infective endocarditis/congenital cyanotic ht.ds.
- Splinter Hemorrhage → Infective endocarditis
- Long fingers; check for Marfan`s syndrome →AR, MVP
- Press on nail and observe for quink`s sign → AR

8-Ask Him To Turn His Hand And Examine Palms

- Jane way (painless)=IEC
- Osler (painful)=IEC

9-Examine His Pulse In 15 Sec.s X 4 for:

- **Rate**
- **Rhythm** (Regular , Irregular , Irregular irregular)
- Volume (Small , Average , Large)
  - o Low Volume in stenotic Lesions
  - o Large volume in VSD, AR
- **Character**
  - o No special CCC
  - o Collapsing =AR , PDA
  - o Bisferiens =Double Aortic valve lesion
  - o Slow rising =AS
- **Equality on both sides**

- **Radio-femoral delay**
- **Intact/impaired peripheral pulsations**
- If you found **MIDLINE STERNOTOMY SCAR** try to **LISTEN TO ANY AUDIBLE CLICKS** of valve replacement , IS IT *ONE* OR *TWO* (double valve replacement) , if **ONE CLICK IS PRESENT, TIME IT WITH THE CARDIAC APEX** while you palpate the Apex to see if it is Aortic or Mitral.

10-Ask Him If He Has Any Pain In Shoulder And Examine For

Water Hammer Pulse By:

- Suddenly elevating the arm feel with both hands (feel with four fingers of Rt.hand over radial artery and Left hand fingers over brachial)

11-Examine Axilla for:

Skin wrinkling & plucked chicken appearance & pseudoxanthomas

- Pseudoxanthoma elasticum=AR, MR

12-Ask Him To Look Up And Examine Eyes

- Xanthelasma
- Corneal arcus
- Pallor

13-Ask Him To Open His Mouth And Examine Mouth for

- High arched palate → AR if Marfan`s , AS if HOCM
- Cyanosis

14-Inspect The Neck For Vigorous Pulsations = AR (Corrigan signs)

15-Ask Him To Turn His Head And Examine JVP for elevation:

- Venous pulsation are seen better than felt , obliterated by pressure on root of neck ,Wavy in CCC
- If external Jugular is congested, pulsating you can measure it
- If you can`t asses JVP on Rt. Side , you can look at the Lt. Side
- Elevated or not.
- Normally < 5cm (measure from sternal angle and your hand tangantialy)
  - Prominent waves (time it with the opposite carotid pulse)
  - Prominent V wave (systolic) = TR
  - Prominent A wave (diastolic) = PH , PS , RVH
  - If the patient is in AF and u see a prominent wave → Its for sure V wave; A waves are absent in AF

16-Feel The Carotid Artery For CCC Of Pulse (any pain in your neck?)

17-Inspect The Pericordium for

- Bulge
- Apex Beat
- Scars
  - Midline sternotomy scar = MVR , AVR, CABG
  - Lt.Subclavicular scar = pace maker / ICD
  - Lt.Submamary scar = Mitral valvuloplasty

18-Palpate The Apex for:

- **Site** (normally in the 5th ICS MCL) the outmost pulsation
- **Character**
  - No special CCC (doesn't elevate your finger)
  - Heaving =AS (elevates your finger & stays for a second before descent)
  - Hyperdynamic = MR , AR (elevate your finger & rapidly descends)
  - Tapping = MS (Tickling under your finger)
- **Thrills**
  - Diastolic = MS
  - Systolic =MR

19-Palpate Lt.Parasternal Edge for:

- Lt. parasternal heave =RVH=PH (Pulmonary HTN)

20-Palpate Pulmonary Area for

2nd LT. ICS just lateral to sternal edge

- **Palpable S2** =PH
- **Thrills** (Time with the carotid pulse)
  - o Systolic = PS
  - o Diastolic =PR

21-Palpate Aortic Area Together With The Neck for:

- **Thrills** (Time with the carotid pulse)
  - o Systolic=AS
  - o Diastolic = AR

22-Auscultate The Apex With Bell for:

- **Irregular Irregular Pusle**
- **S1**
  - o Accentuated =MS (Normally S2>S1 slightly)
  - o Muffled=MR
  - o Variable intensity =AF
  - o Clicky sound → valve replacement
- **S2**
  - o Accentuated =PH , HTN (Compare P2 & A2)
  - o Muffled = AR , AS
  - o Normally S2 is slightly louder > S1
  - o Clicky sound → Valve replacement
- **Murmurs :**
  - o Low Pitched Mid diastolic rumbling murmur with an opening snap → MS
  - o Soft blowing pan systolic murmur radiate to axilla → MR
- If you hear systolic murmur on apex move with your stethoscope to see where it increases towards:
  - o Axilla =MR
  - o Tricuspid (Lt. Sternal edge) =TR
  - o Aortic area = AS

23-Auscultat The Apex With Diaphragm For The Same

24-Ask The Patient To Turn On His Left Lateral Position

25-Relocate The Apex And Assess Site & CCC & Thrills With Palpation

26-Auscultate With Diaphragm For The Same

27-Ask The Patient To Breath Out And Listen Again

28-Lie The Patient Supine Again

29-Auscultate The Tricuspid Area For Murmurs

- Soft blowing pan-systolic murmur (TR)= prominent V wave in JVP
- Mid diastolic rumbling murmur (TS)

30-Ask Him To Take A Deep Breath In While Listening

31-Auscultate Pulmonary Area (2nd Lt.ICS) note

- **S2**
  - o Accentuated = PH (Compare P2 with A2=pulmonary & Aortic area)
- **Murmurs**
  - o Early diastolic murmur = PR or Graham steel murmur with PH in MS (Mitral stenosis)
  - o Harsh Ejection systolic murmur= PS or PH

32-Ask Him To Take Deep Breath In While Listening

33-Auscultate Aortic Area (2nd Rt. ICS) for:

- **S2**
  - o Muffled S2 =AR ,AS
  - o Accentuated S2 = HTN

Important Notes

- Prosthetic Valves are Heard Best On The Tricuspid Area
- If You Find Thoracotomy Scar Go To See The Legs; Look For Scar Of Saphenous Vein Harvest Of CABG, If No Scar On The Leg = Valve Replacement
- Lt. Parasternal Thrill may be due to VSD, PS
- Always examine Medic alert bracelet or Necklace
- Differential cyanosis (Cyanosis only in lower limbs = PDA with reversed shunt)
- Central cyanosis = Heart or Lung disease

- **Murmurs**
  - High pitched early diastolic murmur = AR
  - Harsh ejection systolic murmur=AS

34-Ask Him To Exhale While Listening

35-Auscultate The Base Of The Neck For Transmited As Murmur

36-Auscultate The Carotids For Bruit=Atheroma

37-Ask Him To Stop Breathing

38-Ask Him To Sit Forward

39-Feel The Base Of The Heart Again (Aortic Area)

40-Auscultate Left Sternal Edge For Soft Early Diastolic Murmur Of AR, Ask The Patient To Breath Out

41-Ask If He Has Any Pain In His Back

42-Feel For Sacral Edema

43-Listen To Bases Of Lungs

44.-Examine The Legs For

- Pitting edema at malleoli , then shins , then patella , then ASIS
- Dorsalis pedis pulsation (bilaterally)
- Saphenous graft harvest scar
- Eccymosis = Anticoagulation

45-Formulate Your Comment & Diagnosis

- **Diagnosis** (MR , MS , AR , AS)
- **Complications** (HF , AF , PH)
- **Cause** (Rheumatic Fever, Infective endocarditis , Myocardial infarction)

46-If It Is Infective Endocarditis → Examine The Spleen & Fundus

47-If You Find Abdominal Distension Examine It (Ascites)

48-If You Find AR Search For Its Signs

- Pistol shot in femoral artery
- Corrigan in neck (vigorous neck pulsations)
- Quinke`s sign (capillary pulsations in nails)
- Dorroizier sign: (systolic & diastolic murmur over femoral artery when it is gradually compressed)

49-Thank The Patient & Cover Him

50-Wash Your Hands Again

Cardiology Case Presentation

This gentleman is lying comfortable in bed with average built , he has no L.L edema , no stigmata of IEC , no signs of HF , no cyanosis , his pulse is 80 BPM , regular , average vol. , no special CCC , equal in both side , no radio-femoral delay , and intact peripheral pulsations , he has midline sternotomy scar , the apex is in the 5th ICS with no special CCC , S1 is normal , S2 is clicky , there is harsh ejection systolic murmur heard best in the aortic area with patient holding breath in expiration radiating to the base of the neck/ MS complicated by AF & Pulmonary HTN

I would like to complete my examination by measuring Bl.pressure , doing a urine dipstick , looking at the observation charts

Cardiology Examination Common Pitfalls

1-Failure to spend 30 secs for general survey

2-Forgetting to examine the pulse; the pulse will give you very important signs to help you with your diagnosis

3-Failure to detect the highest intensity of a murmur and accept its source where you first heard it.

4-Failure to locate the apex and recognizing its character; if you can't feel the apex ask the patient to roll on his left side and feel for it again ; locate it and observe its character.

5-Omitting infective endocarditis in a cardiology case with clubbing and a heart murmur.

6-Overlooking an obvious present sign; just because it is in another system; e.g.; not examining for ascites in a cardiology case with a very distended abdomen & evidence of heart failure.

7-Forgetting to examine the carotid pulse for CCC of pulse and depending only on the radial pulse.

Cardiology Cases

Mitral stenosis

Clinical Examination

- Low volume pulse
- Might be in AF
- Tapping cardiac apex
- ? Diastolic thrill at the apex according to severity
- Muffled S1
- Low pitched mid-diastolic rumbling murmur with an opening snap heard best on the apex with the patient on the Lt. lateral position holding breath in expiration
- If the patient is in AF, with MS, there is no opening snap
- Might be complicated by PH
- Might be in CCf or Right sided Heart Failure.

Look for a cause:

- *Carcinoid syndrome:* wheezing, facial flushing, rhinophyema
- *Rheumatic heart disease:* if no obvious cause

Quick Discussion

What Are The CXR Signs Of Pulmonary HTN ?

Lung oligemia + straightening of the heart border + prominent pulmonary artery

What Are The Indications For Mitral Valve Replacement?

1-Mitral Stenosis

- Severe pulmonary hypertension (pulmonary artery systolic pressure >60 mm Hg) & valvotomy is contraindicated
- Left atrial thrombus (Despite anticoagulation)
- Mitral regurgitation (MR) is present
- Abnormal valve morphology

2-Mitral Regurgitation

Elevated LVESD >45 mm with ejection fraction <60

What Treatment You Will Offer This Patient?

- Diuretics & ACE
- Treatment of AF
- balloon valvutomy
- valve replacement as indicated

What Are The Causes Of Absent Opening Snap In MS?

- Calcific Mitral valve

What Are The Causes Of Mitral Stenosis?

- Rheumatic heart disease & mucopolysacharidosis
- Carcinoid Syndrome

What Are The Complications Of MS?

- pulmonary HTN
- AF →Embolization & Stroke
- CCF
- Increased susceptibility of having Infective endocarditis

What Are Signs Of Severity Of Mitral Stenosis?

- Soft S1
- PH
- Early opening snap
- Duration of Murmur
- Thrill

What Investigations You Would Do For This Patient?

- Echo with Doppler
- ECG → P Mitral, AF, RAD, RVH
- X-ray → Calcific, Enlarged LA, Increased Broncho-vascular markings (before PH)

What Are The Signs Of Eisenmenger`s Syndrome?

- Pt. Is Cyanotic (central & peripheral), Clubbing, Tachypnea, Elevated JVP , Lt. Parasternal heave, Palpable P2
- L.L edema
- S2 is loud & single
- Murmur of TR, PR, PS.

What Are The Causes & Ttt Of Eisenmenger`s Syndrome?

ASD, VSD, PDA

<u>TTT:</u> heart & lung transplantation

Aortic stenosis

Clinical Examination

- Low volume pulse
- Slowly rising pulse
- Heaving apex
- ? Systolic Thrill over Aortic area (2nd Rt. ICS)
- Systolic murmur over aortic area
- Muffled S2
- ? S4
- Harsh Ejection Systolic Murmur Heard Over The 2nd Rt. ICS With The Patient Leaning Forward Holding His Breath In Expiration Radiating To The Base Of The Neck
- Might Be in CCF

Look For A Cause:

- Turner facies
- Senility/Calcification
- William syndrome: facies
- *HOCM:* Young, double apex.

Quick Discussion

What Are The Differences Between Aortic Stenosis & Aortic Sclerosis?

Aortic Stenosis	Aortic Sclerosis
Thrill	No Thrill
Small pulse volume	Normal Pulse volume
Murmur is Radiating to neck	Murmur is Not radiating to neck

Both AS & Aortic Sclerosis have ejection systolic murmur over Aortic area

What Are The Causes Of AS?

- Rheumatic & Bicuspid aortic valve (Turner)
- Aging → sclerosis ,calcification
- Supra-valvular →William
- Sub-valvular → HOCM

What Are The Complications Of AS?

- CCF
- IHD
- Cardiac dysrhythmias
- Infective endocarditis

What Investigations You Want To Do For This Patient?

- Echo & Doppler
- X-ray → calcification , cardiomegaly
- ECG → Lt. Ventricular hypertrophy with strain pattern
- Cardiac catheterization
- Basic investigations

What Treatments You Want To Offer This Patient?

- Beta blockers for angina pain
- Replacement if indicated

Mitral regurgitation

Clinical Examination

- Large volume pulse
- Might be in AF
- Apex might be shifted outside 5th ICS MCL
- Hyperdynamic apex
- Systolic thrill over the apex
- Muffled S1
- Soft Blowing Pan-Systolic Murmur Heard Best At The Apex With The Patient On The Lt. Lateral Position Holding Breath In Expiration Radiating To The Axilla
- Might Be Complicated By PH.
- Might be in CCF or Right Sided Heart Failure

Look for a cause:

- *IEC:* stigmata of IEC
- *IHD:* old, Arteriopathy signs
- *Rheumatic fever:* no obvious cause
- Pseudoxanthoma elasticum: peripheral signs
- *Ehler's danlos:* peripheral signs
- *Marfan's syndrome:* peripheral signs
- *Ankylosing spondylitis:* Kyphoscoliosis, Tender sacroiliacs
- *SLE:* butter fly rash
- *RA:* Joint changes

Quick Discussion

What Are The Causes Of Mitral Regurgitation?

- Rheumatic fever (young age)
- Infective endocarditis (patient is dyspneic , clubbing)
- Myocardial infarction
- Dilated cardiomyopathy
- Marfan's, Ehler danlos , Pseudoxanthoma elasticum , ADPKD, MD → (MVP)
- Previous Mitral Valvotomy

What Are Signs Of Severity Of Mitral Regurgitation?

- Thrill
- Shifted Apex
- Pulmonary HTN
- CCF
- S3

What Are The Complications Of Mitral Regurgitation?

- Pulmonary HTN → Core-pulmonale
- Infective endocarditis
- AF → Embolization

What Are The Investigations Of Mitral Regurgitation?

- Echo with Doppler
- CXR → Calcific valve, Dilated LA (double shadow in Rt. Cardiac silhouette), Cardiomegaly , Congested lungs in in CCF
- ECG → LV dilatation and hypertrophy, P mitral , AF

What Treatment Would You Offer This Patient?

- Diuretics & ACE Is to dec. Pulmonary HTN
- TTT of AF
- prophylaxis to infective endocarditis
- Replacement if indicated

What Are The Causes Of MR With Preserved S1?

- Mixed Mitral valve lesion
- Posterior leaflet MR
- Mild MR

What Are The Signs Of Mixed Mitral Valve With Predominantly Stenosis?

- Signs of MS (low volume pulse, Accentuated S1, Non-displaced apex , Tapping ,murmur)
- Murmur of MR

What Are The Signs Of Mixed Mitral With Predominantly Regurgitation ?

- Signs of MR (low volume pulse, hyperdynamic apex, Soft S1, displaced apex, murmur, thrill)
- Murmur of MS

What Are The Signs & Causes Of MVP?

- Mid systolic click, with late MR murmur
- Marfan`s syndrome, pseudoxanthoma elasticum, Osteogenisis imperfecta, Ehler danlos, ADPKD, HOCM, MYOTONIA
- ECHO for diagnosis

Aortic regurgitation

Clinical Examination:

- Large volume pulse
- Collapsing pulse
- Water hummer pulse
- Quink's sign
- Corrigan sign
- Hyperdynamic Apex
- Apex shifted outside 5th ICS MCL
- Diastolic thrill at 2nd Rt. ICS
- Soft S2
- ? S3 Gallop
- High Pitched Early Diastolic Murmur Heard Best On The Lt. Sternal Edge With The Patient Leaning Forward And Holding Breath In Expiration
- ? Pulmonary HTN
- ? CCF

Look For A Cause:

- *Ankylosing spondylitis:* Kyphoscoliosis
- *IEC:* peripheral signs
- *Marfan's syndrome:* Peripheral signs
- *Pseudoxanthoma elasticum:* Peripheral signs
- *SLE*: Facial signs
- *Rheumatic Heart Disease*: No Obvious cause or Precordial Bulge
- *Ehler's Danlos*: Peripheral signs

Look for Peripheral Signs:

e.g. Pistol Shot Sign

Quick Discussion

What Are The Causes Of Aortic Regurgitation?

- Rheumatic Fever & Infective Endocarditis
- Syphilis
- Marfan's Syndrome
  - Autosomal Dominant
  - Fibrillin gene defect On Chr. 15
- Pseudoxanthoma Elasticum
- Ankylosing Spondylitis
- Seronegative Arthropathies
- Bicuspid
- Turner's Syndrome
- Dissection Of The Aorta

What Are The Peripheral Signs Of Aortic Regurgitation?

- Corrigan's → Visible Neck Pulsation
- De Musset → Head Nodding
- Quinkes → Capillary Pulsations
- Muller's Sign → Uvula Motion
- Drouzier's sign → Diastolic Murmur Of Femoral Artery When Pressing With Stethoscope
- Pistol Shot In Femoral Artery

What Are The Signs Of Severity Of Aortic Regurgitation?

- Austin Flint Murmur (Functional Mitral Stenosis)
- Duration Of Murmur
- Soft S2
- Presence Of S3
- Wide Pulse Pressure

- Hills Sign
  - L.L Pr > UL Pr. 20-40 = Mild, 40-60 = Moderate, >60 = Severe)
- Peripheral Stigmata Of AR
- HF
- Shifted Apex

What Investigations You Will Do In AR Case?

- Echo with Doppler
- X-ray → Cardiomegaly
- ECG
- Cardiac catheterization

What Is The Treatment For AR?

- ACEIs
- Valve replacement if indicated

Rheumatic Heart Disease

Clinical Examination

- Any valvular lesion or valve replacement
- Pulse might be in AF
- There might be associated complications e.g. AF, PH, CCF
- Usually presents with more than one valve lesion.
- No stigmata of IEC
- No Obvious cause for the Valvular lesion
- Developing Countries

Quick Discussion

What Are The Signs Of Mixed Aortic Valve Ds With Predominentaly Regurgitation?

- Signs of AR (collapsing pulse or bisfiriens , large volume pulse , peripheral signs of AR, Apex displaced, thrusting Apex, murmur of AR)
- Murmur of AS
- Diastolic Thrill , may be a systolic thrill

What Are The Signs Of Mixed Aortic Valve Predominantly Stenosis?

- Signs of AS (Low Volume Pulse, Slow Rising, Apex Not Displaced, Heaving, Murmur)
- Murmur of AR
- Systolic or diastolic thrill

VSD (Ventricular Septal Defect)

Clinical Examination:

- Cyanosis if Eisenmenger's Develops
- Pulse Is Low Volume.
- Apex Is Displaced
- Thrusting (Hyperdynamic)
- S1 Normal
- S2 Normal
- Lt. Parasternal Systolic Thrill
- Harsh Pansystolic Murmur On Lt. Lower Sternal Edge Radiating All Over The Precordium
- Mid Diastolic Rumbling Murmur Lt. Parasternal Area (Functional TS)
- Signs Of PH
- Signs Of CCF

Look for a Cause:

- Congenital (Down) → Facies
- Myocardial Infarction
- Maladie De Roger → Small Insignificant , With Loud Murmur →Will Close Spontaneously

Quick Discussion

What Are The Complications Of VSD?

- Pulmonary HTN → Eisenmenger
- LVH
- RVH
- CCF

What Investigations You Do In VSD Case?

- Echo with Doppler
- X-ray → Lung Plethora, Cardiomegaly
- ECG → RVH, LVH

What Is The Treatment For VSD?

- Surgical (percutaneous transcatheter closure) if affecting growth or causing CCF

Infective Endocarditis

Clinical Examination:

- ? Valve replacement signs with valve failure (Regurgitation murmur)
  - o Mid Line Sternotomy Scar
  - o One or both of the heart sounds is metallic
  - o Regurgitation murmur
- ? Needle marks of IV drug abuse
- Stigmata of IEC:
  - o Clubbing
  - o Splinter hemorrhage
  - o Janeway Lesion (Painless erythema of fingers, Hands, Toes)
  - o Osler`s Nodules (Painful Nodules)
- Regurgitation Murmur
- Peripheral signs according to the regurgitation murmur
- ? Splenomegaly
- ? CCF

Quick Discussion:

What Are The Criteria of Diagnosing Infective Endocarditis?

Modified Duke`s Criteria

- One of these combinations of clinical criteria:
- 2 major clinical criteria
- 1 major and 3 minor criteria
- 5 minor criteria

Major Criteria

1-**Positive blood culture** with typical IE microorganism:

- o Viridans-group streptococci, or
- o Streptococcus bovis including nutritional variant strains, or
- o HACEK group, or
- o Staphylococcus aureus, or
- o Community-acquired Enterococci, in the absence of a primary focus

2-**Evidence Of Endocardial Involvement With Positive Echocardiogram** defined as

- Oscillating Intracardiac Mass On Valve Or Supporting Structures, In The Path Of Regurgitant Jets, Or On Implanted Material In The Absence Of An Alternative Anatomic Explanation, Or
- Abscess, Or
- New Partial Dehiscence Of Prosthetic Valve Or New Valvular Regurgitation (Worsening Or Changing Of Preexisting Murmur Not Sufficient)

Minor criteria

- Predisposing factor: known cardiac lesion, recreational drug injection
- Fever >38 °C
- Embolism evidence: arterial emboli, pulmonary infarcts, Janeway lesions, conjunctival hemorrhage
- Immunological problems: glomerulonephritis, Osler's nodes, Roth's spots, Rheumatoid factor
- Microbiologic evidence: Positive blood culture (that doesn't meet a major criterion) or serologic evidence of infection with organism consistent with IE but not satisfying major criterion

What Investigations You Want to Do for This Patient?

- Echo: TTE first then TOE to visualize vegetations
- Blood Cultures
- RF
- Urine dip for Blood & Proteins
- Fundoscopy for Roth`s spots

How Will You Treat This Patient?

- IV Antibiotics according to hospital Protocol & Blood cultures

Metallic Valve Replacement

Metallic Mitral Valve Replacement:

- There is midline sternotomy scar
- Apex Might be Shifted if due to Mitral regurgitation
- Might be in AF
- There is a click at the 1st Ht sound (Best Heard on tricuspid area)
- S2 is normal
- Mid-diastolic flow murmur (mild stenosis is a common finding)
- Stenotic murmurs are ok with MVR & AVR

Look for Signs of Valve Failure

- Regurgitation Murmur (PanSystolic Murmur) in the affected valve
- Signs of CCF

Metallic Aortic Valve Replacement

- There Is Midline Sternotomy Scar
- Paex Might Be Shifted Outwards if due to Aortic Regurgitation
- 1st Ht. Sounds Is Normal (Unless Accompanied By MS)
- Ejection Systolic Murmur,
- Followed By A Click In 2nd Ht. Sound (Best Heard in Tricuspid area)

Look For Signs of Valve Failure

- Regurgitation Murmur (Early Diastolic)
- CCF
- Peripheral Signs of Aortic Regurgitation

Dual Valve Replacement

- Mid-Line Sternotomy Scar
- First heart sound is metallic
- Second heart sound is metallic

Quick Discussion:

What Are The Indications For Aortic Valve Replacement?

1-AORTIC STENOSIS

- Symptomatic With Severe AS (Anginal Pain, Syncopes)
- Undergoing CABG
- Systolic Pressure Gradient 60 mmhg

2-AORTIC REGURGITATION

- EF < 50 LVESD > 55 mm

What Are The Complications Of Metallic Valvular Replacement?

- Thrombus formation & embolization (anticoagulants dec. This)
- Hemorrhage from excessive anticoagulation
- Infective endocarditis (Suspect if leakage)
- Failure (suspect if dec. Click & Regurgitation murmur & S3 & hemodynamic instability)
- Valve obstruction from thrombus or fibrosis
- Hemolysis (Aortic Valve more commonly) → Anemia, Jaundice

How Will You Manage A Patient With Metallic Valve Replacement?

1-INVESTIGATIONS

- Basic investigations
- INR
- CXR

- ECHO

2-TREATMENT

- Anticoagulation (Warfarin or Clexane) ; follow up Warfarin by INR , TOE
- Prophylaxis to infective Endocarditis (Ampicillin or Ampicillin + gentamycin for GIT/GU surgery)
- Treatment of heart Failure

Atrial Fibrillation

Clinical Examination:

- Irregular Irregular Pulse In Rate & Volume
- Pulse Deficit >10
- Absent A Waves On JVP
- ? Mitral Valve Murmur
- S1 Variable Intensity
- ? CCF
- ? PH
- ? Hemiplegia

Look for A Cause:

Mitral Valve disease

Thyrotoxicosis: Wt.Loss ? Grave`s disease signs

Quick Discussion

What Are The Causes Of AF?

- MR or MS
- Thyrotoxicosis
- IHD
- HTN
- Alcohol
- Lone AF
- Cardiomyopathy

What Is The Management Of AF?

Investigations:

- ECG: Absent P waves, Irregular rhythm
- Echo looking for structural heart disease
- TSH, T4, T3

Treatment:

- Anti-coagulation if the CHADSVASC score is > 1
- Rate control
  o BB, Digoxin, CCB
- Rhythm control
  o Lone , young patient , <48hrs , TOE normal
  o Dc or amiodarone
- If hemodynamically unstable →DC cardioversio

HOCM

Clinical Examination

- Young Patient
- Jerky pulse
- Double apex
- Systolic Thrill
- S4
- Subvalvular AS: harsh ejection systolic murmur of AS

Look for a Cause

- Associated with friedrich`s ataxia (Pes Cavus, Hammer toe, Spastic Paraparesis)
- Autosomal Dominant

Quick Discussion

What Investigations You Would Like To Do?

Echo: Asymmetrical septal hypertrophy, SAM (Systolic anterior motion) of Mitral leaflet

ECG → LVH, T wave changes, Q waves inferior & Lateral leads, LAD

What Treatment You Would Like To Offer This Patient?

Implantable DC or BBs

What Are The Poor Prognostic Factors For HOCM?

- History of syncope
- Family History of sudden death
- Abnormal pressure records on Exercise testing
- Ventricular arrhythmia on Holter
- Out flow gradient >40 mmHg
- Septal thickness >18 mm

What Are The Signs Of PDA (Patent Ductus Arteriosus)?

- ? Young Patient
- Large Volume Pulse
- Collapsing Pulse may be Water Hammer Pulse
- Lt. Infra-clavicular Machinery Murmur
- Thrusting Apex
- Lt. Parasternal Heave
- Differential Cyanosis if Eisenmenger`s syndrome develops
- Causes
  - Congenital
  - Prematurity

What Are The Signs Of Fallot Tetralogy With Blalock Shunt?

- Central Cyanosis
- Clubbing
- Lt. Pulse Weaker Than Rt.
- Thoracotomy Scar
- Lt. Parasternal Heave
- Thrill In Pulmonary Area
- Ps Murmur (Ejection Systolic)
- Continuous Machinery Murmur
- AR (murmur)

What Are The Causes Of Elevated JVP?

Pulsatile

- Eisenmenger
- Pulmonary HTN
- PE

- Complete heart block
- Core Pulmonale
- CCF
- TR
- Constrictive pericarditis
- large pleural effusion

Non-pulsatile: SVCO = Mediastinal syndrome

What Are The Signs Of Coarctation Of Aorta?

- Radio-femoral Delay
- Large Volume In Arms
- Low Volume In Legs
- Visible Pulsations
- Bruits Around Scapula
- Lt. Sternal Border
- Heaving Apex
- Systolic Murmur 4TH IC Space Posteriorly

Look for a Cause

- Turner's Facies & body habitus

Do MRI for diagnosis

Association:

- Rib Notching
- Turner
- Bicuspid Aortic Valve
- Berry Aneurysm

What Do You Know About Dextrocardia?

Cardiac Apex at Rt. Side, might be associated with:

- Situs Inversus Totalis → Liver Is on the Lt. Side
- Kartagner'S Syndrome → Bronchiectasis, Infertility, Sinusitis, Otitis Media

What Do You Know About ASD?

- Defect in the Septuc between both atria can presents with:
  - AF + Wide Splitting Of 2nd Ht. Sound + PS Murmur → ASD With Little Hemodynamic Significance
  - AF + Lt. Parasternal Heave + Systolic Thrill Over Pulmonary Area + Widely Split S2 + Ps Murmur + TS Murmur = ASD with significant hemodynamic significance
- Ostium Secondum is the most common it causes RAD on ECG
- Ostium Primmum leads to MR causes RBB, LAD on ECG
- Diagnosis → TOE
- Treatment → Surgery if symptomatic or Pulmonary to systemic ratio 2:1
- Complications:
  - Eisenmenger
  - Paradoxical emboli
  - CCF
  - Infective endocarditis

What Do You Know About Noonan Syndrome?

- Proportionate Short Stature; Height Is Equal To The Span
- Low Set Ears, Triangle, Smiling Face
- Ptosis, Flat Nasal Bridge
- Preserved Beard & Moustache
- Cubitus Valgus
- Webbed Neck
- Pectus Excavatum
- AD
- Chromosomal analysis: 44+ XY

Station III Upper Limbs Neurologically

1-Wash Your Hands

2-Greet The Patient and Shake Hands, note if he has **Myotonia** And note his **Speech**

- Slurred (loss of some letters)=UMNL → Stroke, Bulbar, Pseudobulbar palsy (note if crossed hemiplegia or not)
- Staccato (Interrupted explosive) → Cerebellum
- Scanning (UMNL + Cerebellar lesion)

3-Expose Arms And Legs

4-Postion The Patient Either Sitting Or Lying On The Bed

5-General Survey from the end of the bed for:

Bed side clues → Walking aids, Orthotics

State Of Muscles of both U.Ls, L.Ls, Face

Tremors

- Static=Parkinsonism
- Intentional =Cerebellum

Fasciculations = LMNL

Nystagmus → Cerebellum affection

Facies

- **Myotonia** (Triangular face + bilateral Ptosis + Frontal baldness)
- **Myxedema** (puffiness around eyes + loss of outer 1/3 of eye brow)= PM
- **Grave's disease** (exophthalmous)=PM (proximal Myopathy)
- **Hemiplegic** (UMNL VII (lower face) same side of hemiplegia with flexed Arm)
- **Facial nerve palsy** (LMNL VII)=Pons lesion
- **Myopathic** (unlined face, loss of nasolabial fold and wrinkles)=PM , MG
- **Myasthenia gravis** (Bilateral Ptosis, Unlined face , +ve Jaw support sign)
- **Parkinsonism** (dec. facial expressions)
- **Wasted muscles of the Neck** =Fascioscapulohumeral
- **Acromegaly** = PM (Proximal myopathy)

Deformities (pes cavus, hammer toe = Long standing Neurological disability E.g.: Friedrich`s ataxia, Charcot-marie tooth.

Characteristic posture (Flexion of upper limb in Hemiplegia, Dystonia)

6-Examine Muscle State "Any pain in Your arms?"

Inspect for:

- Wasting, Disuse atrophy
- Fasiculations
- Hypertrophy
- Tremors

Palpate for Fasiculations & Tenderness by tapping on Muscles.

7-Examine The Tone

- Hold hand, Circumduction of wrist, Flex & Extend elbow , then Circumduction of shoulder, then repeat on other side
  - Cogwheel rigidity (In Wrists because Of Tremors) or Lead pipe (Elbow) = Parkinsonism
  - Clasp knife= UMNL
  - Hypotonia = LMNL , Cerebellum

8-Examine Muscle Power

- Both shoulders Abd. (C5), Add (C5,6), Flexion , Extension
- Each Elbow Flexion (C5,6) & Extension (C 7,8) repeat on other side
- Each Wrist flexion & Extension (C6,7) , repeat on other side

- Ask him to Squeeze Your hands
- Fingers flexion (C8) & Extension(C7), repeat on other side
- Ask him to make a Circle with Thumb & Little (C8-T1) & repeat other side
- Then abduct fingers (T1) , then adduct with card then repeat other side then
- Abduct thumb (toward ceiling) (median nerve) , then Adduct with card test (ulnar nerve) , then Extend (radial) repeat on other side
- Interpret the Sites of the weakness
  - Weakness of EXT> FLEX, Abd> Add, Distal>Proximal =UMNL
  - P>D , ADD >ABD = Proximal myopathy=look at facial Muscles & Neck; FASCIOSCAPULOHUMERAL
  - D>P , EXT>FLEX , ADD>ABD =LMNL

9-Examine Reflexes

- Biceps, Triceps, Brachioradialis note: **"Clench on your teeth"**
  - Hyper reflexia = UMNL
  - Hyporeflexia =LMNL
- *Hoffman sign* =(UMNL) (Hold Middle finger between your index & Middle, flick middle finger distal phalynx by thumb If flexion of distal phalynx of thumb & index fingers = +ve = UMNL)
- Don't assume the reflex is absent without doing jandrasek maneuver = Ask the patient to CLENCH ON HIS TEETH
- MID-CERVICAL REFLEX (INVERTED REFLEXES)= lost biceps , brachioradialis, exaggerated triceps, or when tapping biceps , triceps contracts, when tapping brachioradialis the fingers contract=Cervical myelopathy (C5,C6) = Cervical spondylosis

10-Examine Co-ordination:

- **Finger to nose**, then finger to doctor finger with doctor moving his finger = over shooting, dysmetria, intention tremors, past-pointing
- If You suspect P.N, Or Dorsal Column affection (You can ask him to do this with closing eyes = impaired coordination = Sensory ataxia
- **Dysdiadokinesia** "Can You Tap over your hands, Faster"
- **Rebound** (support his arms not to hit his eyes) = ask him to extend both arms in front of him, gently push one arm down, you will notice rebound pull back of the arm which is exaggerated more than normal
- **Staccato speech**

11-Examine Sensations

Pin Prick:

- using pin, touch the chest ask him what he feels = prick
- then ask him to close his eyes
- Then prick him from distal to proximal, **"What Do You Feel? Is It The Same As On Your Chest?"**
- And compare on other side (bilaterally)
- If he can feel move proximal it could be dermatomal
- If he still can feel = no loss of spinothalamic tract
- If he cannot feel it the same ask him when it becomes the same as his chest to tell you , while you r moving from down upwards
- Move up pricking in medial & lat. Areas of both sides
- If he feels at level on arm/Legs then Examine it circumferential (in a circle) if all are same & less sensation from the areas above= P.N **"Is It The Same All Around?"**
- If when you do the circle (Circumferential) it is not the same then it is dermatomal , or nerve affection then check dermatomes and nerves
- If he doesn't feel the whole arm then it is hemiplegia sensory loss
  - C5=Deltoid + lateral arm , C6=lateral form arm & hand , C7=Middle 2 ring fingers, C8=Medial hand , T1=medial forearm , T2=medial arm
  - Median = lateral 3.5 fingers + lateral 2/3 palm
  - Ulnar = medial 1.5 fingers + medial 1/3 of palm
- In L.Ls, if he doesn't feel at level in legs move up to upper part of leg move up to trunk and note sensory level on trunk = spinal cord problem, if no sensory level → Hemiplegia.

Light touch with a cotton the same as pin prick

- Touch on chest 1st, **"Do You Feel It, Close Your Eyes, When You Feel It On Your Arms Say Yes"**

Vibration

- Start on head ask him what he feels = Vibration
- Then start at the *fingers*, Then *radial bone, olecranon,* sternum , *clavicle* , *mastoid*
- L.Ls: Big Toe, Medial Malleolus, Shins, Patella, ASIS, Sternum , Clavicle & Mastoid

Position Sense

- Show him first **"That's your finger is up , down , now close Your eyes"**
- Move finger while supporting up and down and ask him where it is

12-Thank The Patient And Cover Him

13- Wash Your Hands Again

Station III Lower Limb Neurologically

1-Wash, Greet, Introduce, Explain, Expose, Position; Note: Myotonia & Speech

2-May I Ask The Patient To Walk? note Gait, Balance, Do Romberg's

3-General Survey: from the end of the bed, Take your time

- Walking aids
- Wasting & Fasciculations =LMNL
- **Facies**
- **Nystagmus**
- **Scars** = frequent falls
- Tremors
- **Flexed U.L Posture**
- **Externally rotated hips and flexed knees** (frog sign)= Hypotonia = LMNL or cerebellum
- **Pes cavus + Hammer toe** = Friedrich`s ataxia , HSMN (Charcoat Marie tooth)

4-Muscle State

- Wasting (LMNL)
- Disuse atrophy(UMNL)
- Fasciculation=LMNL
- PALPATE FOR TENDERNESS, FASICULATIONS (by tapping) **"Any Pain In Legs?"**

5-Tone

- Rolling, Lifting (with both hands in popliteal fossa)
- Circumduction of ankle
- Knee Flexion & Extension
  - Hypotonia
  - Hypertonia
    - Clasp knife
    - Lead pipe /Cog wheel

6-Power

- Hip flexion (L1,2,3) & Extension (L5,S1)
- Abd (L4,5,S1) , Add (L2,3,4)
- Knee flexion (L5,S1) ,Ext. (L3,4)
- Foot dorsiflexion (L4, L5) , Foot plantar flexion (S1 , 2)
- Eversion & Inversion
  - Weaknes P>D = Proximal Myopathy
  - Weakness D>P , E>F , Add>Abd = LMNL
  - Weakness D>P , F>E , Abd >Add = UMNL

7-Reflexes

- Knee
- Ankle
- Plantar reflex
  - Equivocal =Normal or LMNL
  - Extensor plantar = UMNL
  - Flexor plantar =Normal
- Pathological reflexes (if u find hyperflexia)
  - Adductor
  - Patellar (Exaggerated)
  - Clonus (90 degree)
  - Abdominal (scratch toward umbilicus in 4 quads)
    - Normally present
    - If spinal cord lesion = absent at level, exaggerated below level
    - If No reflex=Do Re-enforcement "pull your fingers against each other"

8-Coordination

- Heel to knee

- Toe to finger
- Tapping heel on your hands (tell him to do it faster)

9-Sensation

- **Pin Prick**
  - Prick the patient first in chest, what he feels?
  - Then examine from distal to proximal asking him to close his eyes , then what he feels? Is it the same as in chest?
  - If he doesn't feel , move up until it is the same as on chest
  - If he feels at a level in the limb=P.N
  - If not the same at level search for dermatome or nerve distribution
    - *ANT:* L1 below inguinal ligament , L2 between L1 & L3 , L3 above knee , L4medial lower leg , L5 , lateral lower leg with big toe
    - *POST:* S1 lateral leg and lower leg , S2 medial leg & lower leg
  - If doesn't feel until high thigh go up to the abdomen to examine for sensory level = Focal spinal cord lesion (confirm with umbilical reflexes)
    - Nipple T4, Xiphsterum T8, Umbilicus T10, Symphisis pubis T 12
- **Light Touch**
- **Vibration sense**
- **Position sense**

10-Thank The Patient And Cover Him

11-Wash Your Hands Again

Station III Cranial Nerves Examination

1-Wash, Greet, Introduce

2-Positon (Sitting)

3-General Survey

- Walking aids
- Myopathic facies = Ptosis = MG, Fascioscapulohumeral
- Parotid Enlargement Look for facial nerve palsy of parotid tumor
- Zoster in ears=facial nerve palsy (Ramsay hunt)
- Cushingoid facies + Bilateral facial palsy = Sarcoidosis Listen for Crackles & Feel for L.Ns
- Nystagmus = Cerebellar affection
- Tremors = Cerebellar affection if intentional
- Scars=Trauma
- Flexed upper limb = Hemiparesis

4-Ask Him If He Can Smell "May I Ask The Pt. About Smell Sir?"

5-Examine His Visual Acuity (II –Optic)

- Counting fingers form one meter
- Complete acuity (Snellen`s chart form 6 meters , if cannot read 6/60 move one meter closer, until he can't 1/60, then counting fingers form 1 meter, then counting fingers form 30 cms, then perception of light)

6-Visual Fields (II-Optic)

- With the patient standing in front of you 1 Meter, Same Level as yours, Remove your glasses: close his eye and your opposite, test temporal fields first; in upper, lower quads, then horizontal, when the patient sees your finger ask him to say then, test nasal fields, then repeat the same with the other eye.

7-Never To Do Field Examination Without Acuity Testing Before It

8-No Field Examination If There Is Defect In Acuity

9-Fundoscopy ask the examiner: "Is It Possible To Dim The Light ?"

10-Examine Eye Movements In H Shape (II, II-Occulomotor, IV-Trochlear, VI-Abducens)

- "Look At My Finger , Move With Your Eyes, Fix Your Head, If You See Double Or Feel Any Pain Tell Me"
- Note Double vision (Eye can't move) = Cr. N.Palsy
  - All mucles of eye movements supllied by 3rd (occulomotor) except:
  - Superior oblique=4th (Trochlear)=move eye down & medical
  - Lateral rectus = 6th (Abducens)=move eye laterally
  - Inferior oblique moves eye superior & medial
- Note Nystagmus = Cerebellum
- Note Internuclear opthalmoplegia=MS (one eye is not adducting the other eye has nystagmus , by covering the eye with nystagmus the non-adducting eye adducts normally, lesion is in the MLB of the non adducting eye)

11-Examine Pupils Make Sure Its Dark = put the patient hand over his midline of face

- Inspect: Size, Equality, Regularity
- Reaction to light (direct and consensual when moving torch in arc , and note if there is relative afferent papillary defect=Marcus Gunn Pupil=Optic neuritis=MS)

12-Examine Pupils For Accommodation

- Any eye problems = check pulse & auscultate pericardium, carotid artery, feel the temporal artery, ask; "I'd like to examine the pericardium & auscultate the heart"

13-Examine Sensations Of Head (V-Trigeminal): FRONTAL BONES (Opthalmic), MAXILLA (Maxillary), MANDIBLE (Mandibular) Of Both Sides

- prick the patient in chest , ask him if he feels , what he feels , then examine both ophthalmic division , together in comparison, the maxillary together and mandibular together

- If you find loss of sensation in face, examine sensations behind the ear (C2) if lost =hemiplegia sensory loss , if not lost and intact in C2 = V lesion (Midbrain Lesion, Internal Capsule)

14-Ask The Patient To Clench Teeth And Feel Masseter & Temporalis

- Note Any Weakness of Muscles supplied by V nerve.

15-Tap On The Jaw (JAW JERK) = Exaggerated in bilateral UMNL of V nerves.

16-Ask Him To Open Mouth And Note Any Deviation (V)

- JAW deviates to side of lesion = lesion of V

17-Ask The Patient To Raise Eye Brows, Close Eyes Tightly, Show You His Teeth, Blow His Cheeks; All Against Resistance

- Mouth deviates to healthy side = **Lesion of VII**

18-Test Hearing By Asking The Patient Name In One Ear And Age In Other Ear While Making Noise With Your fingers In The Unexamined ear (VIII-Acoustic Vestibular)

19-Ask Him To Open His Mouth And Says Ahh, See With Torch Note Deviation Of Uvula

- Uvula supplied by vagus deviates to the health side

20-Test Power Of Trapezius & Sternomastoids (XI-Spinal Accessory)

21-Ask Him To Open Mouth And Put His Tongue Out (XII-Hypoglossal)

- Deviates to the side of the lesion (Note Fasciculations, Wasting or spasticity)

22-Ask Him To Push On Cheeks With Tongue From Inside

23-Thank The Patient And Cover Him

24-Wash Your Hands Again

Station III Full Neurological Examination

1-Examine L.Ls Completely (Motor & Sensory & Coordination)

2-Examine U.Ls Motor & Coordination

3-Examine For Nystagmus

4-Examine Cranial Nerves (VII, XII) And III, V

5-May I Ask The Patient To Walk?

Neurology Case Presentation

This gentle man is comfortable at rest, average built, using a walking aid, walking with a **High Steppage gait**, **+ve Romberg sign**, he has **Sensory loss of light touch, pin prick, vibration, Position sense, in stocking distribution** (High Stocking distribution), and some extent glove, there is **LMNL signs in lower limb** in the form of Weaknes D>P, Extensor>F, Add > abd, Wasting, Decreased tone, Lost ankle reflex, Equivocal planters. Coordination is intact.

Station III Examination For Disequilibrium

<u>1-Wash, Great, Introduce, Explain, Expose, Position The Patient Lying In Bed Or Sitting On A Chair</u>

- General Survey

<u>2-Examine the Patient`s Gait:</u> "May I Ask The Patient To Walk?"

- Stamping gait = Dorsal column, P.N. (Peripheral Neuropathy)
- High steppage gait = P.N
- Circumduction gait = hemiplegia
- Ataxic gait = Cerebellar lesion
- Scissoring gait=spastic paraparesis
- Waddling gait = proximal weakness
- Shuffling gait = parkinsonism

<u>3-Ask Him To Walk Heel To Toe</u> for Equilibrium ? Cerbellar lesion

<u>4-Ask Him To Walk On Heels</u> for L5 weakness

<u>5-Ask Him To Walk On Toes</u> for S1 weakness

<u>6-Romberg Test</u>

<u>7-Ask Him To Sit & Stand For Proximal Myopathy</u>

<u>8-Ask Him To Sit On The Bed</u>

<u>9-Examine Eyes For Nystagmus</u> (your finger 30 cm away moving 30 degree rt. & lt.)

<u>10-Complete Neurological Examination Of Lower Limbs</u>

<u>11-Tests For Coordination In U.L</u>

<u>12-Thank The Pt. & Cover Him</u>

<u>13-Most Important Sign Is Nystagmus For Cerebellar Cause</u>

ROMBEG TEST

- Ask The Patient To Stand With Feets Together Holding His Arms Flexed At Shoulders Infront Of Him And Supinated And Note:
  - Pronator drift (one arm start pronating & falling =UMNL)
  - Desequilibrium = Cerebellar lesion
  - Then ask him to close eyes, if he has desequillibrium on closing the eyes = Sensory Ataxia =P.N or Dorsal column affection

---

Common Pitfalls

1-Not Appreciating The Importance Of General Survey Of The Patient (Very Important In A Neurology Case; Pes Cavus & Hammer Toe In HSCD, Flexed Adducted U.L In Hemiplegia When Asked To Examine Lower Limbs Only.

2-Examining The Superficial Sensation Of The Patient With Bias; By Directing The Patient To Say What You Want; Let The Patient Say What He Feels.

3-Forgetting To Ask The Patient To Walk If He Is Complaining Of Weakness Or Disequilibrium

4-Forgetting To Read The Instructions For The Case And Proceeding Directly To A Full Neurological Examination.

5-Not Observing Any Bedside Clues

6-Hurting The Patient While You Do The Pin Prick Test.

7-Testing The Pin Prick Test Very Gently That The Patient Does Not Feel It, And You Think He Has A Problem With Sensations.

8-Formulating Your Diagnosis Relying Only On One Modality Of Sensation; Keep In Mind All Modalities Together.

Neurological Case Findings Scheme

- **SURE SIGNS OF UMNL**
  - Exaggerated reflexes with Pathological reflexes
  - Clasp Knife Spasticity
  - Extensor plantar
  - Hoffman sign
- **SURE Signs of LMNL**
  - Hypotonia with intact coordination
  - Distribution of weakness (Add>Abd, E>F)
- **LMNL Causes**
  - P.N (Distal weakness)
  - MND (Distal weakness)
  - Myopathy (Proximal weakness)
  - MG (Proximal weakness)
- **Always keep in mind the LEVEL OF loss of sensation to all modalities Together** (Vibration, Cotton, Pin prick) → To determine if Dissociated Sensory loss
- **If You Find LOSS OF VIBRATION SENSE** on big toe= examine it over medial malleolus, shins of tibia, tibial tuberosity, ASIS, sternum, clavicles the mastoid
- **To say DORSAL COLUMN lesion** →Loss of vibration sense at least to the level clavicles or Mastoid not only peripherally
  - if loss to a level on leg = P.N
  - If loss to a level on trunk = Focal spinal cord lesion
  - If u find the level at ASIS level = P.N not dorsal column affection
- **To say CEREBELLAR lesion** you must recognize → Nystagmus, Dysmetria, Intentional Tremors, Overshooting or Dysdiadocokinesia
- **To say P.N.** = Lost Ankle reflex + Loss of pin prick & Cotton + Loss of Vibration to a level on a limb (Might affect the whole Limb, but no level on the trunk)
- **To say UMNL** → Clasp Knife Spaciticity + Distribution of weakness Or Hyper reflexia + Pathological reflexes OR Upgoing plantars (not the weakness only)
- **Bilateral UMNL** (Asymmetrical weakness, Reflexes, Tone)=MS
- **If You Find CEREBELLAR SIGNS** = Look for Nystagmus, Suspect MS, HSCD
- **DORSAL COLUMN** = Suspect MS, HSCD
- **If suspecting MS**= look for inter-nuclear ophthalmoplegia=MLB lesion
- **If You Find ASSYMETRICAL SIGNS** (especially with tone & reflexes)= MS
- **Multiple Sclerosis Never Cause Peripheral Neuropathy**
- **MS** can present with no sensory loss
- If You Find A Sensory Level In Limbs = **Peripheral Neuropathy**
- If You Find Sensory Level On Trunk = **Focal Spinal Cord Lesion**
- **MND Never Causes Sensory Affection**
- **If INTACT SENSATIONS** D.D. is
  - Myopathy
  - MND
  - MS
  - MG
  - HSMN purely motor
  - Internal capsule hemiplegia
- **FROG SIGN** (hypotonic externally rotated legs) =
  - Cerebellar lesion
  - LMNL
- **LOST ANKLE REFLEX, PRESERVED KNEE** =
  - P.N
  - HSMN
  - S1 Lesion
- **LOST KNEE, WITH PRESERVED ANKLE REFLEX** = Proximal Myopathy
- **LOST ANKLE, KNEE REFLEX, WITH SENSORY LEVEL on LIMB** =P.N
- **Hypotonia With Exaggerated Reflexes, Intact Sensation And Coordination** = MND (UMNL + LMNL + Intact sensation + intact cerebellum)

- **Hypotonia + Exaggerated Reflexes + Impaired Coordination + No P.N** =MS (UMNL + Cerebellar Hypotonia)
- **Hypotonia + Exaggerated Reflexes + Impaired Coordination + P.N** = HSCD (Hereditary spinocerebellar degeneration = Friedrich`s ataxia and others)
- **Hypertonia + Exaggerated Reflexes+ Up going Planters + Pathological Reflexes + Weakness Of L.Ls F>E, D>P, Abd>Add** = UMNL
- **Hypotonia + Lost Reflexes + Weakness Of Ext>Flex, D>P, Add > Abd** = LMNL
- **Bilateral UMNL** (up going planters) + **P.N** (lost ankle, hypotonia, loss of sensations in stocking) + **DORSAL COLUMN** (lost position & vibration to mastoids) + **CEREBELLAR Signs** (impaired coordination)= **HSCD**
- **Bilateral UMNL + P.N + DORSAL COLUMN** = SCD (Sub Acute Combined degeneration)
- **If You U Find Focal Spinal Cord Lesion** =Examine the back for scars
- **Multiple sclerosis Presentations**
  - o Cerebellar signs + Bilateral UMNL Only or
  - o Bilateral UMNL + Dorsal Column Lesion Only or
  - o Bilateral UMNL + No Sensory Loss =Ms
  - o Cranial Nerve Affection
- **Differences Between MS & HSCD** (Friedrich`s)
  - o MS Has no P.N, while HSCD has P.N
  - o MS Is patchy and Asymmetrical while HSCD is Symmetrical
  - o Pes Cavus & Hammer toe are only in HSCD (Friedrich`s)
- **UMNL In L.Ls** (Spastic Paraparesis) **With Sensory Level in Trunk To All Modalities** = Focal Spinal Cord Lesion
  - o Transverse Myelitis
  - o MS
  - o Trauma
  - o Tumours
  - o Infections
- **Hemiplegia + Ipsilateral Facial, Hypoglossal Lesion** = Internal capsule lesion
  - o Rt. side Hemiplegia + Mouth deviated to left side + Tongue deviates to Rt. side
- **Hemiplegia With Contralateral Occulomotor** (Ptosis , mydriasis , eye is down & out) = **MID BRAIN LESION**
- **Hemiplegia With Contralateral Facial & Abducens Nerve Palsy** = Pons lesion
- **Hemiplegia With Contralateral Hypoglossal Lesion**=Lesion in the Medulla
- **Brain Stem Hemiplegia Is Crossed Hemiplegia** = Hemiplegia On A Side And Cr.N. Lesion On Opposite Side
- **Weak Flexed Arm And Weak Leg With UMNL On One Side & Weak Leg On The Other Side With UMNL** = Hemiparesis With Monoparesis = Internal Capsule & Cortical Infarcts = Hypercoagulable state or Sickle cell anemia; look for jaundice
- **UMNL FACIAL nerve palsy** (Lower face affected)= Internal Capsule Lesion
- **MONOPARESIS** =Cortical infarction
- **DIPLEGIA** = Paralysis of Both U.Ls or Both L.Ls
- **HEMIPLEGIA** May Be:
  - o **Crossed Hemiplegia**= Brain Stem Lesion
    - ▪ Hemiplegia With Hemianaethesia
    - ▪ Cr.Nerve Lesion On Opposite Side Of The Hemiplegia
    - ▪ Uncrossed Hemiplegia
    - ▪ No Cr. Nerve Lesion
    - ▪ Cr. Nerve Lesion On The Same Side Of The Hemiplegia
  - o **Non Crossed** =Internal Capsule Lesions:
    - ▪ With Ipsilateral Cr. N (VII , XII) (VII Only Lower Face Is Affected)
    - ▪ Without Cranial Nerve
    - ▪ With Sensory Loss
    - ▪ Without Sensory Loss (Pure Hemiparesis With No Hemianaesthesia)
- **In A Hemiplegia Case:**
  - o Examine for III
    - ▪ Look for ptosis & eye down & out Opposite to hemiplegia = Mid Brain Lesion
  - o Examine VII

- Ask him to elevate eye brow , close eyes & open his mouth
  - Loss of all of these opposite to hemiplegia deviation of mouth to hemiplegia =Pontine lesion
  - If mouth deviates opposite to hemiplegia =Internal capsule Lesion
- Examine XII
  - Ask him to put his tongue out
    - If it deviates to hemiplegia = Internal capsule Lesion
    - If tongue deviates opposite to hemiplegia =Medulla

Neurological Cases

Peripheral Neuropathy

Clinical Examination

- Using A Walking Aid
- Walking With A High Steppage Gait
- +ve Romberg Sign
- Sensory Loss Of Light Touch, Pin Prick, Vibration, Position Sense, In Stocking Distribution (High Stocking Distribution)
- Glove Distribution sensory loss
- LMNL Signs In Lower Limb In The Form Of Weaknes D>P, Extensor>F, Add > Abd, Wasting, Decreased Tone, Lost Ankle Reflex, Equivocal Planters

Look for a cause

- _D.M_: Dermopathy, Necrobiosis Lipoidica, Insulin Injection Sites, Charcoat Joint, Amyotrophy
- _Alcohol_: Parotid Enlargement, Stigmata Of CLD, Palmar Erythema, CCF
- _HSMN:_ For Long Time+ Pes Cavus & Hammer Toe
- _SCD:_ UMNL , Dorsal Column , Pallor)
- _HSCD_: UMNL+P.N + Cerebellar signs + Dorsal Column lesion signs + Pes Cavus
- _Guillian Barre_: Acute Onset, Preceding Viral Illness, Tracheostomy, Central Lines for plasmapheresis.
- _RA_: Hand Signs

Quick Discussion

What Are Other Causes Of Peripheral Neuropathy?

- Para-proteinemia
- Amyloidosis (HSM)
- Drugs (INH, Metronidazole, Amiodarone, Vincristine, Nitrofurantoin)
- Dapsone =Motor Only
- Carcinoma (Cachexia, Clubbing, 1ry Tumor)
- Idiopathic
- PAN
- HIV
- Uremia
- Predominantly Motor Causes
  - Diphtheria
  - Lead
  - Porphyria
  - Charcot Marie Tooth
  - Dapsone

What Investigations You Would Like To Do For This Patient?

- NCS=Loss of conduction velocities in Demylinating causes, Dec. Amplitiude in axonal lesions
- EMG
- Investigations for causes

How Would You Treat This Patient?

- Non pharmacological
  - Physical therapy
  - Orthotics
- Medical therapy
  - Managing Blood sugar
  - Stopping alcohol
  - Gabapentin & TCA for pain

Charcoat Marie Tooth Disease

(Common Peroneal Muscle Disease, HSMN)

Clinical Examination:

- Wasting of Distal muscles of leg with Preserved thigh muscles (Inverted Champain Bottle Appearance)
- Pes cavus & Clawing of toes
- Hypotonia D>P
- Weakness D>P , EXT.>FLEX , ADD>ABD
- Weaknes of plantar flexion (EXTENSION) more than dorsiflexion
- Weakness of inversion more than eversion
- Lost Ankle reflex, Equivocal plantar
- Intact coordination, lost when eyes closed (sensory ataxia)
- Lost all modalities of sensations to level on leg (Vibration to ASIS)
- High steppage gait
- Wasting of small muscles of the hand
- Palpable lateral popliteal nerve, Ulnar nerve

Quick Discussion

How Would You Treat This Patient?

- Surgical correction of deformities
- Physiotherapy (Strengthening , ROM)
- NSAIDS for pain
- Orthotics
- Referral to neurology department

What Is The Cause Of This Condition?

- Autosomal dominant

N.B: In common peroneal Nerve lesion (lateral popliteal nerve) or L5 lesion Ankle jerk is preserved

Myotonia Dystrophia

Clinical Examination

- Myotonic facies (Temporalis Wasting, Long face, bilateral ptosis & cataracts, frontal baldness, Drooping of mouth due to facial muscle weakness)
- Myotonia during greeting (after he made a fist he was unable to quickly open it)
- Distal muscle weakness (LMNL)
- Reflexes lost even with re-enforcement
- D.M (insulin injection sites, necrobiosis lipoidica, diabetic dermopathy)
- MVP

Quick Discussion

What Are The Causes Of This Condition?

- AD
- DM1 =DMPK gene (CTG repeat) on chr. 19
  - Characterized by anticipation, M>F
- DM2=ZNF Chr. 3

What Are Other Associations With MD?

- D.M, MVP, Cardiomyopathy, Slurred speech
- Nodular thyroid enlargement, intellectual disorders

How Would You Treat this condition?

- Referral to neurologists
- Physiotherapy

What Do You Know About Myotonia Congenital (Thomsens Disease)?

- Myotonia only with no other features of Myotonic dystrophy
- AD, or AR dt. Defect in ion channels

Hemiplegia/Hemiparesis

Clinical Examination:

- Using walking aid
- His arm is held in a flexed & Adducted position
- Circumduction gait
- Disuse atrophy of muscles
- Weakness U.L = D>p, Ext.>Flex, Abd>Add
- Weakness L.L = Flex > Ext
- Increased tone in a Clasp knife spasticity
- Exaggerated reflexes on affected side
- + ve babiniski (Upgoing Planters)
- Hoffman sign
- Clonus
- Patellar tap
- Adductor reflex
- Lost / no loss of Sensations at the affected side
- ? Slurred speech
- If Pons (LMNL Of Facial Contralateral To Hemiparesis)
- If Internal Capsule (Lower Part Of VII, XII Affected On Same Side Of Hemiplegia/ Or No Cr. Nerve Affected Or No Sensory Loss)

Quick Discussion

What Are The Causes?

Middle / Old Age

- Thrombosis, Hemorrhage, Embolism, Tumors

Young Age:

- Trauma, Tumors, Infection (Meningitis, Encephalitis)
- Hypercoagulable State
  - PNH, Behcet, Antiphospholipid Ab ,
  - Myeloprolefrative Disease
  - Factor V Leyden
  - Sickle Cell Anemia (Look For Jaundice)
  - Patent Foramen Ovale

What Investigations You Would Like To Do For This Patient?

- Basic blood tests
- Bl. Glucose & Lipid profile
- ECHO
- ECG
- CT Head (infarction is hypodense) + MRI
- Carotid Doppler

How Would You Treat This Patient?

- Physiotherapy
- Prophylaxis for further episodes
  - Clopidogrel 75 mg
  - Statins
  - Treat HTN =130/80
  - Treat D.M
  - Stop smoking
  - Control reversible causes

Motor Neuron Disease

Clinical Examination

Amyotrophic Lateral Sclerosis

- Distal muscle Weakness, Wasting, Fasciculations in U.Ls muscles but exaggerated reflexes
- UMNL spastic weakness in the legs with exaggerated reflexes , extensor (up going) plantar
- Sensation Are Intact
- No Cerebellar Signs

Progressive Bulbar Palsy

- Tongue fasciculation
- Dysarthria
- absent palatal movement
- Sensations are Intact

Progressive Muscle Atrophy

- Distal muscle weakness of U.L & L.Ls showing
  - Wasting
  - Weakness
  - Hypotonia
  - Absent Reflexes With Fasciculations

Quick Discussion

What Are The Causes For This Condition?

- Unknown = Glutamate Toxicity
- Familial = AD (super-oxide dismutase defect)

What Investigations You Would Do For This Patient?

- EMG , NCS=fasciculation , fibrillation potentials
- Routine blood tests , FVC
- Brain , spinal MRI=exclude other conditions

What Treatment Can You Offer Him?

- Riluzole (glutamate antagonist)
- Ventilatory support

What Is The Differential Diagnosis Of This Condition?

- Cervical cord compression
- Syphilitic Amyotrophy
- Spinal muscular atrophy juvenile type 3
- MS

Spastic Paraparesis

Clinical Examination:

- Walking aid / Wheel Chair
- Scissoring gait
- UMNL signs of L.Ls
  - Disuse atrophy
  - Weakness Abd> Add, D>P , F>E
  - Clasp Knife Spacticity
  - Exaggerated Reflexes
  - Upgoing Plantars
  - Clonus
  - Patellar & Adductor Reflexes
  - Sensory Loss According To Cause
  - Cerebellar Affection According To The Cause

Look for a Cause

1-Multiple Sclerosis

Clinical Examination:

- Nystagmus
- Staccato Or Slurred
- Cerebellar Signs
- Inter-nuclear Opthalmoplegia
- Spastic Paraparesis (Pyramidal Signs)
- Dorsal Column Signs
- Lhermet Sign (Tingling Or Pain On Neck Flexion
- Uhtoff Phenomenan: Transient Visual Obscuration Dt. Hot Bath, Meal
- Signs Are Asymmetrical & Patchy
- No peripheral Neuropathy
- No Pes Cavus/Hammer toe compared to HSCD

Quick Discussion:

What Are The Causes Of This Condition?

- Autoimmune disease attacks myelinated axons in CNS causing demyelination
- Unknown cause may be viruses (EBV) & environmental causes

How Would You Investigate This Case?

- MRI = Demyelinated plaques
- VEP = Delayed latency
- CSF = Oligo clonal bands

How would you treat this patient?

- Physiotherapy
- Disease modifying agent for MS (Natilzumab, INF beta, glatiramar acetate)
- High dose steroids in acute patients with predominantly movement disorder
- Symptomatic treatment
  - Fatigue = amantadine ,
  - Spasticity = baclofen (# ISHD) or diazepam ,
  - Bladder problems = prazosin or oxybutynin if residual urine vol. after U/S <115 , if >115 =surgery ,
  - Pain= TCA ,
  - Optic neuritis= high dose IV steroids
- Benign course if: pure sensory, long remission & infrequent relapses , onset with optic neuritis , sensory or motor signs in contrast to cerebellar & brainstem

2-HSCD (Friedrich`s Ataxia)

Clinical Examination:

- Spastic paraparesis (UMNL)
- Scanning Speech
- ? Visual loss
- Pes cavus, Hammer toe
- High Arched Palate
- P.N
- Dorsal column affection
- Cerebellar signs
- HOCM signs on CVS examination

Quick Discussion:

What Are The Associations With This Condition?

- HOCM
- O.A.
- D.M
- High arched palate
- Kyphoscoliosis
- Dementia
- Scanning speech

What Are The Causes Of This Condition?

- Autosomal recessive (GAA repeat) on Chr. 9
- part of hereditary spinocerebellar degeneration

What are the D.D for HSCD?

- MS
- Abetalipoprotinemia (acanthosis, steatorrhea, retinal pigmentation, Freidrichs like ataxia)
- Refsum`s (elevated serum phytanic acid due to. Defective lipid alpha oxidase= Optic atrophy, pigmented retina, deafness, friedrichs like Ataxia)
- Roussy –levy syndrome (HSMN 1 as Charcot's Marie Tooth + friedrich`s)

How Would You Investigate This Case?

- Genetic counseling for prenatal diagnosis, exclude other causes

How would you treat this case?

- High dose propranolol & Vit E for HOCM
- Surgery for foot deformities
- Physiotherapy

3-Motor Neuron Disease

No sensory signs, +ve fasciculations

4-Focal Spinal Cord Lesion

Clinical Examination:

- Spastic Paraparesis
- Sensory level on the trunk

Look For a cause:

- T.B, Brucellosis, Abscess
- Tumors
- Anterior Spinal Artery occlusion
  - Dissociated sensory loss sparing the Dorsal column
- TRAUMA (look for scar on the back) Site of scar determined by

- o Root = cervical – 1 upper thoracic -2 lower thoracic -3
- o If T7 root affected u will find scar at T4 spine

5-Anterior Spinal Artery Occlusion

- Spastic paraparesis
- Dissociative sensory loss up to a sensory level on the trunk.
- Loss of pain & temp, with preserved dorsal column (position, vibration)

6-Transverse Myelitis

- Inflammation in spinal cord → axonal demyelination dt. Previous viral inf. (CMV) or Idiopathic
- **Investigations:** MRI

7-Syringomyelia

Clinical Examination

- Kyphoscoliosis
- Wasting of small muscles of the hands
- ? Horner's
- Spastic Paraparesis
- Dissociated sensory loss
- Destruction of spinothalamic (Loss of pain & temp.) {shawal like distribution in arms}
- Preserved dorsal column (light touch , vibration , position)
- Cranial Nerve affection if Syringobulbia

Quick Discussion

What Are The Causes Of This Condition?

- It is fluid filled cavity in the spinal cord syrinx
- Bony abnormalities (small posterior fossa)
- Meningioma of foramen magnum
- Chiari formation
- Cerbellar tonsils herniation
- Idiopathic

What Investigations You Would Like To Do For This Patient?

- MRI & CT = Cyst
- CSF pressure elevated
- Myelography

What Treatment You Would Offer This Patient?

- Physiotherapy
- Surgery (Lamnectomy & Syringotomy)
- Ventriculo-Peritoneal Shunt

8-SCD (Subacute Combined Degeneration)

Clinical Examination

- Spastic Paraparesis
- P.N. (Absent Ankle Reflex)
- Dorsal Column Affection (Lost Vibration & Position & Romberg +ve)
- Pallor + Glossitis
- Examine The Abdomen (Gastrectomy Scar Or Splenomegaly)

Quick Discussion

What Are The Causes Of This Condition?

- Pernicious anemia

- Partial or total gastrectomy
- Ileal resection or crohns
- Congenital intrinsic factor deficiency
- Tropical sprue

What Investigations You Would Like To Do For This Patient?

- Vit.B12 Levels
- Antiparietal Cells Antibodies
- Intrinsic Factor Abs
- Schilling Test

What Treatment Will You Offer Him?

- Vit B12 IM
- Physiotherapy

9-Cervical Spondylosis (Cervical Myelopathy)

Clinical Examination:

- Spastic Paraparesis
- Loss Of Dorsal Column Affection Below The Level (C5, C6) With Preserved Spinothalamic (Or May Be Affected)
- U.Ls= Inverted Reflexes (Lost Biceps, Tapping Biceps → Triceps Contraction & Lost Brachioradialis, Tapping Brachiradialis → Finger Contraction
- Abnormal Sensation In Hands
- No Muscle Wasting Of Small Muscles (T1)

Quick Discussion:

What Is The Cause Of This Condition?

C5,C6 spondylosis

How Would You Investigate This Case?

- X-ray → Spondylotic changes (narrow disc space , osteophytes formation)
- MRI → Spinal cord roots compression at C5 , C6

How Would Would You Treat This Patient?

- Physiotherapy

What Are The Causes Of Absent Ankle Reflex + Extensor Planatar Causes?

1-SCD

2-Freidrich`S Ataxia

3-MND

4-D.M +Cervical myelopathy

5-D.M + MS

10-General Paralysis Of Insane

- Neuropsychiatric Disorder dt. Syphilis
- Seizures+ Dementia+ Aryl Robertson+ Abnormal Reflexes

11-Other Causes of Spastic paraparesis

- Hereditary Spastic Paraplegia
- Parasagittal Cranial Meningioma
- AIDS Myelopathy

Summary of The Spastic Paraparesis Case

- **With Cerebellar Signs** = MS, HSCD

- **With Peripheral Neuropathy** = HSCD, SCD
- **Sensations are Intact** = MND, MS, Parasagittal Meningioma, Heriditary Spastic Paraparesis, Tropical Spastic Paraparesis, Cerebral palsy
- **With Sensory Level** = Focal Spinal Cord lesion

Old Poliomyelitis

Clinical Examination

- Short Leg (Unequality Suggest Childhood Illness)
- WASTED
- Weakness
- FLACCID
- REDUCED ANKLE REFLEX & Normal Plantar Reflex
- NORMAL SENSATION
- Normal Coordination
- ? BULBAR SIGNS
- No Pyramidal Signs.

Quick Discussion

What Are The Causes Of Unilateral Short Limb?

- Old polio
- Infantile hemiplegia (sensory affection + pyramidal signs): dt. Measles , pertussis, scarlet fever

1-Cerebellar Ataxia (Cerebellar Syndrome)

Clinical Examination:

- Wide base, Arms held wide, U.L & L.L tremble & shake, intention tremors, staccato speech, impaired coordination & equilibrium esp. With heel to toe test, -ve Romberg signs
- Examine eyes for Nystagmus, L.L complete neurologically to determine cause & perform signs of impaired coordination in U.L
- Lobe Affection = Limb Ataxia
- Vermis Affection =Truncal Ataxia
- Always Ask The Pt. To Walk

Look for a cause

Quick Discussion

What Are The Causes Of Cerebellar Ataxia?

- MS (Internuclear Ophalmoplegia)
- HSCD
- Ataxia Telangectasia
- Alcohol Misuse
- Cerbello-pontine angle tumors
- Posterior fossa stroke
- Meningitis/Encephalitis
- Brainstem Vascular Lesion (Lateral Medullary Syndrome)
- Posterior Fossa Space Occupaying Lesion
- Paraneoplastic
- Alcoholic Cerebellar Degeneration=Examine Liver
- Phynetoin (Epileptics)

How Would You Investigate This Case?

Investigations Of the cause:

- MRI, MRI with contrast
- LP
- *Anti-purkinji cell Ab* in paraneoplastic

How Would You Treat This Patient

- Gait training, Coordination exercises
- Treatment of cause

2-Sensory Ataxic Gait

Clinical Examination:

- Gait Is Ataxic, Stamping, Walking Widely Based, Watching The Ground , Difficulty Walking Heel To Toe , +Ve Romberg Sign
- Look For Argyl Robertson Pupil & Pallor = Syphilis
- Examine L.L Complete Neurologically
- No Cerebellar Signs
- No Intentional Tremors Whilst Eyes Are Open
- Intentional Tremors & Dysmetria While Eyes Are Closed.

Look For A Cause

Quick discussion

What Are The Causes Of Sensory Ataxia?

- MS
- SCD
- P.N.

- HSCD
- **Tabes Dorsalis**
  - o Facies, Argyll Robertson Pupils (Bilaterally Small, Not Responsive To Light But Responsive To Accommodation)
  - o Pyramidal Signs (Spastic paraparesis)
- **Cervical Myelopathy**
  - o Mid-Cervical Reflex
  - o Spastic paraparesis

3-Spastic Paraparesis

- Scissoring
- Stiff Gait
- ? Dysarthria

4-Circumduction

Clinical Examination:

- Rt. Leg is stiff & with each step he tilts the pelvis to the other side , trying to keep the toe off the ground, Rt leg describes semicircular with toe scraping the floor & the fore foot flops the ground before heel
- Rt. Arm is flexed & held tightly to his side
- ? Slurred Speech
- ? Cranial Nerve palsy

Quick Discussion

What Is The Cause Of This Gait?

- Hemiplegia → Stroke, Infection, Tumor

5-High Steppage Gait

Clinical Examination

- He Raises His Foot High To Avoid Scrapping His Toes, Has Foot Drop And Unable To Walk On Heel
- He Has Loss Of Sensation In Stocking Distribution

Look For A Cause

Quick Discussion

What Are The Causes Of This Gait?

- **P.N**. (Alcoholic, D.M)
- Lead Poisoning
- **Lateral Popliteal N. Injury** (common peroneal) = Look for scar just below & lat. To knee
  - o Wasting of ant. Tibial & peroneal muscles group, can't dorsiflex or evert foot, impaired sensation in outer side of the calf
  - o He can stand on toes but not on heels
  - o Ankle jerk is preserved
  - o Plantar reflex normal
  - o _Causes:_ splints , casts , trauma at head of fibula
  - o _Treatment_ physiotherapy & Orthotics
- **Charcot`s Marie Tooth** (HSMN1), common peroneal atrophy

6-Shuffling Gait (Parkinson`s Disease)

Clinical Examination:

- Walking Aid
- Depressed, expressionless, unblinking Face
- Slurred low volume Monotonous speech

- He is drooling, and has titubation
- The patient stoops, his gait initially hesitates, shuffling , hands shows pill rolling tremors
- Static tremors (pill rolling) Assymetrical
- Test Bradykinesia by counting fingers or tapping
- Test for Micrographia
- Impaired motor coordination
- Cog Wheel rigidity on hands
- Lead pipe rigidity of arms & legs

Look For A Cause

Quick Discussion:

What Are The Causes Of This Condition?

- Post encephalitic
- Anoxic Brain Damage
- Neurosyphilis
- Tumors Affecting Basal Ganglia
- Drug Induced e.g. Metoclopramide

What is The D.D ?

- Normal pressure hydrocephalus (Ataxia, Dementia, Urinary incontinence
- Srteriosclerotic parkinsons (broad based gait , pyramidal signs)
- Alzeheimer, Wilson`s, Jakob-creutzfield

How Would You Treat This Condition?

- Stop Offending medications
- Dopamine receptor agonist (bromocriptine, cabergolide)
- Anticholinergics for tremors (benztropine, benzhexol)

7-Waddling Gait (Proximal Myopathy)

Clinical Examination:

- Lumbar lordosis, walks on wide base with waddling gait, his trunk moving from side to side & his pelvis drooping on each side as his leg leave the ground
- There is proximal weakness of muscles
- patient unable to sit up with U.Ls outstretched (Gowers signs)
- Signs of proximal myopathy (weakness, wasting, hypotonia)

Look For A Cause

DUCHENE , BECKERS MUSCLE DYSTROPHY (XL-R)

- Hypotonia proximally
- Weakness proximally with normal distal power
- lost reflex proximally (knee)
- Normal power , Normal Tone , Normal Reflexes distally
- Weakness P>D , Adductors > Abductors , Ext>Flexors
- Pseudo-hypertrophy of shoulder & calf
- Selectivity test (some Ms affected more than others)
- Winging of scapula
- Intact sensations
- Weak abdomen muscles (protruding abdomen)
- +ve Gower`s sign
- Sensations are intact
- No cerebellar signs
- **Investigations:** EMG=Dec Amplitude , CpK MM, muscle biopsy
- **Death from:** Cardiac involvement , Respiratory infection
- **Management:** Social , occupation , financial support & physiotherapy

FASCIOSCAPULOHUMERAL SYNDROME (AD)

- Myopathic facies: dull, unlined , loss of wrinkles, expressionless face, open slack lips, ptosis

- Wasting of facial & Limb girdle muscles
- Facial & neck movements are impaired (smiling, whistling, closing eyes)
- Weakness of LMNL of Arms , Shoulder , Neck , Face
- Winging of scapula
- *Small scapula*: superior margin of scapula viewed from front above the clavicle
- Legs=Foot drop = LMNL
- Sensations are intact
- **Causes** : AD inheritance
- **Investigations:** CK MM , exclude other causes , Muscle biopsy (EMG guided biopsy) , EMG , NCV
- **Treatment:** Creatine monohydrate therapy , physiotherapy

DIABETIC AMYOTROPHY
- Weakness & Wasting of Thigh Muscles (Proximal Neuropathy)
- Assoc. peripheral neuropathy
- Necrobiosis Lipoidica
- Dermopathy
- Insulin injection marks (Lipodystrophy)
- Fundus Examination

LIMB GIRDLE SYNDROME
- Limb girdle wasting , weakness affecting some groups of muscles , more than others (Deltoids are usually preserved)
- face is spared
- AD, more benign if upper limb affected 1st

POLYMYOSITIS
- Tender muscles
- LMNL S/S Proximal muscles
- Lost reflexes
- Autoimmune (Anti Jo)
- Raised CK
- Respiratory muscle involvement
- Ocular involvement is rare
- Limb girdle affected more than shoulder
- ? Hidden Malignancy

DERMATOMYOSITIS
- Same As Polymyosistis with
- heliotrope rash & gottron Papules
- May be Cushingoid features

OTHER CAUSES
- **Cushing Syndrome** (Moon Face ,Axial Obesity , Striae)
- **Thyrotoxicosis** (Eye Signs , Large Thyroid)
- Osteomalcia
- BB, AMIODARONE, ALCOHOL, INH
- **Mcardle Syndrome** (HSM ,Cramps After Excersis)
- **Mitochondrial Myopathies** (muscle biopsy =ragged red ribers)

What Is The Stiff Man Syndrome?

Progressive muscle stiffness of spine and L.L.s, muscle spasm =unable to feel , +ve anti GAD ,assoc with D.M1, Addison , hyper-hypothyroidism, pernicious anemia.

What Is The Differential Diagnosis Of Proximal Myopathy?

1-INFLAMATORY
- Polymyositis
- Dermatomyosistis =tender muscles , sensations are intact.

2-HEREDITARY

- Becker`S, Duchene (X-LR)
- Limb-Girdle (AR)
- Fasciscapulohumeral (AD)

3-ENDOCRINAL & METABOLIC

- Hyper-hypothyroid
- Cushing
- Acromegaly
- Drugs
- Alcohol
- Hypo-Hyperkalemia
- Osteomalacia

Homonymous Hemianopia

- Lesion Is Opposite To The Side Of The Lesion
- Right Homonymous Hemianopia Means Patient Has Visual Defect In
- Right Temporal Field & Left Nasal Field

Causes:

1-Optic Tract Lesion

2-Occipital Cortex Lesion (Hemiplegia, AF)

Bi-Temporal hemianopia

- Loss of Temporal Field vision on both eyes usually Dye to Chiasmal Lesion.

Causes:

1-Pituitary Adenoma

2-Craniopharyngeoma

3-Aneurysm

4-Suprasellar Meningioma

Tunnel vision

Causes:

1-Glaucoma

2-Retinitis Pigmentosa

3-Choroidoretinitis

Homonymous upper quadrantanopia

Lesion in the Temporal cortex (PITS) of contralateral side

Homonomous lower quadrantanopia

Lesion in The Parietal cortex (PITS) of contralateral side

1-Unilateral Ptosis

A-HORNER`S SYNDROME
- Ptosis, Miosis, Apparent Enophtalmous , Anhydrosis

Causes:

1-Neck trauma

2-Pancoast tumor of lung (wasting of small muscles of hand T1 , clubbing , L.Ns, tracheal deviation , chest signs)

3-Carotid artery aneurysm or dissection / Vertebral artery dissection

- Triad of hyperextension or rotation of neck (Vomiting, Sneezing, Coughing) + Pain On One Side Of The Face + Horner`s +Cerebral Or Retinal Ischemia)
- Investigations: Arteriography, Contrast enhanced CT
- Treatment: anticoagulation (to prevent thrombo-embolism) except if dissection spread intracranial.

4-Brainstem vascular ds (Wallenberg Syndrome / Lateral Medullary Syndrome, Post.Inf.Cerebellar Syndrome)

- Vertigo + Ipsilateral Face Anesthesia + Horner`s + Palatal Dysfunction ,+ Cerebellar Syndrome + Contralateral Limbs Anesthesia (Pain & Temp)
- Due to Occlusion of Posterior Inferior Cerebellar artery
- Treatment: pain (gabapentin), physiotherapy, protection of aspiration pneumonia)

5-syrigomyelia

6-Brain stem demylination

B-THIRD NERVE PASLY
- Ptosis, Lifting Eye Lid Shows Divergent Strabismus, Dilated Pupil, Eye Fixed In Out & Down Position

Causes:

- Posterior Communicating Artery Aneurysm
- Mononeuritis Multiplex
- Myasthenia Gravis
- MS
- Vascular Lesions
- Meningitis
- Opthalmoplegic Migraine

C-OTHER CAUSES
- Myotonia
- Myasthenia Gravis
- Congenital

2-Bilateral Ptosis

A-MYASTHENIA GRAVIS
- Ptosis increase by upward gaze , eye lashes not buried when completely closing eyes
- 6th nerve palsy signs
- lack of expressions on face
- facial weakness
- proximal muscle weakness which increase by repetitive movements
- Normal reflexes
- positive jaw supporting sign (Pt. Put hand under chin to support jaw &neck)
- ? Other autoimmune disorders
- Sensations are intact.

Investigations

- Anti Acetyl choline receptor Abs
- FVC
- Chest CT (Thymoma)
- Edrophonium (Tensolin test)

Myasthenic crisis

- Infections, emotions, drugs (gentamycin, Streptomysin , procainamide, Quinine) → paralysis of respiratory muscle

Treatment

- Pyridostigmine , neostigmine , plasmapherisis ,IVIG , thymectomy

B-TABES DORSALIS

- Patient is Underweight
- *Argyl-Robertson Pupil*
  - o Bilateral Small
  - o One Might Be Smaller Than Other
  - o Irregular
  - o React To Accommodation But Not Light
- Wrinkled Forehead
- Ptosis
- Stamping Gait, +Ve Romberg, Loss Of Joint & Vibration Sense
- Absent Knee Jerk
- Charcot`S Knee
- Aortic Incompetence.

Causes

- syphilis (Demylination)

Investigations

- Syphilis serology= TPHA ,VDRL (active infection)

Treatment

- IV penicillin
- Carbamazepin, opiates for pain

C-OTHER CAUSES

- Myotonia
- Congenital
- Bilateral Horner
- Occulopharyngeal Muscular Dystrophy (Fascioscapulohumeral)

Holmes-Adies-Moore Pupil

Clinical Examination:

- Young Lady
- Unilateral Dilated Pupil
- Fails To React To Light
- No Ptosis
- No Diplopia
- Eye Movement Is Normal
- Constricts Slowly To Accommodation Until It Becomes Smaller Than The Normal
- Dilates With Mydriatics
- Absent Tendon Reflexes

Quick Discussion

What Are The Causes of this condition?

- Viral or bacterial destruction of ciliary ganglion

What Investigations You Would Like to do?

- responds to pilocarpine rapidly

How Would You Treat it?

- Pilocarpine & Reading glasses

Horizontal Nystagmus

- Nystagmus Greater On One Side., With Fast Component To The Same Side
  - Ipsilateral cerebellum lesion =look for cerebellar signs
  - Contralateral vestibular lesion
- Ataxic Nystagmus, More in The abducting Eye With dissociation of conjugate eye movement; on looking Rt., Rt. Eye abducts normally, but impaired adduction of Lt. Eye , when the abducting eye is covered , adduction of other eye is normal
  - Diagnosis : Inter-nuclear opthalmoplegia , lesion in medial longitudinal fasciculus of eye failing to adduct; look for cerebellar signs =MS

6ᵗʰ Nerve Palsy (Abducens)

Clinical Examination

Convergent Strabismus

Impairement Of Lateral Movement Of One Eye

Diplopia Worse On Looking Lateral To The Side Of The Affected Eye.

Quick Discussion

Causes:

- **Mononeuritis Multiplex** (D.M, PAN, Granulomatosis Polyngiitis, Churg Strauss, RA , SLE, Sarcoidosis, Amyloidosis, Lyme)
- MS
- Raised ICP (Intracranial Pressure)
- Myasthenia Gravis
- Vascular Lesion (Weber)
- Basilar Artery Aneurysm →Compression
- Aids

Complete 3ʳᵈ Nerve (Occulomotor)

- Ptosis, Lifting Eye Lid Shows Divergent Strabismus, Dilated Pupil, Eye Fixed In Out & Down Position

Jugular Foramen Syndrome

- IX , X , XI Nerves lesions
- Neurofibroma , Meningioma , Metastasis , CPA lesions

Lower Motor Facial Nerve Palsy

Clinical Examination

- Paralysis Of Upper & Lower Face On One Side
- Pt. Can`t Elevate Eye Brow on the affected side
- Cant (Weakly) Close Rt. Eye Completely (Easly Opened By The Examiner) , Eye Ball Turns Upward In Attempt Of Closure (Bell`S Phenomenon)
- Has Smooth Nasolabial Fold
- He Is Unable To Blow Or Whistle
- With Deviation Of The Mouth To The Opposite Side Of The Affected Nerve.
- Examine Ear For Herpes
- Examine For Crossed Hemiplegia

Look For A Cause

Quick Discussion

What Are The Causes Of LMNL Facial Nerve Palsy?

- Bell`s Palsy (Idiopathic)
- Parotid Tumors
- Cerebellopontine Angle Compression (Acoustic Neuroma , Meningioma 5,6,7,8 Nerves Palsy + Cerebellar Syndrome)
- Trauma
- Mononeuritis Multiplex
- Causes Of Bilateral Facial (Lyme , Polio , Sarcoidosis ,Guillian Barre , MND , Myasthenia)
- Ramsay Hunt Syndrome (Herpes Zoster Auditory Canal)
- Millard Gubbler Syndrome
- Multiple Sclerosis

Tardive Dyskinesia

- This Schizophrenic pt.
- Has tic-like Orofacial dyskinesia
- Include lip smacking
- Chewing
- Grimacing
- Choreo-asthetosis of limbs & trunks

Causes:

- Phenothiazines , butrophenones , reserpine
  Other side effects of these drugs =Acute dystonia (occulogyric crisis), Akasthesia , Parkinson

Dystonia

- Twisting and Repetitive movements or abnormal postures.
- **Generalized dystonia** = AD , affecting most of the body , arms , legs
- **Focal Dystonia**
  - o Blepharospasm
  - o Occulogyric crisis
  - o Oromandibular dystonia
- **Meig Syndrome (Cranial Dystonia)**
  - o Combination of Occuloguric & Oromandibular dystonia
- **Segmental Dystonia** = Foot , Arm

Choreo-Athetosis

- Brief, Jerky, Abrupt, Irregular , Semi-purposful, Involuntary movements , movements flit from one part to other part of body ,
- present at rest, accentuated with movement, he is restless
- Patient is unable to keep his tongue out (it darts in & out)
- there is abnormal posture of the hand , Wrist is flexed , fingers are hyperextended MCP , when upper limb is raised,there is pronation of forearm

Causes:

- Sydenham chorea (Rheumatic fever , pregnancy , OCP)
- Hutington (lower limbs more than upper limbs→AD)
- Drug-induced (L-dopa)
- Encephalitis ,SLE , Wilson , thyrotoxicosis

Treatment

- Neuroleptics (causes of tardive dyskinesia)

1-Guillian Barre Syndrome

Clinical Examination

- Young adult
- Predominantly Motor Neuropathy
- Weakness is Distal
- Hyporeflexia (Ankle+/- Knee)
- Bilateral LMNL facial weakness
- loss of all sensations distally
- tachycardia
- Signs of Previous Ventilatory support e.g. Tracheostomy
- Signs of Plasmaphereses e.g. Central Lines
- Ascending Neuropathy

Quick Discussion

What Are The Causes Of This Condition?

Demylination dt. Previous viral illness

How Would You Investigate This Case?

NCS= demylination (decreased conduction velocity)

What Treatment Will You Offer This Patient?

- Plasmapheresis in 1st 2 weeks
- IV immunoglobulins
- supportive care

What Do You Know About Miller-Fischer Syndrome?

- Ataxla + Ophtalmoplegia + Areflexia
- Abs to GQ1b gangliosides

2-Other Causes:

- MND
- Polio
- Meningitis
- Syrigobulbia (Syringomyelia +Horner & Nystagmus)
- Vascular (Brain Stem Lesions=Crossed Hemiplegia)

Ulnar Nerve Palsy

Clinical Examination

- **Wasting** Of All Small Muscles Of The Hand Except Thenar
- Inability To Adduct (**Palmar muscles weakness**) Or Abduct (**Dorsal muscles weakness**) Fingers
- +ve Froment Sign (**Adductor Polices weakness**)
- Weak Muscles Of Digiti Minimi
- **Partial Claw Hand** (Hyperextension MCP , Flexion Interphalengeal)
- Loss Of Sensation Medial 1.5 Fingers , 1/3 Palm
- If Lesion In The Forearm (Scar)
  - Weakness Of Flexion & Adduction Of Wrist
  - Radial Deviation On Flexion (Fl.Carpi Ulnaris lesion)
  - Weakness Of Flexion Of Distal Phalynx Of 4th &5th Fingers (Ulnar Paradox) due to affection of Medial1/2 Of Fl. Digitorum Profundus
  - Loss Of Sensation On Ulnar Side Of Forearm

Look for A Cause

Quick Discussion

What Are The Causes Of This Condition?

- Fracture , dislocation , deformity elbow=examine the elbow
- Injuries to wrist=examine wrist
- Occupational
- Mononeuritis multiplex (D.M, RA, SLE, PAN, Wegner`s, Churg strauss , Amyloidosis)

What Is Your Differential Diagnosis?

- Syringomyelia
- C8 lesion
- Cervical rib

What Investigations You Would Like To Do?

- EMG
- NCS

How Will You Treat This Patient?

- Physiotherapy
- Closed fracture=spontanous recovery , if no recovery after 6 m → Surgery & graft

Radial Nerve Palsy

Clinical Examination

- Wrist & Finger Drop
- Loss Of Sensation On 1st Dorsal Interosseous
- If Wrist Passively Extended → Can Extend Fingers At Interphalyngeal Joints
- If Wrist Passively Extended Power Of Grip Improves
- If Hand Resting Flat Can Do Abduction & Adduction Of Finger

Quick Discussion

What Are The Causes Of This Condition?

- Saturday night palsy
- Trauma to nerve
- Mono-neuritis Multiplex

How would you treat this patient?

- Physiotherapy
- Treat The Cause

Wasting Of Small Muscles Of The Hands

Clinical Examination

- There Is Wasting, Weakness, Of Thenar & Hypothenar Eminences & Of Small Muscles Of The Hand So That Dorsal Guttering Is Seen
- There Is Extension In MCP Joints, & Flexion Of Interphalyngeal Joints (Complete Claw Hand).

Quick Discussion

What Are The Causes Of This Condition?

1-*C8-T1 Roots Lesion* = Spondylosis, Trauma

2-*Combined Ulnar & Median Nerve Injuries* (Complete Claw Hand + Sensory Loss Except Snuff Box)

3-*AHC Affection At C8*

- Syringomyelia
- MND= No Sensory Loss
- Charcot Marie Tooth

4-*Damage To Lower Trunk Of Brachial Plexus*

- Cervical Rib
- Pancoast Tumor
- Klumpks Paralysis At Birth

Brown Sequard Syndrome

Hemisection Of Spinal Cord

Clinical Examination

- At level LMNL, sensory loss
- Below level= UMNL , loss of dorsal column same side , loss of pain contralateral

Quick Discussion

What Are The Causes of This condition?

- MS
- Injury
- Tumour
- Radiation
- Abscess

Lesion at level of S1

<u>**Clinical Examination**</u>

- LMNL S1
- Weakness Of :
    - Abductionof Hip
    - External Rotation Of Hip
    - Knee Flexion
    - Ankle Plantar Flexion
- Loss Of Sensation S1
- Ankle Reflex Lost
- +ve Straight Leg Raising Test

Look for Cauda Equina Signs

- Saddle Anesthesia
- Loss Of Anal Sphincter Tone

<u>**Quick Discussion**</u>

What Are The Causes Of This Condition?

- Fracture, Prolapsed Disc, Spondylosis, Pagets Disease of the bone
- Tumors
- Haemorrhage (Trauma , Rupture Spinal Artery , Bleeding Tendency)
- Inflamation (T.B,MS,)

How Would You Like to Investigate This condition?

- MRI
- CT
- Myelography
- EMG

Station IV

Law, Ethics & Communication Skills

Introduction

- Effective Communication Skills, Strategies And Etiquette Thus Become Critical Not Only To Avoid Errors, Complaints And Legal Claims, But To Establish The Essential Therapeutic Doctor-Patient Relationship To Ensure Adherence To Medical Therapy And For Good Clinical Outcomes.
- Lack Of Time, Clinician Fatigue, Heavy Workload, And Complexity Of Patient's Clinical And Emotional Problems Are Commonly Implicated As Major Causes Of Poor Doctor-Patient Relationship Building. Although More Time Enables Better Communication, Time Alone Does Not Ensure Better Communication Or Patient Satisfaction With The Clinical Encounter.
- Given The Wealth Of Evidence Linking Ineffective Clinician-Patient Communication With Increased Malpractice Risk, Non-Adherence, Patient And Clinician Dissatisfaction, And Poor Patient Health Outcomes, The Necessity Of Addressing Communication Skill Deficits Is Of The Utmost Importance.
- In Communication, Ethics Work To Enhance Credibility, Improve The Decision-Making Process And Allow For Trust Between The Patients And Physicians.
- Patients' Perceptions Of The Quality Of The Healthcare They Received Are Highly Dependent On The Quality Of Their Interactions With Their Healthcare Clinician And Team. The Connection That A Patient Feels With His Or Her Clinician Can Ultimately Improve Their Health Mediated Through Participation In Their Care, Adherence To Treatment, And Patient Self-Management.
- Communication Among Healthcare Team Members Influences The Quality Of Working Relationships, Job Satisfaction And Has A Profound Impact On Patient Safety.
- Similar To Other Healthcare Procedures, Communication Skills Can Be Learned And Improved Upon. Improvement In Communication Skills Requires Commitment And Practice.
- Respect For Our Patients Includes Respecting Their Wishes, Expressing Concern For Their Welfare, Demonstrating Sensitivity To Their Individual And Cultural Characteristics, And Providing Appropriate Care Regardless Of Patient Characteristics. Displaying Respect Is The Foundation Of Rapport Building.

Ethical Issues

A) THE PATIENT AUTONOMY
- The Patients' Right To Be Told The Truth.
- The Patients Right To Share With You The Decision Of Their Own Management Plan.
- The Patient Right To Accept Or Refuse The Medical Advice.

Respect Patient Autonomy
- Explain to the patient clearly what his medical problem is, explain the management plan and the options and let him decide with you. Do not act as a parent and take decisions on his behalf or force him to take some decisions, just explain the options and let him choose as long as he has capacity (see later).
- If the patient refuses the medical advice which is in his best interest, you must explore the reason for that (see later).
- Be nice and friendly and give him a chance to think and participate in the discussion, e.g.:
  - "What Do You Think We Can Do More For You?"
  - "Here Are The Options; However My Recommendation Would Be…."
  - "So What Are Your Concerns About The Procedure "
  - "I Do Appreciate Your Decision, But Could You Tell Me Why Are You Refusing This Kind Of Medication?"

Taking Decisions

Only the patient should take a decision regarding his treatment as long as he is competent and can understand the information given
For the patient to take a decision the following should apply:
- The Patient Should Receive Full, Complete, Right Information
- The Patient Should Take The Decision On His Own (Not Forced To Take The Decision By Anyone).

The clinician can dishonor some decision if he believes that the patient was forced to take this decision

B) BENEFICENCE
- The Medical Team Works For The Best Interest Of The Patient.
- Not Only The Best Medical Interest, But The Whole Patient's Best Interest; Medical, Social And Mental.
- To Determine The Best Interest You Should Talk With The Patient About His Daily Activities, Work, His Wishes, And If He Is Coping Well.

C) NON-MALEFICENCE
- Always Keep Your Patient`s Care Your First Priority.
- Never Do/Induce Any Harm Intended Or Not.
- Active Euthanasia Is A Criminal Act.

D) JUSTICE
- Never Discriminate Between People For Any Reason.
- Offer The Best Medical Care To The Maximum Number Of People With The Available Resources Regardless Of Their Origin, Religion Or Believes Etc.

Legal Issues

A) CAPACITY (Competence)

- It Is The Ability To Use, Weigh And Understand Information To Make A Decision, And Communicate Any Decision Made.
- Any Person Above 16 Years Of Age Is Considered To Be Competent Until Proved Otherwise.
- If The Patient Lacks Capacity (e.g. In Coma) It Is The Treating Physician Who Should Determine His Best Interest, But In Conjugation With His Family, Carers And Other Members Of The Team.
- In Case That The Patient Has No Family, And No Capacity You Should Contact The (Mental Capacity Advocacy Service) To Assign An Advocate Who Can Propose Opinion About What Have The Patient`s Wishes Been, Not Giving Decisions, Just Opinions.
- Competent Patients Can Refuse Treatment But Cannot Ask For Treatment.

Special Conditions:

Incompetent Patients (Patients Who Lack Capacity)

- Doctors Work For The Best Interest Of The Patients Unless They Left A Living Will Or Nominated Anybody To Take Decisions On Their Behalf.
- The Best Interest Of The Patient Is Discussed With The Multidisciplinary Team, The Family, Carers Of The Patient Or The Mental Capacity Advocate (If No Family Members)
- Lack Of Capacity Is Not A One Off Decision, And Usually It Is Fluctuating In Patients Who Lack Capacity, Regular Review For "Capacity Assessment "Is Very Important.
- In Emergency Situations, Consent Is Presumed Unless Stated Otherwise By An Advance Directive Or A Power Of Attorney.

Causes Of Lack Of Capacity

- A. Coma
- B. Confusion (Temporary Lack Of Capacity)
- C. Dementia
- D. Some Psychiatric Problems
- E. People Committed Suicide
- F. Hypoxic Brain Injury
- G. Children <16 Who Are Not Gillick Competent

 If In Doubt He Should Be Checked By A Psychiatrist

 Best Interest Doesn't Mean The Best Medical Interest, It Means The Whole Patient`s Best Interest, You Should Speak With Family And Other Carers

 In Cases Of Organ Donation, Or Obtaining Consent For Autopsy You Should Seek Consent From The Next Of Kin Of The Patient.

 When Someone Lacks Mental Capacity To Consent To Care Or Treatment, It Is Sometimes Necessary To Deprive Them Of Their Liberty In Their Best Interests, To Protect Them From Harm **(Deprivation Of Liberty Safeguards)** E.G.: Confused Patients, Psychiatric Disorders.

Advance Directive (Living Will)

- In Discussing DNR (Do Not Attempt Resuscitation) Situations, Withholding Treatment Or Organ Donation About A Patient Without Capacity.
- Should Be A Formal Written Witnessed Paper Stating Exactly What Are The Patient`s Decisions
- A Doctor Can Regard It As Invalid If It Is Not Formal, And This Should Be Documented In The Patient`s Notes
- Organ Donation Card Is Not A Formal Advance Directive But Could Be Considered When Taking A Decision About Organ Donation In A Deceased Patient If The Issue Of Organ Donation Was Not Raised In The Past.
- Ask: "Do You Have Any Idea About His Wishes When He Was Alright?"; "Did He Express His Wishes Before?"

The Lasting Power Of Attorney (Nominating Other To Take Decisions On His Behalf)

In Discussing DNR (Do Not Attempt Resuscitation) Situations, Withholding Treatment Or Organ Donation In A Patient Without Capacity

- Ask: *"Has He Nominated Any One To Take Decisions On His Behalf?"*

- It Should Be A Formal Written Witnessed Paper, And The Individual Having This Power Should Act In The Patient`S Best Interest.
- If A Doctor Thinks That The Individual Holding The Power Of Attorney Is Not Acting In The Patient`S Best Interest Should Raise The Issue To The Court Of Protection

People Committing Suicide Are Not Competent Even If He Is Alert, Conscious And Aware

Competent People Don't Commit Suicide.

People Committing Suicide Are Not Competent (Their Decisions Cannot Be Respected)

You Should Treat Them Even Against Their Wish

Advance Directive Is Not Reliable In Suicidal Patients

You Should Ask If They Took The Drug Overdose By Themselves Or They Were Forced To Take Them, Ask:

"Did You Take It By Yourself? Or Any One Has Obliged/Forced You? Did You Leave Any Letter Or Note?"

If Paracetamol Poisoning Ask About:

Type Of Tablets (Co-Codamol)= Opiate Overdose Too

Phenytoin, Rifampicin (Enzyme Inducers)

Alcohol

For Any Person Below 16 You Should Seek Gardian Consent Especially Parental Consent

Any Person Below 16 Could Be Deemed As Gillik Competence And Take His Own Medical Decision If:

- Asking For Contraceptive Advice
- Is Able To Completely Comprehend The Information Given To Him
- If His Decision Is In His Best Interest
- Some Children Are Gillik Competent Regarding Some Decisions But Not Other Decisions.

B) CONFIDENTIALITY

This Is A Part Of Respecting The Patient`S Autonomy.

You Should Keep All The Patient Medical Information And Records Confidential. No One Should Know Anything About His Medical Condition Without His Own Permission.

In Hospitals, Don`T Leave Monitor Screens Switched On With Patient`S Information Displayed On The Screen Unnecessarily.

Situation Where Confidentiality Can Be Breached:

1) If Patient Has Given Consent
2) Best Interest Of The Patient, But Obtaining Consent Is Not Feasible Or Impractical
- Patient Lacking Capacity And You Need Another Specialist Advice.
- Patient Lacking Capacity And You Need To Discuss His Best Interest From His Family And Carers
- Patient In Coma And You Need To Discuss With The Family If He Is Leaving A Living Will Or A Power Of Attorney.
3) Public Interest
- Birth And Deaths
- Court Orders (Don't Breach A Patient's Confidentiality For The Police, Insurance Companies And Lawyers Unless You Obtain His Consent)
- Notifiable Diseases
- DVLA
- Third Party At Risk
- You Should Always Inform The Patient That You Will Breach His Confidentiality And Document Your Discussion With The Patient In His Records.
- Always Keep The Public Interest Reason As A Last Resort, And Try To Obtain Consent From The Patient
4) The Law Does Not Obligate The Clinician To Inform A Third Party At Risk Against The Patient's Will, But Try To Discuss This With The Patient.

5) If A Son Or Relative Of A Competent Patient Wants To Know About The Patient's Condition
   Say: **"*May I Ask, Have You Taken The Patients' Permission To Discuss His/Her Condition*?"**

C) CONSENT FORMS
Proxy Consent
Like A Patient That Agreed To Tell You About His Medical Issues During History Taking, Or Like Taking A Blood Sample From A Patient. There Should Not Be A Written Form For These Tasks.
Informed Consent
It Is A Written Form That The Patient Should Sign Before Any Invasive Procedure. "Informed" Means That The Patient Accepts To Have The Procedure Done After Explaining The Steps Of The Procedure, The Benefits And The Potential Risks That May Happen During The Procedure.

D) DRIVING ISSUES
- You Should Always Enquire And Ask If Your Patient Drives A Car When You Suspect That The Illness The Patient Has Could Affect His Driving.
- Always Ask The Patient To Inform The DVLA And Get Guidance From Them.
- Don't Give The Patient False Information; If You Don't Know For How Long The Patient Will Be Suspended From Driving You Should Check The DVLA Website.
- Here Are Some Examples, But I Would Recommend You Check The DVLA Website.

	Private cars	Public transport cars
MI	1m	6w
1st attack of Epilepsy	6 m	1 year with no medication
Epilepsy	1 year	10 years
Diabetes on insulin	Ok if no hypos	Banned
TIA/CVA	1m	1y

If You Don't Remember Tell The Patient:
"I Will Look It Up For You And Tell You In Our Next Appointment"

- If The Patient Has A Condition That Bans Him From Driving, It Is His Own Responsibility To Inform The DVLA.
- If For Any Reason The Patient Refuses To Inform The DVLA About His Medical Condition That Will Ban Him From Driving, You Need To Explain Politely That This Puts Him And Others At Risk, And This Puts The Medical Team In Responsibility To Inform The DVLA About His Condition And You May *(Break His Confidentiality)*.

E) OTHER LEGAL ISSUES:
Abortion
Is Accepted If Continuation Of Pregnancy Will Result In Physical, Psychological Or Mental Disorders For The Mother Or Child, But The Mother Can Refuse Abortion For Any Reason (Religious). The Patient Should Have Capacity For Such A Decision.

Doctors Can Refuse Doing Abortions But Can't If It Is Live Saving In Emergency Situation.

Illegal Drugs (E.G. Cocaine):
Not Legally Licensed For Prescription

Doctrine Of Double Effect (Distinguish Actions Intended From Actions For Seen)
Giving Morphine To Relief Pain In Terminally Ill Might Shorten Or End His Life

Persistent Vegetative State:
Treated As A Patient Who Lacks Capacity For 6m - 1 Year (Best Interest) Hoping He Might Regain His Normal State.

After 6m- 1 Year Raise The Case To The Court, Only The Court Will Take His Decisions.

Communication Between Healthcare Personnel & Clinicians

Good Communications Is Very Important Between Team Member Using The SBAR Approach; In Hand Overs, Requesting Referrals And Accepting Referrals

S=Situation;
Good Morning, I Am Dr., SHO Of ...Department, I Am Talking Regarding One Of My Patients Mr......, Under Consultant ...... He Is Complaining Of ....

B=Background
He Is 50 Years Old Man, Smoker For 20 Years, With History Of ISHD, COPD

A=Assessment
His Pulse, B.P, Temp., RR, SO2, Chest Examination Reveals

R=Recommendation
I Started Him On IV Tazocin, So Do You Have Any Advice For Me On How To Proceed? / I Think He Needs Urgent Review Within 10 Minutes

Communication Scenario Scheme

1. **Greeting**
2. **Introduce Yourself Including Your Role**
   E.G. "My Name Is Dr......... SHO In The General Medicine Clinic "
3. **Confirm Your Patient Identity**
4. **Establish Rapport (Break The Ice)**
   E.G. "I Hope You Have Not Been Waiting For Long "
5. **Explain The Aim Of The Appointment**
   - Always Remember The Task Written In The Scenario
   - You Must Avoid Saying Medical Terms (Jargon) While Explaining.
   - You Should Be Able To Address The Expected *Legal* And *Ethical* Issues In Your Scenario From The Written Information Provided Before Entering The Station.
6. **Explore The Situation** (Let The Patient Speak In Order To Unify The Agendas)

   - Patient Idea And Expectations
   - Patient Concern
   - Medical Situation
   - Social Issues
   - Financial Issues
   - Situation At Home
7. **My Way** (Clinical Scenarios Would Be One Or More Of These Titles)
8.

> **A. Explaining** (A Disease Or A Procedure Or A Situation)
> **B. Refusal** (Treatment/Advice/Admission/Discharge/...Etc)
> **C. Break In The System**
> **D. Breaking Bad News**
> **E. Difficult Situations**
>   - *Difficult Person* (Angry, Noncompliant Patient , Harmful Doctor)
>   - *Critical Situations* (End Of Life, Organ Donation, Ventilate Or Not To Ventilate)
>   - Difficult Disease (HIV, T.B, Hepatitis B or C,...)

Address Patient Concern (And Manage The Concern)

9. **You Are Not Alone**
   Always Remember You Are A SHO And You Have A Great Team Of Consultants, Senior Doctors, Nurses, Specialist Nurses, Physiotherapists, Occupational Therapists, Oncology, Etc.. And You Need To Seek Their Help And Get Them Involved.

10. **Supportive Information**
    - o Flyers And Patient Information
    - o Supportive Societies
    - o Internet Websites
11. **Recap**
12. **Make Sure Your Patient Understands Your Plans**
13. **End Of Appointment**

- We Should Discuss The Different Prototypes Of Case Scenarios Rather Than Individualized Case Scenarios. If You Pick Up The Main Concept And Idea, Any Case Scenario Should Follow.
- During Your Consultation You Should Show Sympathy And Empathy All Through. You Should Use Verbal Cues And Nonverbal Cues (Body Language) To Show That.
  - o **Sympathy** Means Feelings Of Pity And Sorrow For Someone Else's Misfortune And Sharing Common Feeling.
  - o **Empathy** Is A Higher Degree In Which You Show The Ability To Share Someone Else's Feelings Or Experiences By Imagining What It Would Be Like To Be In That Person's Situation.

- Any Case Scenario Will Include All The Concepts Of Legal Issues (Autonomy, Beneficence, Non-Maleficence And Justice), But Not Necessarily All Legal Issues. That Is Why, You Need To Pick Up The Principles That Suites Your Scenario, And Approach The Patient In A Sympathetic And Empathetic Way. This Is A Definite Question That You Will Be Asked After Finishing Your Conversation With The Patient. ***"So What Are The Ethical And Legal Issues In Your Scenario??"***
- If There Is A Medical Issue In The Scenario, And You Are Not Fully Aware With The Condition, Don't Panic!! But Don't Invent Or Fabricate Information. It Is Not A Problem If You Say That You Don't Know And You Will Seek A Senior Advice, Or Look It Up In A Text Book... Etc. However, This Station Is Not Testing Your Medical Knowledge.
- Keeping **Eye Contact** As And When Necessary Is An Important Aspect In Interpersonal Transaction, As It Shows Interest.
- Conversations shouldn't be Doctor Centered (You speaking most of the time) nor patient Centered (Patient speaking most of the time). The conversation should go in both ways instead.

My Way

A. Explaining

- It Is One Of The Major Principles In Communication And Almost Always You Will Have To Explain Something In Any Case Scenario.
- You May Be Asked To Explain A Disease, Procedure, Or Even A Situation.
- You Must Avoid Using Medical Terms (Jargon) As Lay People Will Have Difficulty Understanding These Terms.
- Use Instead Very Simple Words E.G.
  - o Arteries/Veins→Blood Conduits
  - o Immune System→General Defense System In Our Body
  - o Bacteria→ Bugs
  - o Thrombosis→Formation Of Blood Clots
  - o Occlusion→ Blocking
  - o Myocardial Infarction→Heart Attack
  - o Radiology → Scans
  - o Blood Investigations→Bloods, Blood Tests
  - o Uterus → Womb
  - o Bronchi, Bronchioles → Airways
  - o Esophagus → Gullet
  - o TIA → Mini-stroke
  - o Lung Fibrosis → Scarring of the lungs
  - o Endoscopy → Camera test
  - o Cannula → Venflon
- You Can Use The Paper And The Pencil To Aid You With Explanation Like Drawing The Heart, Brain, Joints, And Biopsy Needles Going Down To The Kidneys Or Between The Backbones...Etc.
- You Must Use Verbal And Nonverbal Cues During The Scenario.

DISCUSSING ANY PROCEDURE SHOULD BE IN DETAILS
- Steps Of Procedure
- Anesthesia (Local/General)
- Indications And Benefits
  You May Stress On That Point If You Need To Encourage The Patient To Go For The Procedure Putting In Your Consideration The Concept Of Autonomy.
- Complications Of The Procedure
  You May Stress On That Point If You Need To Discourage The Patient To Go For The Procedure Putting In Your Consideration Again The Concept Of Autonomy.
  You Also Need To Explore If The Patient Is In A Situation That Puts Her In Risks Of Complications And/Or If There Is Any Contraindications For The Procedure??
- Precautions To Avoid Complications And Management Plan If Complications Happen.
- Give The Patient Time To Digest The Information, Raise His Concerns, And Think About It Or Discuss It With His Family Or Someone He Trusts. It Is Not Necessary For The Patient To Decide About The Procedure In The Same Setting.
- You Need To Let The Patient Sign An Informed Consent After Your Discussion If He Is Happy To Go For The Procedure (Legal Issue).

DISCUSSING ANY DISEASE SHOULD BE IN DETAILS
1. Simple Pathogenesis
2. Clinical Picture And Symptoms

3. Investigations
4. Treatment Modalities
5. Possible Complications And Prognosis Of The Disease.

The Following are examples of simple scenarios of explaining

Explaining Procedure

Scenario:

Mrs. Smith Was Referred To The Renal Clinic For The First Time Last Week For Her Nephrotic Syndrome As Suspected By Her Gp. She Was Reviewed By One Of The Consultants That Looked Up Her Investigations And Feels That She Is A Candidate For A Renal Biopsy. She Is Coming Today To The (One Day Case) To Have Her Renal Biopsy Done, However The Nurse In Charge Feels That The Patient Does Not Have Enough Information About The Procedure.

Your Task Is To Explain The Procedure To The Patient.

How To Deal With That Case Scenario??
Apply The Scheme And Give It A Go.

Action Plan

1. **Greeting** " Hello, Good Morning "
2. **Introduce Yourself Including Your Role**

E.G. "My Name Is Dr........., I'm One Of The Doctors In The Renal Medicine Unit "

3. **Confirm Your Patient Identity** "Are You Mrs. Smith??"
4. **Establish Rapport (Break The Ice)**

E.G. "I Hope You Did Not Have To Wake Up Too Early For This Appointment "

5. **Explain The Aim Of The Appointment**
   Always Remember The Task Written In The Scenario

E.G. "I Understand That You Came Today For A Kidney Biopsy, And I Am Here Today To Answer Your Questions And Concerns About The Procedure "

- You Should Be Able To Address The Expected Legal And Ethical Issues In Your Scenario From The Written Information Provided Before Entering The Station.

6. **Explore The Situation** (Let The Patient Speak In Order To Unify The Agendas)

E.G. "First Of All, Tell Me How Far You Were Told About The Procedure? "

Here You Must Address The Following

- Patient Idea
- Patient Concern
- Medical Situation And Is She Understanding Why Do We Need   To Have The Biopsy Done??
- Any Previous Experiences Or Shared Experiences, Did She Try To Look It Up In The Internet??

7. **My Way (Explaining A Procedure)**

You Must Avoid Saying Medical Terms (Jargon) While Explaining. Try To Reassure The Patient By Saying "It Is A Procedure That We Do On The Renal Ward On Daily Basis, And Almost Always It Passes Uneventful "

Explain The Procedure As Mentioned Before:

a. **Steps Procedure**

"Initially We visualize The Kidney By An Ultrasound Machine To Localize The Points Where We Should Stick The Needle, And The Procedure Will Be Guided By The Ultrasound Machine All Through The Procedure. After Finding This Point We Will Do Good Cleaning Of The Skin For The Procedure To Be Completely Sterile And To Minimize Any Risk Of Infection. After That We Will Put The Local Anesthetic And That Is The Uncomfortable Bit In The Procedure, So Basically You Will Feel A Sharp Scratch Of The Needle, Then When Injecting The Anesthetic You Will Feel Some Stinging. It Would Be There For A Couple Of Seconds, Then Your Skin Will Go Nice And Numb, And You Would Not Feel Any Pain, But You Will Feel Some Pushing In Your Back. Then We Do A Very Small Opening In The Skin To Stick The Needle Through And We Go Down With The Needle All The Way To The Kidneys And Take A Snip Or Two. Again This Should Not Be Painful. These Snips Will Be Sent Straight Away To The Experts To Examine Them Under The Microscope And Then They Should Feedback The Diagnosis"

b. **Indications And Benefits**

"Depending On The Diagnosis, We Will Know Exactly What Is Happening Inside Your Kidneys, And Accordingly We Will Give You The Suitable Treatment For That "

c. **Complications Of The Procedure**

"As Any Invasive Procedure, There Are Some Risks And Unlikely Some Complications May Happen. The Most Serious One Is Bleeding As The Kidney Is A Bloody Organ. It Is Not Uncommon To Find Some Blood In Your Waterworks After The Procedure, However This Should Be Self-Limiting And It Will Clear Up Spontaneously. Other Less Likely Complications Like Pain, Infection, Or Failure To Take The Snip For Technical Difficulties "

d. **Precautions To Avoid Complications And Management Plan If Complications Happen**.

- *Bleeding Risk:*

"Before The Procedure We Will Do Some Basic Blood Tests To Ensure That Your Blood Is Ok With No Medical Conditions That May Put You In The Risk Of Bleeding, And After The Procedure You Will Have To Lie On Your Back For 6-8 Hours To Compress The Wound And Pick Up Bleeding If It Happens As Well As Monitoring Your Blood Pressure. Are You On Any Blood Thinning Medications??

"If Bleeding occurs We Will Carry Blood Transfusion, Till In Stops Spontaneously. If This Does Not Happen We May Ask For Help From Our Colleagues In The Interventional Radiology Or Even The Surgeons To Stop That Bleeding. Again This Is Extremely Unlikely To Happen "

- *Pain:*

"If You Feel Any Pain, Just Let Us Know, We Could Always Put More Local Anesthetic"

- *Infection:*

"We Usually Do Very Good Skin Cleaning And The Possibility Of Getting Any Infections From The Procedure Is Extremely Unlikely"

8. **Give The Patient Time To Digest The Information, Raise Her Concerns, And Think About It Or Discuss It With His Family Or Someone He Trusts.**

Manage Concerns If Raised.

"Could I Bleed To Death?"

"Isn't There Another Way To Catch The Diagnosis Other Than This Invasive Procedure?"

"Do You Need To Biopsy Both Kidneys?"

9. **You Are Not Alone**

Always Remember You Are One Of The Doctors And You Have A Great Team Of Senior Doctors, Specialist Nurses, Or You May Even Use The (Patient Information) Leaflets To Deliver The Message.

10. **Recap**

11. **You Need To Let The Patient Sign An Informed Consent After Your Discussion If He Is Happy To Go For The Procedure (Legal Issue).**

E.G. "I'll Give You Some Time To Digest This Piece Of Information And Will Come Back Later. However, If You Are Happy To Go For The Procedure, You Will Have To Sign A Consent Form. This Form Will State The Conversation We Had Including Benefits And Risks Of The Procedure. "

12. **Make Sure Your Patient Understands Your Plans**

"Is Everything Clear? Do You Have Any Questions For Me? Any Other Concerns?"

13. **End Of Appointment**

Explaining Disease

Your Role: You Are The Doctor In The Rheumatology Clinic
Problem: Explaining Rheumatoid Arthritis
Patient: Mr. Paul Brown, A 52 Year-Old Man

Please Read The Scenario Printed Below. When The Bell Sounds, Enter The Room. You Have 14 Minutes For Your Consultation With The Patient/Relative, 1 Minute To Collect Your Thoughts And 5 Minutes For Discussion. You May Make Notes If You Wish.

Where Relevant, Assume You Have The Patient's Consent To Discuss Their Condition With The Relative/Surrogate.

Scenario:

 Mr. Brown Was Referred To The Rheumatology Clinic Last Month With A Long Standing History Of Painful Small Joints Of The Hands. He Was Seen By Your Consultant And He Ordered Some Investigations And Simple X- Ray On Both Hands. The Results Came Back With A Positive Rheumatoid Factor (RF) And Anti-CCP And The X-Rays Showed Ulnar Deviation With Abnormal Left MCP Joints Which Favors The Diagnosis Of Rheumatoid Arthritis. His FBC, Crp, U&E Were All Normal. Unfortunately, Your Consultant Is Busy Doing His Post Take Round, And He Asked You To See The Patient.

Your Task Is To Explain The Disease To The Patient And Address His Concerns.

Do Not Examine The Patient
Do Not Take A History
Any Notes You Make Must Be Handed To The Examiners At The End Of The Station.

How To Deal With That Case Scenario??
Again, Apply The Scheme And Give It A Go.

<h1 align="center">Action Plan</h1>

1. **Greeting**
2. **Introduce Yourself Including Your Role**
3. **Confirm Your Patient Identity**
4. **Establish Rapport (Break The Ice)**
5. **Explain The Aim Of The Appointment**
   Always Remember The Task Written In The Scenario
   You Must Avoid Saying Medical Terms (Jargon) While Explaining.
   You Should Be Able To Address The Expected *Legal* And *Ethical* Issues In Your Scenario
   From The Written Information Provided Before Entering The Station.
6. **Explore The Situation** (Let The Patient Speak In Order To Unify The Agendas)
   Patient Idea And Expectations
   Patient Concern
   Medical Situation (Quickly, Other Joints Affected That May Affect His   Quality Of Life?)
   Social Issues (Occupation, Mobility, Living Alone?)
   Financial Issues
   Situation At Home (Stairs, Able To Do Simple Hand Tasks,Etc)

7. **My Way: Explaining A Disease**
   a. <u>Simple Pathogenesis Of RA</u>
   E.G. "It Is One Of The (Autoimmune Diseases). To Simplify This Bulky Term, Sometimes Our
   Immune System Instead Of Attacking Germs And Bugs, It Goes Crazy For An Unknown Reason,
   And It Starts Attacking Our Own Tissues. In Your Case, It Is Attacking The Joint And The
   Capsule Surrounding It "
   b. <u>Clinical Picture And Symptoms</u>
   E.G. "The Classic Presentation Of This Disease Is Pain And Inflammation In The Small Joints Of
   The Body Like The Hands And Feet "
   c. <u>Possible Complications And Prognosis Of The Disease.</u>
   E.G. "Sometimes This Disease Hits Hard And Destructs The Joint, Other Times It May Even
   Affect Other Organs Like The Heart, Eyes, Lungs Or The Kidneys. However Our Role As A
   Medical Team Is To Do Regular Follow Up In Order To Make Sure Your Main Symptom Is
   Managed, And To Detect Complications Early If They Tend To Occur."

   d. <u>Treatment Modalities (You Don't Need To Say It In Details, Just Broad Lines)</u>
   E.G. "We Usually Start Treatment In The Form Of Simple Pain Killers To Control Your
   Symptoms, However If The Disease Flares Up Or The Symptoms Persist We May Have To
   Escalate With More Potent Medications Like (Immunosuppressant Medications) Which Are Drugs
   That May Suppress The Crazy Defense System In Our Body."
   **e. <u>Here You May Need To Explain The Side Effects Of The Immunosuppressant
      Medications</u>**
   E.G. Repeated Infections Or The Risk Of Malignancies On The Long Run If The Patient Insists To
   Know All About It. The Rule Here Is Try Not To Go Through That Issue, As The Patient Will Have
   A Lot To Digest In A Single Setting, Loads Of Concerns And As Long As You Are Not Starting Him
   On These Medications, Then It Would Be Appropriate Just To Mention It Without Details.

8. **Address Patient Concern**
   "Would I Be Disabled At Some Point?"
   "Would The Medications Control My Pain?"
   "Would I Need To Inform My Employer?"
9. ***You Are Not Alone***
   You Will Discuss The Case With The Consultant, And Next Time In The Clinic He Will Be
   Reviewed By The Consultant.
   Supportive Information
   Flyers And Patient Information

Rheumatoid Arthritis Supportive Groups

Referral To Physiotherapist/Occupational Therapist If Needed (According To His QOL, Ability To Cope With The Disease And Manage At Home)

Internet Websites

10. **Recap**

11. **Make Sure Your Patient Understands Your Plans**
12. **End Of Appointment**

B. Refusal

- Refusal Means That Your Agenda Is Not Unified With The Patient's Agenda.
- The Patient May Refuse Medical Advice, Treatment, Hospital Admission Or Discharge.
- The Patient Has The Right To Refuse An Issue Even If It Was Not In His Best Interest As Long As He Has "Capacity ". You Have To Respect The Patient Autonomy.
- If The Patient Refuses A Medical Issue That Should Be In His Best Interest And He Has Capacity, You Need To **Approach As Following:**

1. **Why?** You Have To Explore The Reason For His Refusal In Details, And Try To Sort A Plan For Managing That Reason. He May Rethink About It If He Feels That Your Team Would Help!
2. **Is He Aware With His Condition Seriousness??** He May Not Be Aware, And If That Is The Case You Will Have To "Explain" As Before.
3. If He Is Aware And Still Refusing, You Should Explain The **Pros And Cons** Of Insisting To Refuse.
4. If He Is Still Refusing, You Could Offer An **Extra Help** To Decrease The Risk Of His "Inappropriate Decision "E.G. (A Patient Insisting To Be Discharged From Hospital Though Being Septic And On Intravenous Antibiotics. You Try To Find Out The Reason, The Patient Is Aware That He Is Critical, And Accepts The Risk Of Going Home With A Poor General Condition. Don't Just Let Him Go, But Try To Help At Home As Giving Him The Antibiotics At Home – Hospital At Home – Or Seek Microbiology Advice Of Switching His Antibiotics To Oral Forms, Involving Social Services For A Care Package If Needed, And Of Course Let Your Consultant Know About That).
5. Finally, Don't Forget To Cover Any **Legal Issues** E.G. (The Patient Would Need To Sign A Form If Ye Insist To Be Discharged Against Medical Advice).

Common Situations With "Refusal "

REFUSAL OF TREATMENT (RESPECT PATIENT AUTONOMY)

- Patients Have The Right To Refuse Treatment As Long As They Are Competent And Have Capacity.
- You Should Seek And Detect The Reasons Why The Patient Refuses Treatment; Ask:
  - Why Are You Refusing Treatment? Any Problems, side effects or previous experiences before? Any problems with dosing? You Know That Will Risk Your Life?"
- Try To Find Solutions And Suggestions To Overcome His Concerns.
- You Should Explain To Him The Benefits (PROS) Of This Medications And The Risks (CONS) Of Not Receiving Treatment.
- If He Insists Try To Find Him Another Alternative (E.G. Less Toxic Effects Though Less Potent Drug).
- The Treating Physician Should Document The Event, And Let The Patient's GP Know About That.

SELF-DISCHARGE

- Patients With Capacity Have The Right To Self-Discharge Themselves.
- Is The Patient Aware with his Condition And How Serious Is It?
- You Should Explore The Reason For Their Wishes And Try To Convince Them To Stay In The Hospital, And Explain The Risks For Them If They Are Discharged Prematurely.
- Try To Suggest Logic Solutions If Possible, Or Seek Assistance If Appropriate (e.g. Social Works, Smoking Cessation Team, Special Services,..etc).
- If The Patient Insists He Should Sign A Legal Document (Discharge Against Medical Advice).
- Explain To Him That You Will :
  - Inform Your Consultant
  - Send A Letter To Gp , Inorder To Carry On With Treatment.
  - Arrange For A Near Appointment For Follow Up.
  - Advice If Any Complication To Turn Up To Hospital Immediately.

N.B. PATIENTS HAVE THE RIGHT TO SEE THEIR MEDICAL RECORDS & TO BE EXPLAINED TO THEM & CHANGE INACCURATE INFORMATION.

JEHOVAH'S WITNESS

- Jehovah's Witnesses Refuse To Take Blood Or Blood Products For Religious Beliefs.
- If The Patient Is Competent He Should Sign A Legal Document That You Have Explained To Him The Importance And The Risks, And That He Refuses The Treatment Against Medical Advice.
- Always Try To Convince Them To Take The Blood If It Is Indicated By Assuring Him:
  - "No One Will Know You Have Taken Blood"
  - "The Blood Will Make You Feel Better And Save Your Life."
- Suggest Alternatives If Still Insisting To Refuse (e.g. Erythropoietin Injections, Iron Infusions, Folic Acid, ...etc.)
- You Can Never Give The Patient Blood Or Blood Products Against His Will, Even If The Family Insists.

Refusal of Treatment

Your Role: You Are The On-Call Doctor In The Respiratory Ward
Problem: Patient Refusing Medication
Patient: Mrs. Margaret Noon, A 45 Year-Old Woman

Please Read The Scenario Printed Below. When The Bell Sounds, Enter The Room. You Have 14 Minutes For Your Consultation With The Patient/Relative, 1 Minute To Collect Your Thoughts And 5 Minutes For Discussion. You May Make Notes If You Wish.

Where Relevant, Assume You Have The Patient's Consent To Discuss Their Condition With The Relative/Surrogate.

> Scenario:
>
> Mrs. Noon Was Admitted To The Ward With Hemoptysis And Was Diagnosed As Anca Associated Vaculitis. She Had A Massive Lung Consolidation And Mild Renal Impairment. Her Case Was Discussed In The Weekly Multidisciplinary Meeting (MDM) And The Decision Was To Start Her On (Induction Treatment) In Form Of Steroids And Cyclophosphamide, In Addition To Plasma Exchange Sessions. Your Consultant Reviewed Her In The Ward Round And Mentioned The Treatment Plan Briefly To Her. During The On Call, The Staff Nurse Informs You That Mrs. Noon Is Refusing To Take Her Due Steroid Dose As She Feels That It Is A Hazardous Drug To Receive.
>
> Your Task Is To Convince The Patient To Take Her Medications As Per Medical Plan And Address Her Concerns.

Do Not Examine The Patient
Do Not Take A History
Any Notes You Make Must Be Handed To The Examiners At The End Of The Station.

How To Deal With That Case Scenario?

Action Plan

1. **Greeting**

2. **Introduce Yourself Including Your Role**
3. **Confirm Your Patient Identity**
4. **Establish Rapport (Break The Ice)**
5. **Explain The Aim Of The Appointment**

- Always Remember The Task Written In The Scenario
- You Must Avoid Saying Medical Terms (Jargon) While Explaining.
- You Should Be Able To Address The Expected *Legal* And *Ethical* Issues In Your Scenario From The Written Information Provided Before Entering The Station.

6. **Explore The Situation** (Let The Patient Speak In Order To Unify The Agendas)

- Medical Situation (Is She Aware With Her Medical Condition? Is She Having Any Medical Disease That Could Be Aggravated With Steroids (E.G. Uncontrolled Diabetes Or Osteoporosis) Or Cytotoxic Medications (E.G. Malignancies)??

- Patient Idea And Expectations

- Patient Concern (In This Scenario It Would Be Related To The Side Effects Of Medications As Diabetes, Hypertension, Depression And Osteoporosis)

7. **My Way: Refusal**

a. **Why?** You Have To Explore The Reason For Her Refusal In Details, And Try To Sort A Plan For Managing That Reason.

In This Scenario Mrs. Noon Had Previous Bad Experience With Steroids, As It Induced Diabetes To Her Mother That Had Fibromyalgia, And She Was On Long Term Steroids. Her Mother Also Had Steroid Induced Psychosis, And She Did Not Want That To Happen To Her, In Addition To That She Has Bad Osteoporosis And She Is Concerned Of Getting Fractures If She Starts Steroids. Another Concern She Will Rise Through The Scenario Is Cyclophosphamide, As She Read That This Drug Is Used As Chemotherapy, And She Is Not Aware That She Has Any Cancers?? Also, She Read That This Drug Itself Could Cause Cancers.

b. **Is She Aware With The Seriousness Of Her Condition ??**

Mrs. Noon Actually Is Not Aware With The Seriousness Of Her Condition, And That This Condition- Especially With Pulmonary Hemorrhages- Could Be Fatal If Untreated. Progressive Renal Failure Is Another Risk. Here You Would Need To Explain What Vasculitis Is, And The Hazards Of Leaving This Disease Not Treated Properly. You Also Need To Inform Her That Treatment Is Long Term, As After Induction She Would Need A Maintenance Course Of Treatment That May Extend Up To 3 Years With Close Follow Up In The Clinic, However This Disease Is An Autoimmune Disease, And There Is Always A Risk That It Could Relapse Even After Finishing The Treatment Course.

c. **Pros And Cons** Of Insisting To Refuse.

- Explain Honestly The Side Effects Of The Drug And What Are The Steps That We May Take In Order To Prevent Side Effects E.G. Gastric Protection, Bone Protection, Regular Blood Sugar Follow Up And What Would Be The Plan If She Gets Diabetes...Etc.
- Also, Explain The Risks Of Not Taking The Proper Treatment As Intractable Pulmonary Hemorrhage, Renal Failure, And Other Organ Affection.

8. **Address Patient Concern**

- Would I Get Diabetes?
- Would My Osteoporosis Get Worse?
- Could The Cyclophosphamide Give Me Cancers?

9. You Are Not Alone

- You Will Discuss The Case With The Consultant
- Supportive Information
- Flyers And Patient Information
- Internet Websites

10. Recap

11. Make Sure Your Patient Understands Your Plans End Of Appointment

C. Break In The System

- Break In The System Means That Something Went Unfavorable, And It Should Not Have Happened.
- That Issue Doesn't Necessarily Have To Be A Medical Mistake, But It Is Definitely A Problem In The Medical System In General.
- The Patients Always Have The Right To Complain Through The Official Routes For Formal Complains (E.G. Patient Advice And Liaison Service), However With Good Communication And Smart Dealing With Situations Patients May Reconsider That If They Feel That Something Will Change In The Near Future.
- In Such Cases You Need To **Approach As Following:**

1. **Is The Situation A True Break In The System??** Or Just An Over Expectation From The Patient?
   (e.g. A Patient Being Told By His GP That He Would Be Referred To The Rheumatology Clinic To Further Investigate His Long Standing Arthritis, And Then He Phones The Rheumatology Clinic Next Day Asking About His Appointment!!)
2. If The Situation Does Not Appear To Be Break In The System, **Clarify That.**
3. **If The Situation Appears To Be Break In The System:-**
a. **Apologize Clearly For The Mistake.**
b. **Never Point To Anyone Of Your Colleagues** But Reassure The Patient That This Will Be A Matter Of Investigation
c. **Explain To The Patient What Are The Steps That You Will Take, In Order For This Error Not To Harm The Patient**, And Not To Be Repeated For Him Or Other Patients In The Future.
d. You Must Clearly Say That **You Will Fill An "Incident Report/Datix"** And This Error Will Be Investigated, And That You Will Let Your Consultant And Head Nurse Know About The Incident.
e. If The Patient Still Insists To Put A **"Formal Complain "**Despite All The Previous Actions That You Will Take, **You Must Help Him By Letting Him Know The Way Of Doing** So. If You Are Not Sure About The Formal Way Of Placing An Official Complain, Tell Him That You Will Ask One Of Your (Colleagues/Seniors/Head Nurses) And Let Him Know.

COMPLAINTS:

- Only Patients (Not Family/Relatives) Can Make Complaints If They are Competent, Or The Relative If The Patient Is Not Competent.
- Good Communication And Doctor Patient Relationship Should Avoid Any Complaints; All Complaints Are A Result Of Defective Communication Between The Clinician And The Patient.
- If A Patient Wants To Make A Complaint For Any Reason He Has All The Right To Do It.
- Formal Complaint Are Sent To The (Trust Legal Department), Or (The Patient Advice And Liaison Service).
- If A Relative Of A Competent Patient Wants To Make A Complaint; Say:
  "We Will Have To Discuss This First With Mr..... If He Wants To Make A Complaint I Will Help Him To Fill The Form And Send It To The Trust Legal Department".
- Remember That Good Communication Can Prevent A Lot Of Complaints.
- Examples Of Medical Mistakes:
  o Breaking Confidentiality Of The Patient.
  o Not Giving The Patient The Appropriate Care He Needs.
  o Giving Wrong Medications.
  o Not Obtaining Consent Before Proceeding With A Procedure.
  o Complications Of Procedures That Are Due To Mistakes Or Errors (e.g. Ignorance or Malpractice).
  o Delayed/Missed Appointments.
  o Mixed or Wrong Blood Results Or Scans.

Medical Error

<u>Your Role:</u> You Are The On-Call Doctor In The Medical Ward
<u>Problem:</u> Patient Allergic To Penicillin And Received The Drug By Mistake
<u>Patient:</u> Mr. John Edwards, A 69 Year-Old Man

Please Read The Scenario Printed Below. When The Bell Sounds, Enter The Room. You Have 14 Minutes For Your Consultation With The Patient/Relative, 1 Minute To Collect Your Thoughts And 5 Minutes For Discussion. You May Make Notes If You Wish.

Where Relevant, Assume You Have The Patient's Consent To Discuss Their Condition With The Relative/Surrogate.

Scenario:

Mr. Edwards Lives With Harry -His Son- Which Is His Next Of Kin. Mr. Edwards Is Known To Have Uncontrolled Diabetes, Hypertension, Alzheimer Disease And An Ongoing Dementia. Harry Works As A University Tutor, And Lives With His Wife And His Elderly Father. Mr. Edwards Had A Bad Cough For The Past Three Days, And Yesterday Evening He Started To Get Confused With A Raised Body Temperature. He Was Brought To A&E By His Daughter In Law, And Harry Was Traveling Abroad Incidentally. Although Mr. Edward's Daughter In Law Mentioned That He Is Allergic To Penicillin, The Patient Was Admitted To The Medical Ward And Was Prescribed Co-Amoxiclav For His Chest Infection, Most Probably As It Was Not Mentioned In His Medical Notes From His Clerking In A&E Neither In Nursing Handover That He Is Allergic To Penicillin. The Patient Had Anaphylaxis That Was Managed Appropriately And The Drug Was Stopped Immediately, But He Developed A Prominent Skin Rash; Nevertheless Mr. Edwards Turns The Corner And Improves On An Alternative Antibiotic. Harry Arrived Today And Comes To See His Father In Hospital, And He Is Extremely Upset To Hear About That Event, And He Needs To Complain About It As He Feels That This Hospital Is Unsafe. You Are Asked By One Of The Nurses To Speak To Mr. Edward's Son.

Your Task Is To Speak To Mr. Edward's Son And Explain The Situation

Do Not Examine The Patient
Do Not Take A History
Any Notes You Make Must Be Handed To The Examiners At The End Of The Station.

Action Plan

1. **Greeting**
2. **Introduce Yourself Including Your Role**
3. **Confirm Whom Are You Speaking To, And Make Sure He Is His Next Of Kin.**
4. **Establish Rapport (Break The Ice)**
5. **Explain The Aim Of The Appointment**
   - Always Remember The Task Written In The Scenario
   - You Must Avoid Saying Medical Terms (Jargon) While Explaining.
   - You Should Be Able To Address The Expected *Legal* And *Ethical* Issues In Your Scenario
   From The Written Information Provided Before Entering The Station.
6. **Explore The Situation** (Let The Son Speak In Order To Unify The Agendas)
- Medical Situation (Is She Aware With His Father's Medical Condition?)
- The Son's Idea And Expectations
- The Son's Concern (In This Scenario Harry Feels That This Hospital Is Unsafe, And He Does Not Trust The Medical Team Anymore)
7. **My Way: Break In The System**
1) **Is The Situation A True Break In The System??** The Answer Obviously Is "Yes"
2) **The Situation Appears To Be Break In The System, So You Need To:**
a. **Apologize Clearly**
   "On Behalf Of The Medical Team, I Apologies For This Mistake"
b. Harry Will Insist To Know Whose Fault Was That, **However Never Point To Anyone Of Your Colleagues But Reassure The Patient That** This Will Be A Matter Of Investigation
   "I'm Sorry, I Can Not Blame Or Defend Any One Of My Colleagues As This Not My Role Here, However I Need To Reassure You That This Event Raises Our Concerns As A Medical Team, And It Will Be A Matter Of Investigation. The Aim Of Investigating The Event Is To Help Improving The Medical Service And Keep Patients Safe Rather Than Pointing To Someone, As Mistakes Do Happen But We Need To Address How To Avoid Them Happening Or At Least To Pick These Mistakes Early Enough To Avoid Patient Harm."
c. **Explain To The Patient What Are The Steps That You Will Take, In Order For This Error Not To Harm The Patient**, And Not To Be Repeated For Him Or Other Patients In The Future.
   "Once We Discovered The Mistake, We Treated Mr. Edwards Allergic Reaction, And We Wrote Clearly In His Notes And On The Drug Chart With Bold Capital Letters Allergic To Penicillin, In Order For This Error Not To Happen Again"
d. You Must Clearly Say That You Will **Fill An "Incident Form/Datix"** And This Error Will Be Investigated, And That You Will Let Your Consultant Know About The Situation.
   "As I Mentioned Earlier, That This Event Would Be A Matter Of Investigation, So We Filled An Incident Form And It Would Be Investigated As Soon As Possible, And His Consultant Is Aware With The Current Situation"
e. If The Patient Still Insists To Place A **"Formal Complain "Despite All The Actions That You Will Take, You Must Help Him/Her By Letting Him/Her Know The Official Way Of Doing So**. If You Are Not Sure About The Formal Way Of Placing An Official Complain, Say That You Will Ask One Of Your (Colleagues/Seniors/Head Nurses) And Let Him/Her Know.

8. **Address Patient Concern**
- "I'm Sorry But I Feel That My Father Is Not Safe In This Place"
- "How Could You Guarantee That This Will Not Happen To Other Patients In This Hospital?"

9. **You Are Not Alone**
- You Will Discuss The Case With The Consultant

- He Can Visit The Trust Website And Know What Is The Policy Of The Trust, And How Could He Raise His Concerns And Complaints On Line. It Is Always Nice To Give A Feedback That May Help Improving The Service.

10. **Recap**

11. **Make Sure Your Patient Understands Your Plans**
12. **End Of Appointment**

D. Breaking Bad News

- Most Of The Patients Appreciate Facts About Their Health. However, The Truth Telling Practices And Preferences Are A Cultural Artifact To A Certain Extent.
- Honest And Truthful Disclosure Is An Extremely Difficult Task And Physicians Often Find That The Disclosure Of Cancer Diagnosis To The Patient As One Of The Most Difficult. Very Few Health Care Workers Have Received Sufficient Training In The "Breaking Bad News" Tactics.
- Bad News Is Defined As One Which Is Pertaining To Situation Where There Is A Feeling Of No Hope, A Threat To A Person's Mental Or Physical Wellbeing, A Risk Of Upsetting An Established Lifestyle Or Where A Message Is Given Which Conveys To An Individual Fewer Choices In His Or Her Life.
- Another Definition States "Any News That Drastically And Negatively Alters The Patient's View Of Her Or His Future" Is Bad News.
- Truthful Disclosure Of Psychologically Painful Information Not Only Hurts The Patient And Their Relatives But Also Embarrasses The Health Care Worker.
- Feelings Of Mistrust, Anger, Fear, And Blame Are Common Reactions If Bad News Is Broken Poorly.
- This Communication Skill Is Typically Learned Through Trial And Error Or Observation Of Senior Colleagues.
- "Breaking" Means That You Have To Give The News Bit By Bit And Not As One Shot. It Would Be Much Better If You Drag The Patient To The Bad News Rather Than Saying It Yourself. Saying That The Patients Bloods Or Scans Showed An "Unfavorable Abnormality" Or Telling The Patient That He Had A "Complex Investigation Or Test To Look For Serious Rather Than Simple Causes" Is Sometimes Considered As A "Warning Shot" And May Let The Patient Pay Attention That The Situation Now Is Critical And He Is About To Hear Something Unpropitious.
- In Breaking Bad News We Always Should Be Extremely Sympathetic And Empathetic With The Patient.
- Always Think If You Were In The Patient's Place How Would You Feel And How Would You Like The Information To Be Given To You.
- There Are Well Known And Recommended Protocols In Breaking Bad News Like Spikes Protocol, ABCDE Module, And The Break Protocols. Any Of Them With Some Practice Will Make You Master Breaking Bad News. These Are Summarized in the following:

"The SPIKES" Protocol In A Case Of Patient Death

S-Set the stage
1-Clearly introduce yourself
2-Clearly state your role in the patient's care
P-Perception
1-Determined the level of knowledge of the relative prior to arrival in the waiting room
2-Take Note of the News receiver's vocabulary
I-Inform
1-Briefly indicate the chronology of events leading to the death
2-Use language that he can understands
3-Don't use euphemisms
K-Knowledge
1-Allow relative to react, ask questions & raise Concerns
2-Answer all questions in appropriate manner
E-Empathy
1-Use appropriate statements of showing concern for the grieving
S-Summary & Strategy
1-Avoid showing any physician guilt for the death/Poor prognosis
2-Establich your personal availability to answer questions that may arise at later stage
3-End the discussion & depart in appropriate manner

The ABCDE Model

A-Advance Perception

B-Build a Therapeutic environment

D-Deal with patient & Family reactions

C-Communicate well

E-Encourage & Validate emotions

BREAKS Protocol Protocol for Breaking bad news

Background

- The in-depth knowledge of the patient's problem.
- The physician must be aware of the patient/relative who comes after "googling" the problem.
- Cultural and ethnic background of the patient is also very important. The physician has to be sensitive to the cultural orientation of the patient, and it should be respected.

Rapport

- The physician should establish a good rapport with the patient.
- Exploring
- Start from what the patient knows about his/her illness. Most of the patients will be aware of the seriousness of the condition, and some may even know their diagnosis.
- The history, the investigations, the difficulties met in the process etc need to be explored.
- Try to involve the significant other people of the patient in the decision-making process, if allowed by the patient.

Announce

- A warning shot is desirable, so that the news will not explode like a bomb.
- The patient has the right to know the diagnosis, at the same time he has the right to refrain from knowing it.
- Hence, announcement of diagnosis has to be made after getting consent.

Kindling

- Adequate space for the free flow of emotions has to be given.
- Hence, it is advisable to ensure that the patient listens to what is being told, by asking them questions like "are you there?", "do you listen to me?" etc. It involves asking the patient to recount what they have understood.
- Be clear that the patient did not misunderstand the nature of disease, the gravity of situation, or the realistic course of disease with or without treatment options.

Summarize

The physician has to summarize the session and the concerns expressed by the patient during the session.

It essentially highlights the main points of their transaction. Treatment/care plans for the future has to be put in nutshell.

A written summary is appreciable, as the patients usually take in very little when they are anxious.

Breaking Bad news about Serious Disease

Your Role: You Are SHO In The Medical Ward
Problem: Breaking Bad News
Patient: Miss. Sheila Whiteman, A 29 Year-Old Woman

Please Read The Scenario Printed Below. When The Bell Sounds, Enter The Room. You Have 14 Minutes For Your Consultation With The Patient/Relative, 1 Minute To Collect Your Thoughts And 5 Minutes For Discussion. You May Make Notes If You Wish.

Where Relevant, Assume You Have The Patient's Consent To Discuss Their Condition With The Relative/Surrogate.

Scenario:

Sheila Was Admitted To The Medical Ward Because Of PUO For 6 Weeks Duration. On Detailed History And Careful Examination, She Has Cervical And Left Axillary Lymph Nodes In Which An Excisional Lymph Node Biopsy Was Taken Last Week, And Today The Pathology Lab. Rings You Informing That The Diagnosis Is High Grade Non Hodgkin Lymphoma. Sheila's Mother Died Last Year From Cancer Breast, And She Was Her Next Of Kin And Suffered With Her During Her Treatment Course. She Is Married And Recently Gave Birth To A 5 Month Old Girl, And Her Mother In Law Is Taking Care Of Her Baby At The Moment.

Your Task Is To Break The Bad News.

Do Not Examine The Patient

Do Not Take A History

Any Notes You Make Must Be Handed To The Examiners At The End Of The Station.

Action Plan

1. **Greeting**
2. **Introduce Yourself Including Your Role**
3. **Confirm Your Patient Identity**
4. **Establish Rapport (Break The Ice)**

   "How Are You Feeling In Yourself Now Mrs. Whiteman? "

   "Do You Feel Any Improvement Since Your Admission To The Hospital?"
5. **Explain The Aim Of The Appointment**

   Always Remember The Task Written In The Scenario

- You Should Be Able To Address The Expected Legal And Ethical Issues In Your Scenario From The Written Information Provided Before Entering The Station.
- Inform Sheila That You Are About To Tell Her The Biopsy-"Snip"- Result. Offer To Speak Privately In A Quiet Room, And Always Ask The Patient If She Wants Anyone Else To Be Attending. Such An Introduction May Let Her Feel That There Is Something Serious In That Discussion.

6. **Explore The Situation** (Let The Patient Speak In Order To Unify The Agendas)

Here You Must Address The Following

- Patient Idea
- Patient Concern
- Medical Situation And Is She Understanding Why She Had The Biopsy Done??
- Her Expectations In Terms Of The Biopsy Result

7. **(The Warning Shot)**

- Start by explaining the background of the situation and medical condition, which may confirm her understanding to the nature of disease and cascade of events or not. E.G. "As You Said Mrs. Whiteman, You Came To The Hospital With The Problem Of Raised Body Temperature And Then We Discovered Another Problem Which Are The Lumps Behind Your Jaw And Below Your Arm Pits. To Be Perfectly Honest, Our Conventional Blood Tests Failed To Clarify The Exact Reason For That, And Maybe That's Why We Thought About Doing More Complex And Invasive Tests In Order To Find Out What Is Going On, And To Exclude Other Serious Causes"
- Fire The Warning Shot. "I'm Afraid The Result Of Your Biopsy Is Back And It Shows An Unfavorable Abnormality"
- You Must Use Facial Expressions And Non Verbal Cues Here. It Is Mandatory.
- Let The Patient Speak And Raise Her Expectations. The Possibilities are:
  - **Ask For Further Clarification:** e.g. "What Do You Mean By Unfavorable?". Here it is preferred to reply with another vague Answer – another warning shot-as "Unfortunately It Did Not Show Something Simple To Treat As An Infection Or So, But It Showed A Much Serious Condition".
  - **The Patient May Ask A Direct Question:** e.g. "Is It Cancer?". Here You Confirm The Diagnosis By Non Verbal Cues First (Head Nodding And Sympathetic Facial Expressions), Then Say Clearly "Yes", And Keep Silent (The Golden Silence).

8. **Give The Patient Time To Digest The Information, And React To It. The Reactions Could Be (One/Some/Or All) Of The Following:**

- *Denial:* Politely Say That You Understand How She Feels And Confirm That The Result Is Hers'.
- *Anger:* Some Patients May Even Insult The Person Giving The Bad News. It Is Preferred Not To React And Usually Patients Do Apologies For Being Rude Later On.
- *Blame:* The Patient May Blame Someone Else, For Example She May Blame Her GP For Delaying Investigating Her Medical Condition Especially If The Cancer Is Untreatable And Disseminating. Keep Silent And Let The Patient Breath Out.
- *Hope:* Here, You Should Start To Speak Again, As The Patient Would Seek Help As They Will Feel Helpless. It Is Your Duty To Reassure Them But Avoid Giving (False Hopes), E.G. "Mrs

Whiteman, I Need To Reassure You This Is Not The End Of The Road, And I'm Sure That We Could Help You If You Accept That".

9. Concerns

The Patient May Ask You Some Detailed Questions In That Stage And May Rise Loads Of Concerns, You Have To Manage All Of These Concerns. Some Of The Expected Concerns:

- Am I Going To Die Like My Mother?
- Is It Treatable?
- Is It Spreading?
- Am I Having Chemotherapy? Irradiation? Both?
- Will My Hair Fall?
- I Have A Newly Born Baby Girl, Who Will Take Care Of Her?

10. You Are Not Alone

- You will need the help of many health care members in this scenario.
- You will need to involve your consultant, and seek the opinion of Hematologist, Oncologist, McMillan nurse if needed, ...etc. They will give a global picture about the patient's situation, and would answer many of her questions and manage her concerns.

11. Make Sure Your Patient Understands Your Plans And Apologies For Breaking The Bad News.

It Would Be Nice If You Offer Any Type Of Appropriate Help To Show Empathy For The Patient e.g. "Is There Anything I Can Do For You Now? Are You Alright? "

12. End Of Appointment

E. Difficult Situations

I) Difficult Persons

It Could Be A Difficult Patient Being Angry Or Non-Compliant, Or Could Be One Of Your Colleagues Acting Inappropriately.

The Angry Patient:
- Could Be Angry For A Mistake That Harmed Himself Or One Of His Family.
- In Such A Situation You Need To Let Him Speak And Breath Out Without Interruption. You Should Try To Calm Your Patient Down And Put Him At Ease.
- You Need To Explore What Happened And If It Appears To Be A Clear Mistake, Then Deal As (Break In The System). If The Situation Is Not A Clear Mistake, Then It Could Be Either Misunderstanding Or Patient High Expectation.
- Again, Explain Quietly With An Appropriate Voice Tone And Good Nonverbal Cues.

The Non-Compliant Patient:
- This Patient Needs Help. He Definitely Has A *Reason* For His Attitude That Was Not Explored Before, And That Would Be Your Task.
- It Could Be Related To *Medications* As Drug Form, Dosage, Timing, Side Effects, Or That Drug Could Be Affecting His Appearance, Social Issues As His Occupation Or His Sexual Life For Example.
- Noncompliance Could Be Related To Other Aspects Not Necessarily Medications. Some Patients Are Not Compliant To *Medical Advice* As Smoking Cessation, Or They May Not Be Keen To Attend Their Clinic Appointments For Example. If You Manage To Explore Their Reasons You May Suggest Simple Solutions Like Referring A Smoker To The Smoking Cessation Clinic For Example, Or Sorting Clinic Appointments In Another Suitable Time For The Patient Or Even Another Suitable Site Within Your Trust If The Case Turns To Be Related To Long Distance Between Patients' Home And Your Current Hospital.
- When You Talk With A Non-Compliant Patient, Always Ask Him About:
  - How Is He Coping With His Condition?
  - Is He Taking His Medications Regularly?
  - If Not Why?
  - What Does He Expect His Condition To Be Without Treatment?
  - Does He Know The Risks Of Not Taking His Medications/ Doing The Procedure?
- Don`t Confront Your Patient, Or Threaten Him.
- Always Keep Yourself Calm And Polite.
- Always Try To Convince A Non-Compliant Patient By Telling Him Reasons That Could Be Related To Him And His Health, Also To The Public Health.
- If He Is Still Non-Compliant Tell Him More Reasons And Even Serious Ones:
- People Not Taking Important Medications Could Endanger Their Lives
- Doctors With Needle Stick Injuries Who Don`T Inform Their Health Team Could Lose Their Gmc Registration
- Seek, Detect And Manage Any Non-Compliant Concerns; If You Reassure Him About His Concerns He Will Be Compliant.

E.G.1: Patient HIV +Ve, Afraid To Tell His Wife: reply
"Well, I Am Afraid That If She Know That She Is HIV +Ve Because Of You She Could Go The Court And Sue You , Imagine Yourself When You Were First Diagnosed With Having HIV How Did You Feel , Would You Be Happy That Your Beloved Wife Feel The Same Feeling, You Know That You Might Be Risking The Health Of Your Beloved Wife , And The Virus Might Spread In Her Body And Cause Her To Have Low Defense Mechanisms And Get A Lot Of Infections And Die; Because Of You. Instead You Can Tell Her And She Can Get Tested And If She Is HIV +Ve She Can Also Start Treatment".

E.G.2: A Singer Patient With Asthma Afraid To Take Inhalers: reply

"Why Did You Stop Taking Your Inhalers? Are You Worried About Your Voice? Well If You Rinse And Wash Your Mouth Regularly You Will Not Face This Problem, But If You Don`t Take The Inhalers As Prescribed, I Am Afraid That You Might Get A Severe Asthma Attack That Might Obstruct Your Airways Completely, Which I Am Afraid To Say Might End Your Life".

E.G.3: <u>A Taxi Driver With Epilepsy Doesn't Want To Inform The DVLA about his illness:</u> reply

"I Am Afraid That You Could Get This Attack While You Are Driving Which Could Be Very Serious For You And May Put Your Life At Risk.
" "You If You Are Driving, Imagine Yourself Driving Your Child Home And You Got This Fit Which Would Stop You From Thinking And Even Hitting The Brakes, You Will Get An Accident With Your Beloved Son, Which I Am Afraid Might End Your Life".
"So For Your Health And For The Public Health You Should Inform The DVLA"".
If The Patient Still Refuses To Inform DVLA, Tell Him That You As A Doctor Taking Care Of Him And Aware With His Heath Issues Are In A Legal Responsibilty As His Attitude Puts A Third Party In Danger, And That You It Would Be Your Duty To (Breech His Confidentiality) And Inform The DVLA.
If The Patient Seizes During Driving And Injures A Third Party Whilst He Is Banned From Driving, He Will Be Sent To The Court.

E.G.4: <u>A Doctor With Needle Stick Injury Doesn't Want To Inform The Hospital Occupational Health Team:</u> reply

"Well, It Is Better To Inform Them And Stop Dealing With Blood, They Might Arrange For You Another Job Not Dealing With Blood, And You Know That This Carries Risks To Your Patients" I Am Afraid To Say If You Don`t Inform Them I Will Have To Take Advise From A Senior Colleague In A Very Confidential Way But I Am Afraid It Might Reach The GMC".

E.G.5: <u>A Patient With Asthma Concerned To Gain Weight If She Takes Steroids Tablets:</u> reply

"I Assure You We Will Be Giving You The Least Required Dose, And You Will Check With Us Regularly And I Will Arrange For You An Appointment With The Dietician So That You Don`t Gain Any Weight".
"I Am Afraid If You Don't Take Them You Might Get A Severe Asthma Attack That Could Obstruct Your Airways Completely And End Your Life".

E.G.6: <u>Air Hostess With IDDM Admitted With DKA, Doesn't Want To Inform Her Occupational Director:</u> reply

"I Am Afraid You Get Another Attack When You Are On The Plane And There Is No One To Help You, And The Next Airport Will Be Hours Away Which I Am Afraid Might End Your Life".
"Instead You Can Work As A Ground Hostess You Will See The Planes Taking Off And Landing, You Will Wear The Same Clothes And Meet Your Friends".

The Inappropriate Colleague:
- Inappropriate Behavior Is An Attitude That Risks Patient Safety Or Offends The Surrounding Colleagues Physically Or Emotionally. Examples For That Is An Aggressive Colleague, Antisocial Colleague, Unprofessional Colleague, Drunk Colleague, Or A Colleague Watching Inappropriate Sexual Material During His Duty.
- Again Your Colleague Needs Help. He May Not Be Aware That His Attitude Is Risky And Offending, Or He May Not Be Medically Knowledgeable Enough And Is Embarrassed To Ask Others. Sometimes The Situation Could Be Related To Alcohol Dependence Or Even Depression. Other Times He May Be Aware With The Problem But Is Not Able To Solve His

Own Problems. All These Examples Could Be Managed With Simple Solutions Only If Explored Properly.

- He Needs To Understand That His Attitude May Affect Patient Safety And Would Affect His Career, Or That His Attitude Is Offending Other Colleagues As Doctors, Nurses, Healthcare Workers, Etc.
- Approach Him In A Friendly Way, And Always Offer Him A Cup Of Tea Before The Conversation.
- In A Smart Way, Tell Him That You Accidently Discovered His Inappropriate Behavior Without Attempting To Breech His Confidentiality, And That His Behavior Raised Some Concerns.
- He May Have A Personal Reason For His Attitude, And You May Guide Him To A Possible Solution He Is Not Aware Of. Always Offer Help Or Suggest Someone Or Some Service That May Help, And Remember (You Are Not Alone). He May Accept Your Advice Or Act Aggressively.
- If He Insists To Be Aggressive And Keeping The Inappropriate Behavior Tell Him That His Behavior Puts Patients' Safety At Risk, And It Is Your Responsibility To Inform His Consultant Or Supervisor, And That May Threat His GMC Registration.
- If Your Colleague Is Unsafe At The Moment He Is On Duty (E.G. Drunk Or Confused), He Should Leave His Shift Immediately, And The Present Colleagues Should Cover Him.

II) Critical Situations

DISCUSSING RESUSCITATION

- Cardiopulmonary Resuscitation Is A Medical Decision In The First Place.
- Usually Discussed With The Patient To Let Him Know; You Should Convince Him As If You Are Considering Yourself In His Place, But Again This Is A Medical Team Decision
- Can Be Discussed With The Relatives If The Patient Is Incompetent, But Again It Is A Medical Team Decision; You Should Ask About:
  - o The Patient`s Wishes
  - o Any Living Will
  - o Power Of Attorney
- If A Patient Wishes Not To Be Resuscitated You Should Talk With Him If He Is Fit For Resuscitation And Try To Convince Him, But If He Refuses You Should Respect His Wish (Autonomy).
- On The Other Hand Some Patients Are Very Frail With Multiple Comorbidities And From The Medical Point Of View It Would Be Futile To Resuscitate Them If Their Heart Stops. This Needs To Be Explained In Details To The Patient, In Addition To The Steps Of Resuscitation. If You Feel That Resuscitation Is Not In The Patients Best Interest You May Describe Resuscitation As An (Uncomfortable) Maneuver, Like Saying Putting Big Tubes In The Throat, And Jumping On The Chest To Do Forceful Compressions, And Always Remember To Use The Word (Futile).
- If The Patient Goes With Not Attempting Resuscitation, Let Him Know That You Will Form The Red Form Or The (DNAR) Form, And It Will Be Placed In His Medical Notes.
- The Patient May Change His Mind Anytime As Long As He Is Competent.

Ceiling Of Care:

- This Meaning Sorting A Future Medical Plan For The Patient In Terms Of How Far Should We Escalate The Level Of His Care If He Deteriorates?
- It Depends On Patient Premorbid Life Style, Quality Of Life, Mobility And Situation At Home Plus His Comorbidities And Prognosis.

In Patients With Poor QOL And Poor Prognosis It Could Be Just (Ward Based) Which Means That He Will Receive Conventional Treatment, And If He Gets Worse, No Escalating To HDU Or ITU As It would Be Futile.

Discussing DNR

<u>Your Role:</u> You Are SHO In The Medical Ward
<u>Problem:</u> Discussing DNR
<u>Patient:</u> Mr J.B., A 80 Year-Old Man

Please Read The Scenario Printed Below. When The Bell Sounds, Enter The Room. You Have 14 Minutes For Your Consultation With The Patient/Relative, 1 Minute To Collect Your Thoughts And 5 Minutes For Discussion. You May Make Notes If You Wish.

Where Relevant, Assume You Have The Patient's Consent To Discuss Their Condition With The Relative/Surrogate.

Scenario:

An 80 Years Old Patient With Severe COPD, Who Was Admitted To The ITU Twice This Year And The Last Admission He Was Difficult To Be Weaned From The Ventilator. Today he is admitted again with a COPD exacerbation and he is doing very poorly. His Most Recent FEV1 done after last admission is 20%. His ABG is marginally maintained to Non Invasive Ventilation, but the medical team thinks that he may not pull through his illness this time. You were asked to Speak with Him Re: Resuscitation

Do Not Examine The Patient

Do Not Take A History

Any Notes You Make Must Be Handed To The Examiners At The End Of The Station.

Action Plan

1. EXPLORE THE PATIENT'S KNOWLEDGE AND EXPECTATIONS ABOUT CONDITION

- "So Mr..., What Do you Know About your Condition? How Do you Expect It To Be?"

2. EXPLORE THE PATIENT'S WISHES

- "May I Ask If your Condition Deteriorates and your heart stops, What Do you Want Us To Do?"

3. EXPLAIN CPR BRIEFLY

- "Do You have any idea what is cardiopulmonary resuscitation"

4. EXPLAIN CPR, THE TAKEN DECISION AND ITS REASONS

- "I Spoke To My Consultant And The Medical Team, And He We Believe That IN TERMS OF YOUR Current Severe Illness And In Presence Of Your Multiple Comorbidities, If We Manage To Carry Out CPR If Your Heart Stops It Would Be Futile, Moreover CPR At This Stages Will Have Poor Outcomes And Even If It Works It Will Just Be Prolonging Your Days Of Suffering And Would Lead To A Very Poor Quality Of Life ".
- "CPR Is A Maneuver That We Do If The Heart Stops. The Best Outcomes Are For Previously Fit Patients With No Heart Or Lung Problems, However It Is Doubtful If There Is A Background Of Many Comorbidities And Chronic Medical Diseases. We Need To Do Massage For Your Heart And You May Need To Be Exposed In An Undignified Way. Furthermore, We Would Need To Introduce Big Tubes In Your Airways, And Do Forceful Compressions To Our Chest And Heart, And You May Have Fracture Ribs."
- "I Am So Sorry To Tell You That, And That's Why We Think That Its In Your Best Interest To Be Declared Not For Resuscitation."
- "I Assure You That Your Basic Medical & Nursing Care Will Not Be Affected".
- "If You Want A Second Opinion, I Can Arrange For A Second Opinion For You".

Post-Mortem Examinations

A) Post Mortem Autopsy

- Usually Obtaining Consent For Autopsy Is Done When The Patient Dies Under Your Care And You Don`t Know The Exact Cause Of Death.
- Usually You Speak With The Relatives About What Happened And What You Are Suspecting And Try To Convince Them To Do A Post-Mortem For The Deceased To Be Sure About The Diagnosis.
- Unlike The Coroner Post-Mortem, There Will Be No Delay In The Funeral And You Will Sign The Death Certificate For The Family To Arrange For The Funeral.
- You Should Assure Them That The Deceased Person`s Dignity Will Be Respected All Through The Procedure And That No Scars Will Be Evident On The Day Of The Funeral.
- In Obtaining Consent For Autopsy You Should :
  o Break The Bad News As Usual
  o Explain To Them Your Suspicions & Request The Post-Mortem
  o Explain To Them The Procedures And Assure Them About The Death Certificate And That There Will Be No Delay In The Funeral
  o Convince Them About Its Importance
  o Obtain Consent.

Action Plan

BREAK THE BAD NEWS

What Do You Know So Far? Well, I Am Afraid Things Didn't Go As We Hoped?
We Were All Beside Him, We Were Taking Care Of Him, But Suddenly Something Strange Happened, He Had Another Chest Pain , We Gave Him Medications , And We Did For Him Life Saving Maneuvers But Unfortunately He Didn't Respond To Our Maneuvers
So What Do You Expect Your Father Condition Was?

EXPLAIN YOU SUSPICIONS AND REQUEST THE POSTMORTEM

Well, We Are Astonished About What Happened? We Don't Know What Happened To Him? It Could Be Something Hidden Or Other Illness He Had That We Didn't Know About, It Could Be Something Running In The Family , That's Why In order To Get A Firm Diagnosis About What Happened We Need To Do Another Test , Have You Heard About A Postmortem?

EXPLAIN THE PROCEDURE

An Experienced Pathologist With The Help Of A Technician They Will Make A Small Clean Cut In Ur Fathers Body, And Examine The Organs Of Suspicion , Sometimes They May Need To Take A Snip And Examine It Under Microscope , Some Times We Need To Retain Organs For Research Purpose But If U Deny That I Assure U No Organ Will Be Missing, After The Procedure He Will Be Dressed Cleanly And No Scar Will Be Visible On The Funeral Day, U Can Come And Have A Look On Him After The Procedure , There Will Be No Delay In The Funeral , I Will Sign The Death Certificate Now For U / I Will Arrange The Concent For U To Sign /I Can Give U Time To Think About It And To Inform Other Family Members

CONVINCE THEM

The Relative May Say (What Difference Could This Make After His Death); Respond:
- It Could Be Something Running In The Family, A Disease Or A Condition That The Family Doesn't Know About, We Don't Want Any Member Of The Family To Suffer The Same Situation
- Also In order To Be Sure That He Was Not Withheld Any Treatment Could Have Saved Him
- Also Families Deal Better With Bereavement When They Know The Cause Of Death
- And This Will Give The Team Further Experience Which Will Help Them In Any Future Situations

- I Assure You His Dignity Will Be Preserved All Through The Procedure, And After The Procedure He Will Be Dressed Cleanly With No Wounds Visible On The Day Of The Funeral
- There Will Be No Delay In The Funeral And I Will Sign The Death Certificate For You Now

OBTAIN CONSENT

- Shall I Arrange The Consent For You To Sign?
- If They Refuse The Whole Thing; Thank Her And Assure Her That The Procedure Is Not Going To Be Carried On,
- If They Agree, Arrange An Appointment For Her With The Consultant To Discuss The Results Of The Post Mortem

B) CORONER POST-MORTEM

- The Coroner Post-Mortem Is Done By The Coroner Who Is An Independent Officer Responsible For The Legal Investigation Of Death.
- Coroner Post-Mortem Is A Must And No Need For A Proxy Consent In The Following Situations:
  - Death On Table During A Procedure
  - Death During The 1st 24 Hours Of A Procedure
  - Death On Arrival To The Hospital
  - Accidents
  - Suspected Homicide
- You Can`t Sign The Death Certificate, Only The Coroner Will Sign It.
- You Should Explain To The Family What Happened And Slowly Break The Bad News, Then To Tell Them That You Need To Run One More Test To Get A Firm Diagnosis About The Patient`s Death Which Is The Coroner Post-Mortem, Explain The Procedure And Explain That It Is Out Of Your Hands, Only The Coroner Will Sign The Death Certificate.
- Unfortunately There Might Be A Delay In The Funeral
- After The Procedure Is Done A Representative Of The Coroner Will Contact The Family And Discuss With Them The Outcome.
- If The Relative Is Suspecting That Death During The Procedure Was Because The Doctors Were Incompetent And They Did Mistakes And Want To Make A Complaint; Assure The Relative That He Has All The Right To Make A Complaint, But To Do The Complaint We Should Know First The Exact Cause Of Death And That's Another Reason Why We Need The Post-Mortem.
- If The Relative Insists On Not Accepting The Procedure; Tell Her That This Is Out Of Your Hands And Now This Is A Legal Issue, And You Can`t Sign Any Death Certificate.
- You Don't Need The Relatives` Consent.

Action Plan

BREAK THE BAD NEWS

As Above

Well, He Had Bleeding From His Gullet Which Was A Massive One , He Lost A Lot Of Blood And We Needed To Do This Emergency Procedure To Stop This Bleeding, We Discuss It With Him And He Accepted The Procedure With Its Risks.

Actually The Procedure Was Done Successfully And He Was Transferred To The Ward, But After 30 Mins. Something Strange Happened; He Suddenly Lost Consciousness; We Tried To Give Him Medications To Support His Blood Pressure And Circulation But Unfortunately This Didn't Help, I Am So Sorry To Tell You This.

Then Suddenly We Noticed That His Heart Stopped, We Tried To Do For Him Life Saving Measures And Did For Him Chest Compression But I Am Sorry To Tell You That He Didn't Respond To Our Maneuverers.

EXPLAIN YOU SUSPICIONS AND INFROM THEM ABOUT THE DECISION TAKEN FOR POST-MORTEM

Well, We Are Astonished About What Happened? We Don't Know What Happened To Him? The Patient's Relative Might Say This Is Due To This Nasty Procedure, You Killed My Father, What Have You Done! I Want To Make A Complaint, I Will Sue You!

Actually We Are Not Sure About What Happened, It Could Be A Complication Of The Procedure And It Could Be Due To Another Illness That He Had And We Didn't Know About, Also It Could Be Something Running In The Family, That's Why In order To Get A Firm Diagnosis About What Happened And In order To Make A Complaint We Need To Know The Exact Cause Of Death **That's Why A Decision Has Been Made To Do A Coroner Postmortem,** Have You Ever Heard about It?

EXPLAIN THE PROCEDURE

The Coroner An Independent Officer Responsible For The Legal Investigation Of Death With The Help Of An Experienced Pathologist With The Help Of A Technician They Will Make A Small Clean Cut In Ur Fathers Body, And Examine The Organs Of Suspicion , After The Procedure He Will Be Dressed Cleanly And No Scar Will Be Visible On The Funeral Day, After The Procedure Is Done A Representative From The Coroner Office Will Contact You To Discuss With You The Outcomes And To Sign For You The Death Certificate.

CONVINCE THEM

The Relative May Say (What Difference Could This Make After His Death); Respond:

It Could Be Something Running In The Family, A Disease Or A Condition That The Family Doesn't Know About, We Don't Want Any Member Of The Family To Suffer The Same Situation Also To Be Sure That He Was Not Withheld Any Ttt Could Have Saved Him

Also Families Deal Better With Bereavement When They Know The Cause Of Death

And This Will Give The Team Further Experience Which Will Help Them In Any Future Situations

I Assure You His Dignity Will Be Preserved All Through The Procedure, And After The Procedure He Will Be Dressed Cleanly With No Wounds Visible On The Day Of The Funeral

Unfortunately This Is The Only Way To Get A Death Certificate, Only The Coroner Will Sign The Death Certificate

In Order To Make A Complaint We Need To Know First What The Cause Of Death Is.

I'M Sorry Its Out Of My Hands, I Cant Sign The Death Certificate, Only The Coroner Can Sign It And There Might Be Some Delay In The Funeral

My Deep Condalescence On Behalf Of Me And The Hospital Team

No Need To Obtain Consent, You Are Convincing The Relative Because If You Were In His Situation You Would Like To Be Convinced Rather Than Being Forced.

Brain Stem Death

The Diagnosis Of Brain Stem Death Is Done By 2 Consultants (Anaesthesia) Who Are Not Members Of The Organ Transplantation Team, Examining The Patient 24 Hours Apart By Examining The Following Reflexes And Diagnosis Brain Stem Death.

- Absent Pupillary Light Reflex
- Absent Corneal Reflex
- Absent Vestibule-Ocular Reflex
- Absent Cough Reflex
- Absent Gag Reflex
- Positive Apnea Test (Stopping The Ventilator Until The Pco2 Reaches 8 Kpa With No Attempts Of Breathing)

Usually The Patient Is Put On A Ventilator, And The Relatives Sees His Chest Is Moving Up And Down Which Makes It Hard For You To Convince Them That Their Beloved Relative Has Passed Away.

Usually You Have To Break The Bad News To The Patient And Convince Them You Are Going To Stop The Machines.

Off Course Stopping The Machines Is A Medical Team Decision, But You Should Put Yourself In The Relatives Place, You Would Like To Be Convinced Rather Than Being Forced With What Is Going To Happen.

Sometimes The Task Is More Difficult; When You Should Break The Bad News, Convince The Relatives You Will Stop The Machines And Ask For Organ Donation.

The Brain Stem Death Scenario Is Going To Be Discussed In The Following Scenario Of Asking For Organ Donation & Withholding Machines.

Withholding Machines

- This Is A Medical Team Decision. Document The Decision In The Patient`s Notes, No Need For An Informed Consent.
- Done When A Patient Is Diagnosed Of Having Brain Stem Death
- Discuss The Diagnosis Of Brain Stem Death With The Patient`s Family, And Inform Them That This Means The End Of Life And That It Is Unwise To Keep Him On Machines.
- Give The Family Time To Have A Last Look On The Patient And Take Spiritual Guidance.

Action Plan

ASK ABOUT THE PATIENT`S WISHES, ADVANCE DIRECTIVE, POWER OF ATTORNEY

- What Were His Wishes? Did He Express His Wishes Before?
- Has He Discussed With You If His Condition Deteriorates What Does He Want Us To Do?
- Has He Nominated Anybody To Take Decision On His Behalf? Is He Leaving A Living Will?

EXPLAIN HIS SITUATION

- Well, He Came To Us With ...., We Did ..., We Are Giving Him The Maximum Treatment He Could Have, We Are Giving Him Medication To Support His Heart And Increase. Its Performance, And Putting Him On Machines, But Unfortunately He Is Not Responding, So What Do You Expect Your Father Condition To Be?

EXPLAIN BRAIN STEM DEATH

- Well, Our Team Believes He Is Not Going To Regain His Consciousness Because The **Maestro Of The Brain Is Not Working Anymore; The Maestro Of The Brain Is The Vital Part Of The Brain Which Is Responsible For Our Breathing And Controlling Our Heart Beating**.

So It Is Unwise To Keep Him Suffering Anymore.

EXPLAIN THE DECISION OF WITHHOLDING THE MACHINES

- I Know It Is Very Hard Time For You Know, I Know It Is Very Difficult For You To Adsorb All This.
- I Will Give You Time To Tell Other Family Members To Come And Have A Last Look On Him.

Treatment Withdrawal

- Some Patients Especially Those With Multiple Comorbidities Respond Very Poorly To Treatment, And Instead Of Improving With The Full Medical Care They Continue To Deteriorate And Continuing To Treat Them Becomes Futile.
- If The Medical Team Tried Their Best Treating A Patient And They Feel That The Patient Is Extremely Poorly And Will Not Benefit Any More From Medical Treatment, Death Becomes Certain And We Usually Think About The **(Palliative Pathway)** And To Start The **(End Of Life Medications)**.
- If The Patient Is Competent He Must Take This Decision For Himself, And If Not Then The Next Of Kin And The Family Members.
- If The Patient And/or His Family Agree With The Medical Team About The End Of Life Decision, The Consultant Usually Fills A Special Form In The Patient Notes, And The Patient Will Be Referred To The (Palliative Nurse) That Will Assess Him And Sort A Plan For The Few Remain Days.
- The Patient May Stay In The Hospital In A Side Room To Allow His Family Spend As Much Time As Possible With Him, Or The Family May Prefer To Take Him Home Or Place Him In A Hospice If The Team Thinks That He May Last For A Bit Longer.
- The End Of Life Medications Are Medications That Should Keep The Patient Comfortable, Avoiding Agitation Or Excessive Respiratory Secretion, And Controlling Pain. These Medications Are Not Killing The Patient i.e (Not Active Euthanasia), But Keeping The Patient Comfortable Till His Time Comes And Makes Him Die In Peace.
- The Patient Then Is Withdrawn From Any Form Of Active Treatment, And In Most Cases The End Of Life Medications Are Given Subcutaneously By A Syringe Driver.

E.G. A COPD Patient With Poor Lung Functions Presents With A COPD Infective Exacerbation. Started Conventional Antibiotics But Continues To Deteriorate. She Developed Type 2 Respiratory Failure And At The Moment She Is On Non Invasive Ventilation On The Medical Ward. ABGs Not Improving On (NIV). Antibiotics Has Been Escalated With No Improvement. CT Chest Shows Right Sided Consolidation With Bilateral Effusions More On The Right Side With No Evidence Of Hidden Malignancy. The Patient Has A Background Of CKD Maintained On HD And CCF Secondary To IHD With 2 Coronary Stents. Today He Started To Get Confused And CRP And WBCs Going Up. Assessed By ITU Doctors And They Feel He Is Not For ITU. Your Consultant Feels That The Patient Is For (End Of Life Pathway). You Will Speak To The Wife (NOK) And The Daughter.

<u>Action Plan</u>

Explore The Family Knowledge About The Seriousness Of The Patients' Condition.

- How Did You Find Him Today?
- Do You Think There Is Any Progress In His Condition?
- What Do You Know About His Current Illness?

Explore The Patients Situation At Home, Life Style, Mobility, And Premorbid Status. You Need To Confirm His Comorbidities As Well.

- Can You Tell Me More About The Situation At Home?
- How Did He Manage To Cope At Home?
- Was He Able To Help Himself At All?
- Was He Managing Dialysis? How Did He Go For Dialysis? Any Chest Pains Recently Or Recurrent Hospital Admissions?

Explain The Current Episode Of Illness And The Medical Efforts To Cure Him But That Turned To Be Futile.

- As You Know, He Is Having A Nasty Infection In His Lungs And It Seems That We Are Not Winning.
- We Tried Many Types Of Antibiotics, And Recently He Is On One Of The Most Potent Ones, But He Is Failing To Improve On The Contrary He Is Getting Worse.
- We Tried To Put Him On A Breathing Machine To Help His Lungs Recover But Unfortunately, Even On The Machine His Lungs Are Failing! And He Is Now Confused And Helpless To Help.
- We Think The Reason For That Is His Multiple Medical Comorbidities That Kept His Body Very Weak And Frail, Not Able To Cope With The Nasty Infection.
- He Was Seen By The ITU Doctors, And They Feel That He Won't Even Benefit From Escalating To ITU Or Even Resuscitation If His Heart Stops.
- We Believe At The Moment That He Is Really Struggling.

Find Out Any Previous Wishes Or Wills For The Patient, And Engage The Family In The Decision Making.

- Did He Have Any Wishes? Wills?
- Did He Nominate Someone To Take Decisions For Him If He Is Not Able To Do So?
- Is There A Power Of Attorney For You At All?

Tell Them About The "End Of Life Pathway" And That The Patient Will Be Comfortable.

- What Are Your Concerns And Expectations Now?
- In Such Cases We Think That We Reached The End Of The Road, And The Chances To Get Him Back Home Are Very Slim.
- The Medical Team Thinks That It Would Be Futile To Continue Giving Active Treatment And We Believe That Its best For Him To Let Him In Peace and start Putting Him On The (End Of Life) Pathway Would Be In His Best Interest. Do You Know Anything About End Of Life Pathway?
- When Patients Are Doing Very Poorly, Not Responding To Treatment And When They Seem To Be At The Edge Of The Cliff, We Put Them On That Treatment Protocol, Which Is Not Active Treatment But Some Kind Of Medications That Would Keep Them Comfortable And Allows Them To Spend The Remaining Days In Their Life Peacefully And Comfortably With No Pain At All.
- So At The Moment, We Are Aiming To Stop All Forms Of Active Treatment Including Medications, The Lung Machine, And Hemodialysis And Just Keep Him On These Palliative Medications I Mentioned Earlier.
- We Will Refer Him To The Palliative Nurse And She Will Come Shortly And Have A Chat With You About All The Other Details You May Like To Know About The Palliative Treatment.

Give Them Time To Think About The Issue, And Raise Their Concerns

- Is There Any Other Concerns?
- Any Questions For Me?
- Sorry For Giving The Bad News.
- Would You Like To Have Some Time Thinking About It And Speaking To Other Family Members?
- I Will Arrange Another Meeting Soon With My Consultant Until You Take A Decision, Until Then We Will Continue To Give Him The Full Active Medical Care.

Organ Donation

- An Organ Donation Card Is Not Considered As A Living Will.
- Organ Donation Will Do No Delay In The Funeral.
- HIV Testing Is Done Before Organ Donation.
- When Talking With Relatives Regarding An Incompetent Patient (A Person Who Lacks Capacity) Always Seek The Following:
  - o The Patient`s Wishes
  - o Is He Leaving A Living Will?
  - o Does Any One Of The Family Members Have A Power Of Attorney?

E.G. An 18 Years Old Patient Came Severely Injured In A Road Traffic Accident And Admitted Straight Away To ITU. His Father Was Told About The Accident And He Is On His Way To The Hospital. He Lives 500 Miles Away And Is Expected To Come Within The Coming 12 Hours. The Patient Develops A Respiratory Failure Secondary To ARDS, And Shortly He Had A Brain Stem Death. The Father Arrived Now And Your Task Is To Break The Bad News Of His Son's Death And Explore The Possibility Of Organ Donation.

Action Plan

BREAK THE BAD NEWS AS BEFORE AND EXPLAIN WHAT HAPPENED
- So What Do You Know So Far Mr.?
- What Do U Expect His Condition To Be?
- I Am Afraid Things Didn't Go As We Hoped?

FIRE AN INTRODUCTION PHRASE TO WHAT YOU WILL SAY
- Was Your Son A Kind Person?
- Did He Love To Help Other People?
- Did He Mention Anything About Organ Donation Before?
- And Have You Ever Thought About It?
- *If The Patient Is Holding An Organ Donation Card In His Pocket;*
  "Do U Know What We Have Found In His Pocket? Has He Mentioned Anything About Joining An Organ Donation Society?"

CONVINCE THE RELATIVE
- Your Sons Kidney Can Help Another Person To Have A Near Normal Life, A Lot Of People Are Having Kidney Damage, They Are Depending On Machines, They Are Not Leading A Normal Life And They Are Struggling, And There Is A Very Long Waiting List For Organ Transplantation.
- *If he is holding Organ Donation card:* This Was the Wish of You Son, He Was Looking Behind Life To Helping Other Sick People. Do You Want To Fulfill The Last Wish Of Your Beloved Son?

EXPLAIN THE PROCEDURE
- Well Our Experienced Team Of Organ Transplantation Will Make A Small Clean Cut And Take The Kidneys, And The Wound Will Be Closed Cleanly, And He Will Be Dressed Cleanly, His Dignity Will Be Respected All through The Procedure And No One Will Notice Any Wounds.
- There Will Be **No Delay In The Funeral**

- We Will Have To Do An HIV Testing For Your Son Before The Procedure

ARRANGE CONSENT
Ok I Will Arrange The Consent Form For You To Sign

N.B: *If The Relative Refuses The Procedure, Assure Him Nothing Will Be Done*

Counselling for Live Organ Donation

> **E.G.:** A Young Girl With CKD, Dialysis Dependent, Waiting For Cadaveric Renal Transplant For More Than 3 Years Now, And You Should Speak With The Mother To Explore Her Possible Intentions In Terms Of Coming Forward For A Live Kidney Donation.

EXPLORE KNOWLEDGE

- So Mrs..., What Do You Know About Your Daughter's Condition?
- Is She Coping With Dialysis?
- Do You Think That Dialysis Is Affecting Her Mood Or Her Life Style At All?
- Do You Know That Transplantation Is The Modality Of Choice For Renal Replacement If It Is Available?

EXPECTATIONS AND CONCERNS

- And What Do You Think We Can Do More For Her?
- Well, Waiting For A Cadaveric Transplant may take many Years, So We Are Thinking About Living Donation That Gives Even Better Results On The Long Term.

FIRE INTRODUCTIVE QUESTION

- Whom Do You Think Might Be Willing To Give Her A Kidney?
- What About You?
- Did You Ever Think About That?
- Do You Think That You May Be A Suitable Candidate For Organ Donation?
- Is There any Reason That Could Prevent You From Having A Major Surgery?
- Do you have any Serious Medical Conditions? Any Known Kidney Problems?

CONVINCE HER IF POSSIBLE

- You Will Give A Loved One Almost A Near Normal Quality Of Life
- It Will Be The Most Precious Gift Ever For Your Poor Daughter.
- Do You Know That Her Chances To Get Pregnant And Have A Safe Delivery Are Much Higher With Transplantation Than With Hemodialysis?

EXPLANATION OF THE PROCEDURE

- If That's Ok, You Have To Know Some Aspects About Donation
- You Will Have To Discuss It With Your Insurance.
- You Will Spend Some Time In The Hospital About 8-10 Days And 8-10 Weeks Off Work
- And You Are Going To Undergo Some Tests For Example Cross Matching, tissue typing, as well as a HIV Test, and Tests To Make Sure That You Don't Have Any Hidden Renal Disease And That Donation Would Be Safe For You In The First Place.
- Any Way I Will Arrange An Appointment For You With Our Renal Consultant And Our Transplant Surgeon Consultant To Discuss This Better With you, and another appointment with our Transplant Coordinator.

New Therapy

(Enrolment In Clinical Trials)

EXPLAIN CONDITION AND TREATMENT OPTIONS
- So What Do You Know ABOUT YOUR Condition & Treatment Options

EXPLAIN THE NEW RESEARCH
Explain That The Hospital Is Conducting A Study On A Drug That Decreases Acid Secretion For Example, Which Might Be Better Than The Other Drugs Used And Of Superior Benefit In Controlling his Symptoms, If He Wants To Enroll Himself In This Research , Also This Research Would Be Conducted Under Supervision Of Your Consultant

So Do You Wish To Enroll Yourself In This Study?

You Should Explain

- Efficacy
- Why Is It Superior To Other Drugs
- Side Effects

OBTAIN CONSENT
So Shall I Arrange The Consent For You To Sign?

Medical Researches
- Should Be Done For The Sake Of Human Material & Data, With Maintain The Wellbeing Of Human Subjects.
- Only Done If The Importance Outweigh The Risks & Burdens Of Subjects
- Always Discuss Everything With The Patient An Obtain Consent

Patient Requesting Genetic Testing For A Well Known Inherited Disease Running In The Family

- If The Disease Is Manageable And Treatable E.G. (Adult Polycystic Kidney Disease), Then It Could Be Helpful To Aid Diagnosis, Try Avoid Reaching ESRD As Much As Possible And Early Follow Up And Planning For Renal Replacement Therapy.
- In This Case, You May Refer The Patient To The Outpatient Renal Clinic For Further Assessment And Proper Investigations.
- On The Other Hand, If The Disease Is Untreatable E.G. Huntington's Chorea, And The Patient Is Asymptomatic At The Time Of Consultation You Need To Explore The Reason For That And Warn The Patient That If The Test Turns To Be Positive It May Affect The Mood And May Have A Bad Psychological Impact.
- Inform the patient that his insurance may be affected if the test turns to be positive.
- You May Advice The Patient To Live Life In A Normal Way And Avoid Thinking Negatively, However If The Patient Insists To Have The Test For Personal Reasons Say That You Will Have A Word With Your Consultant And Specialist Nurses About The Nature Of The Test And That You Will Go Back To The Patient Either By Contacting Him Or Sorting An Appointment In The Clinic.

Patient Requesting New Form Of Treatment

- Check The Source Of Information E.G (Internet, Other Patient, Family Recommendation, Second Medical Opinion).
- Explore How The Patient Is Coping With His Current Treatment Form And If There Are Any Modifiable Difficulties.
- The Treatment May Not Be Suitable For This Patient Individually For A Reason Or Another E.G. (Rheumatoid Arthritis Patient Not Fit For Biological Therapy Due To Latent T.B, APKD Patient Not Fulfilling Criteria For Tolvaptan Therapy, Drug Is Under Trial Or Very Expensive And Funding Would Be Very Difficult).
- It Is Better To Refer The Patient To The Specialist As In Most Cases You Will Not Be Fully Aware With The New Form Of Treatment.

Counselling About Needle Stick Injury

- Needle Stick Injuries Are Common
- There Is A Risk Of Transmission Of:
  - HBV 30 %
  - HCV 3%
  - HIV 0.3 %
- Assure Him That A Lot Of Doctors Are Exposed To Needle Stick Injuries Throughout Their Career And Most Of Them Are Free From Blood Born Pathogens.
- Always Ask About:
  - Type Of Needle
  - If He Was Wearing Gloves
  - If He Washed His Hands
  - His HBV Vaccination Status
  - The Patient`s HBV,HCV,HIV Status
- Never Accept That The Healthcare Worker Exposed To Needle Stick Injury To Do Blood Tests For The Patient For HIV, HBV, HCV Without His Consent. It Could Be A Proxy Oral Consent But Should Be Documented In His Notes.
- If The Patient Is Known To Be HIV +Ve Give Post Exposure Prophylaxis = Zidovudine + Lamivudine For 28 Days)
- If Pregnant= Zidovudine & Lamivudine Are Safe , Do Ceserian Section , Never To Breast Feed , Risk Is 30% For Vertical Transmission And Use Safe Sex Methods

Action Plan

LET HIM EXPLAIN WHAT HAPPENED AND REASSURE
- Could You Explain To Me What Happened?
- Calm Down and Don't Panic, It Is Manageable. No worries.

ASSESS CIRCUMSTANCES AND THE RISK
- What Kind Of Needles?
- Sharp Or Blunt Needle?
- Did You Bleed A lot?
- Were You Wearing Gloves?
- Did You Wash Your Hands?
- Did You Take HBV Vaccine In The Past?
- Have You Measured Your Antibody Response Before?
- Did You Complete The Course?
- Do U Know The HIV, HBV, HCV Status Of The Patient?

KNOWLEDGE AND RISKS OF NEEDLE STICK INJURIES
- So What Do You Know About Needle Stick Injuries, And Its Risks?

INFORMING THE HOSPITAL OCCUPATIONAL HEALTH TEAM
- Well, You Have To Inform The Hospital Occupational Health Team For Further Advice, As It Could Be Risky For The Mean Time To Continue To Practice As A Surgeon. I Think Infection Control as well should be involved.

EXPLAIN THE MANAGEMENT PLAN
- Well , We Will Have To Measure Your Antibodies Now Then In 3 Months , Then In 6 Month , Then You Will Be Claimed Clear To Go To Work Again , And If The Hospital Occupational Health Team and Infection Control Team Are Suspecting The Patient Is High Risk For HBV,

Or HIV We Will Have To Start Post-Exposure Prophylaxis, *In The Form Of* Zidovudine, Lamivudine , Indinavir For HIV For 28 Days ,HBV Immunoglobulins + Vaccine , If Known Responsive To Vaccine =One Shot Of Vaccine .

- We Can Always Check The Doses And Forms Of Prophylaxis With The Microbiologist As Well.
- Also Meanwhile You Will Need To Use Barrier, And Don't Attempt to Donate Blood.
  You Will Have To Stop Working As A Surgeon In The Mean Time, And Inform The Hospital Occupational Health Team , Might Find You Another Medical Job For The Mean Time Not Dealing With Exposure Prone Procedure Or With Patients Until You Are Declared Clear To Work .
- I`M Sorry To Tell U That The GMC Guidance Enforces Me To Take Advice From My Consultant In A Strictly Confidential Way, But I`M Afraid It May Reach The GMC.
- A lot Of Doctors Are Exposed To Needle Stick Injuries Through Out Their Career, And Most Of Them Are Free.
- If +Ve Results You Can Claim For Compensation.

Surgeon +Ve HIV/HBV

HISTORY OF THE INFECTION
- How Did You Get It? For How Long?
- If It Is From Needle Stick Injury Did You Inform The Occupational Health Team And Did An Incident Report To Claim For Compensation?
- Have You Received HBV Vaccination
- Do You Have Any Symptoms For HIV/ HBV?

MANAGEMENT
- Same As For Needle Stick Injury Regarding Doing Blood Tests For Other Viruses
- Do Specific Investigations For The Virus He Has
- Give Specific Therapy For The Virus He Has
- Same Precautions As Previously Mentioned
- Informing The Occupational Health Team
- You Can Disclose Your Concerns About A Doctor Practice Under The Public Interest Disclosure Act

Notifiable Diseases

Notification To Health Protection Agency Who Will Trace The Patient's Contacts, Test And Treat Them.

Notifiable Diseases Are:

- Acute Encephalitis
- Acute Infectious Hepatitis
- Acute Meningitis
- Acute Poliomyelitis
- Anthrax
- Botulism
- Brucellosis
- Cholera
- Diphtheria
- Enteric Fever (Typhoid Or Paratyphoid Fever)
- Food Poisoning
- Haemolytic Uraemic Syndrome (Hus)
- Infectious Bloody Diarrhoea
- Invasive Group A Streptococcal Disease
- Legionnaires' Disease
- Leprosy
- Malaria
- Measles
- Meningococcal Septicaemia
- Mumps
- Plague
- Rabies
- Rubella
- SARS
- Scarlet Fever
- Smallpox
- Tetanus
- Tuberculosis
- Typhus
- Viral Haemorrhagic Fever (Vhf)
- Whooping Cough
- Yellow Fever

Pregnancy

- You May Come Through A Pregnant Female With An Underlying Medical Condition And Your Task May Be Anything From The Previous Ways Mentioned Before.
- If You Are Able To Memorize The Safe Medications During Pregnancy Then Well Done, However If You Couldn't You Could Always Go Back To A Senior Collegue Or Your BNF, And Then Inform The Patient.

DRUGS & PREGNANCY

Before Prescribing Any Medication To A Pregnant Or Breast Feeding Women You Should Be Aware About Its Safety First; Here Are Some Examples:

Thyrotoxicosis
- Carbimazole/Propylthiouracil , B-Blockers Are Safe
- Carbimazole = Agranulocytosis = Sorethroat , Do Regular FBC

Tuberculosis
- Rifampicin/Inh/Pyrazinamide Are Safe
- Streptomycin/Ethambutol Are Contraindicated

HIV
- Zidovudine /Lamivudine Are Safe

Asthma
- All Are Safe Except Montelukast

Antiepileptic
- Carbamazepine / Phenytoin/Phenobarbitol = Neural Tube Defects
- Lamotrigine Is Safe

SLE
- Steroids , Azathioprine , Bbs , Calcium Chennel Blockers = Safe
- Methotrextae , ACE Inhibitors , Cyclophosphamide Are Contraindicated

Myasthenia Gravis
- Neostigmine & Atropine Are Safe
- Pyridostigmine , Muscle Relaxants Are Not Safe
- Plasma Pharesis Is Safe

Anticoagulants
- Warfarin Contraindicated In 1st And 3rd Trimester

Hepatitis
- Ribavirin Is Safe
- Interferon is Contraindicated

The Epileptic Pregnant

- If a female is controlled on a teratogenic medication and gets pregnant then the situation is very tricky.
- You would need To Involve a Consultant Neurologist, to maintain the patient on the least effective dose of the teratogenic antiepileptic, or to switch her to a different one if he feels that is appropriate.
- An Obstetrician Should Be Involved Early As Well, Not Only The Midwife.
- This patient will need close monitoring.

- However, the risks Hazards that may affect the mother and her fetus if she seizes during pregnancy are life threatening. So avoiding antiepileptics during pregnancy is not an option.
- If You Are Counselling A Female In The Child Bearing Period And She Is About To Start Antiepileptics For A Reason Or Another Remember That Most Antiepileptics Are Drug Inducers, And May Affect The Dose Of Oral Contraceptive Drugs. Barrier Contraception Is Always A Good Solution If You Are In Doubt, Or Until You Seek Help From An Expert.

Tuberculosis

- You Need To Explore Some Aspects If Your Task Is To Approach A Tuberculous Patient. You Need To Find Out:
  o Is The Patient Symptomatic?
  o Ethnic Background?
  o Risk Factors E.G. (DM, Immunosuppressed, Smoker)
  o Contact With Sick Patients Or Sick Family Members?
  o Occupation? In Close Contact With Public?
  o Accommodation Issues? Shared Accommodation?
  o Is The Patient Contagious? Is He Risky In The Community? Open T.B?
  o Will He Need Admission? Isolation?
  o You May Need To Screen Contacts.
- Some Patients Are Not Aware That Tuberculosis Is A Serious Disease, And They Deal With It As A Normal Chest Infection. You Must Rectify This False Idea.
- Tuberculosis Is Fatal If Left Untreated.
- Remember That Patients Should Be Admitted As Long As They Are AFB Positive.
- Antituberculous Medications Have Lots Of Side Effects And Drug Interactions. Be Aware Of Them If Possible.
- Treatment Course Is Long (At Least 6 Months) And Compliance Is Important To Avoid Recurrence Or Resistance.
- Direct Observed Therapy Is Always An Alternative If The Patient Is Non-Compliant To Conventional Treatment Regimens.
- In Complicated Cases You May Need To Involve An Infectious Disease Specialist Or A Respiratory Specialist.
- Tuberculosis is a notifiable disease

HIV and AIDS

- This Is Not An Uncommon Scenario In The Exam.
- It Could Be A Scenario Of Breaking Bad News, Refusing To Tell The Partner Or A Difficult Non-Compliant Patient Continuing To Practice Unprotected Sex.
- You Need To Explore Knowledge And Expectations Before Going Through The Task In Your Scenario.
- You Will Need To Go Very Quickly Through The Sexual History And To Get Some Information About The Partner.
- HIV Infection Is Not Curable, But With The HAART Treatment It Is Controllable.
- With Proper Treatment Patients May Live A Near Normal Life.
- Many Patient Do Mix Between HIV Infection And AIDS. You Need To Explain And Clarify That Especially If Breaking Bad News.
- HIV Is A Non-Notifiable Disease, However The Patient Should Act Responsibly And Avoid Spreading The Infection. You May Need To Explain The Routes Of Transmission (Sexual, Blood Borne And Vertical).
- If You Feel That The Patient Could Be Acting Irresponsibly And A Third Party Is At Risk, You Need To Counsel The Patient And Let Him Know That Others Are In Danger, And He Could Be In A Difficult Legal Situation If That Was Discovered.
- Some Patients Act Irresponsibly As They Feel Angry Or Have Rage Against Society Or Even They Could Be Depressed. Some Other Patients Are Scared To Lose Their Beloved Partners, Feel Shameful Or Have Lack Of Confidence. These Kind Of Patients May Benefit From Psychiatric Referral And Assessment.
- If The Patient Still Insists To Act Recklessly, You May Then Threat Him Politely That You Will Breech His Confidentiality And Let Your Consultant Know About His Inappropriate Behavior.
- Always Seek The Specialists' Advice (Infectious Diseases Consultant, HIV Specialist Nurse), And You May Give The Patient Written Information About The Disease Or Guide Him To Society Groups.
- Remember The Side Effects Of Anti Retrovirals And Their Drug Interactions Especially With OCs.

Managing Problems And Concerns

ALWAYS REMEMBER THAT JUST ASKING ABOUT THE PATIENT CONCERN IS NOT ENOUGH. YOU NEED TO MANAGE THESE CONCERNS AND REASSURE THE PATIENT OR SORT A PLAN FOR HIM.

IS IT CANCER DOCTOR?
- That's an early question to ask now, You don't have any symptoms suggesting bowel cancer, but i think it is better to be checked
- It's unlikely, it doesn't look like a cancer, this will be in the bottom of my differentials
- I'm afraid to say, it is a possibility, It's Better To Be Checked Out

IS IT SERIOUS DOCTOR?
- I am afraid to say, it could be serious if left untreated
- I'm sorry to tell u it is serious, but the good news it is controllable

IS IT REVERSIBLE DOCTOR?
- Yes, it is completely reversible
- Well ... it will improve but not completely reversible, i am sorry to tell you this.

IS IT CURABLE DOCTOR?
- Yes
- I'm sorry to tell u it is not curable, but it is controllable, and researches are still going on, hoping one day we find a solution for it

I CAN NOT DO MY JOB ANY MORE BECAUSE OF MY ILLNESS:
- We can contact the occupational therapist, and u can inform Your occupational health team They Could Do You A Replacement With Another Suitable Job In The Same Company. Do You Like Us To Write To Them?

WILL I BE ABLE TO WALK AGAIN DOCTOR?
- With treatment and physiotherapy, You will feel better, and Your weakness will improve hoping one day You get a complete recovery, but we cannot predict this now

A SON WANT TO SEND HIS MOTHER TO A RESIDENTIAL HOME
- At the moment our assessments recommend that she could manage at home with a care package. However, if you feel its more appropriate to send her to a care home or a residential home, i'm afraid you will have to fund that yourself. Again, we think that she will be safe at home and that was her wish. We don't want to let her down.

WILL I NEED TO BE ADMITTED DOCTOR?
- Well, first we need to confirm that You have this blood clot, so we will do some blood tests, some Imaging to Your Chest, a Heart Tracing, And a Scan To Your lungs then according to the results we will take that decision either You will be admitted or not

I HAVE A CHILD AT HOME AND I AM HIS ONLY CARER, I CAN NOT BE ADMITTED
- We can contact the social worker and arrange for a baby sitter

FOR STD CASES
- Refer to sexual health department
- Investigate for other STDs
- Trace contacts

I Am Afraid Of Insulin Needles
- We Have Insulin Pen Now, You Will Not See The Needle And Even You Will Not Feel Any Prick

I Am Afraid Of Mri (Closed Chamber)
- We Have Open MRI

I Can`T Give Myself The Medications/ Clean The Colostomy(STOMA) Bag By Myself
- We Can Contact The (Stoma Nurse) She Will Show You How To Take Care Of The Stoma Bag. It Is Quite Simple And Most Of The Patients Find It Easy.
- If You Still Feel It Difficult We Could Arrange For A District Nurse Who Will Help You How Cleaning It And Give You Your Medications.

I Am Afraid To Gain Weight
- We Can Contact A Dietician Who Will Help You To Control Your Diet To Prevent Any Excess Weight

I Am concerned To Take Medicine All My Life
- Well That's An Early Question To Answer Right Now, We Need To Confirm First Your Problem And We Will Discuss That Later
- I Am Sorry To Tell You That You Will Have To Take It Through Your Life, Unfortunately This Is The Only Way To Control Your Problem, But You Will Visit Us Regularly To Observe You Are Controlled And Detect Any Side Effects And Deal With Them If It Happens, And Researches Are Still Going On, Hoping One Day We Find A Solution For This Problem

I Am Concerned About The Side Effects
We Will Give You The Minimal Dose To Control Your Symptoms, And You Will Visit Us Regular To Monitor Your Response And Any Side Effects That Could Develop Would Be Picked Up.

I Am Worried That My Kids Would Be Affected By The Same Condition
Well We Can Do A Prenatal Genetic Testing For Your Baby Inside Your Womb To See Any Possible Affection, Then You Can Decide Whether To Keep Them Nor Not

Dr. If They Told Me It's A Lung Cancer 9 Months Ago It Would Not Have Spread
I'm So Sorry For This, But Cancer Lung Is Aggressive From The Start

I Am Afraid To Lose Hair With Chemotherapy
You Can Wear A Wig , You Will Look Very Pretty , No One Will Notice Your Hair Has Fallen

I Am Worried About Infertility If I Take Immune-Suppressants
Don't Worry About That, We Can Take Your Ova / Sperms, Store Them In A Special Bank, And When You Finish The Course Of Treatment, You Can Use It And Do Artificial Fertilization And Have Lovely Babies, In Order Not To Disturb Your Fertility

Inherited Disease , I Am Worried About My Children
Well Mrs... Im Sorry To Tell You That ..% Might Be Affected By Your Condition , However Nowadays With The Advanced Researches Of This Diseases We Can Do A Prenatal Genetic Screening For The Babies To See If They Are Affected Or Not And Then You Can Decide Whether To Keep Them Or Not

How Much Time Left To Me?
It Is Difficult To Answer This Question? Well, We Are Multi -Disciplinary Team, Taking Care Of You, We Are Beside You Miss..., We Will Not Leave You Suffer Alone, We Are Doing The Best For You, I Can't Tell You Now As No One Knows, But Its A Matter Of Months Rather Than Years

Young Girl Committing Suicide, CONSCIOUS, Refusing Treatment, (Unconscious Leaving A Living Will Not To Treat Her)

Living Will Here Will Not Be Approved In Case Of Suicide And She Should Take Treatment And Be Helped , Also If Conscious She Will Receive Treatment Against Her Will (Competent Patients Doesn't Commit Suicide)= I`M Deeply Sorry , I Understand Things Went Very Hard To Let You In Such Situation , I`M Here As Well As All The Team To Help , We Want You To Overcome This Difficult Situation , You Shouldn't Be Here , I See You A Young Bright Girl , It's Absolutely Difficult To See You In Such Situation , Bright Life Is Waiting For You , If You Give Me A Chance To Gain Your Trust We Can Discuss Your Problem And It Will Be Strictly Confidential , No One Will Know Even Your Family, Do You Know The Name Of The Tablet? , Where You Alone? Did You Take Other Drugs? Have You Been Suffering Of Any Psychiatric Illness? Is That Your First Time? (Clarify Situation), This Isn't The End Of The World , We Can Ask A Psychiatrist To Come , He Can Help You Overcome Your Situation , Now We Want To Get Rid Of This Drug Out Of Body Which Can Harm You , We Will Give You The Treatment Through Your Blood Conduits For Some Days To Get Rid Of That Drug , You Are Lucky Enough , You Came In The Right Time

How Long Will I Take These Medications?

If Not Sure: I Will Check With My Consultant And I Will Tell You In Our Next Appointment

If A Patient Asks You About Your Personal Issues

It Would Be Very Inappropriate To Discuss My Personal Issues With You.

Talkative Patients

I Only Have Short Time Left With You, So What Is The Most Important Thing We Need To Discuss?

Your Consultant Made A Mistake

I Am Not In A Position Of Judgement To Judge Other Doctors Performance

Why Did U Give Him This Nasty Medication?

It Was A Live Saving Treatment And Fortunately Your Father Responded To It, It Was The Best Medication For Him

Unpredictable Diseases

MS (Multiple Sclerosis) Is A Highly Unpredictable Disease, We Don't Know When Or Where Will Be The Next Attack

Why your Consultant Did Not Inform Him About Side Effects?

I'm Not Sure If The Consultant Inform Him Or Not, But It Is Our Usual Practice That We Explain How The Medications Work And Their Side Effects Before We Prescribe Them. Usually We Inform The Patient About The Most Common And Most Serious Side Effects, I Will Speak With My Consultant About That.

Alcohol Issues

Well Its Better To Cut Down Your Alcohol Consumption, You Can Join A Self Help Group

Smoking Issues

I Will Refer You To A Smoking Cessation Clinic

Need Support At Home

Contact The Social Worker Who Will Arrange For House Keeper /Baby Sitter/ Care Package

Contact The Occupational Therapist

LAB TECHNICIAN POSITIVE HIV
Inform Hospital Occupational Health Team, Continue Job, But No Deal With Patients

SURGEON WITH HBV
Can Return To Work If PCR < 10^3

AIR HOSTESS WITH IDDM / CROHNS
Its Better To Inform Your Occupational Health Team ,For Your Health And The Sake Of The Public , Try To Change Your Job From An Air Hostess To A Ground Hostess/Control Tower (Pilot) , You Will Wear The Same Clothes And Meet Your Friends And Crews , You Will See Planes Taking Off And Landing , We Are Afraid That You May Have Another Attack Of Loss Of Consciousness / Another Attack Of This Severe Bloody Diarrhea With This Severe Pain In The Plane , You Will Be Very Weak & Dehydrated With No Body There To Help You , And The Next Airport Would Be Hours Away , Which I Am Afraid Would Be Very Serious & Might Threat Your Life

RECENTLY DIAGNOSED WITH IDDM AND HAVE NEEDLE PHOBIA
After Breaking The Bad News , We Have An Insulin Pen , You Will Hardly See Any Needle And Its Going To Be A Very Simple Sharp Scratch Which You Will Hardly Feel It , You Will Need To Change The Site Of Injection Regularly , I Will Refer You To The Diabetic Clinic , Where The Nurse Could Show You How To Use This Pen , Also She Will Give You A Small Device To Measure Your Blood Sugar Regularly And Make A Diary Of It , To Show It To Us On The Follow Up , She Will Explain For You Any Sudden Complications That You Might Face Such As Hypos , Always Keep A Piece Of Sweets Inside Your Pocket

IDDM CONCERNED WITH COMPLICATIONS
With Regular Treatment And Our Regular Follow Up You Will Lead An Active Life, U Will Not Face Any Complications, But If U Forget To Take Your Shots/Tablets, If You Miss Our Follow Ups You May Face Some Complications, D.M Can Be Your Intimate Friend, But Sometimes Could Be Your Worst Enemy

WORRIED ABOUT A SCAR OF A PROCEDURE
I Assure You In The Best Experienced Hands Of Our Doctors And The Advanced Technologies Of This Procedure It Will Be A Very Minimal Line Scar That Could Hardly Be Seen By Anybody

CONVINCING A PATIENT ABOUT AN IMPORTANT PROCEDURE/SURGERY
I Am Afraid That Your Condition Didn't Respond To Treatment/ You Are In A Critical Stage Now, I'm Sorry But Your Condition Went To The Worst / We Are Afraid If You That Your ...... (Heart Valve Will Be Completely Blocked/Bleeding Will Not Stop....) , So What Do you Think The Team Can Do For You? Well The Team Have Decided That You Need ......, I Assure You That In The Best Experienced Hands Of Our Doctors And The Advanced Techniques Of This Procedure Complications And Risks Will Be Very Minimal As............. , I Can Give You Time To Think About It , Also If you Want I Can Let You Join A Support Group In The ... Clinic , To See How People Are Coping With Their Conditions , You Will Cope Better With You Daily Activities , You Will Lead An Active Life , It Will Not Be A Burden Anymore , And There Are Some Precautions I Would Like To Tell You About ..... So Do You Accept The Procedure? I Will Arrange The Consent For You To Sign.

SHALL I TELL MY HUSBAND
It's Up To You, But I Think He Will Be Very Supportive If You Tell Him.

If A Relative Doesn't Want You To Tell The Patient The Truth About The Condition

May I Ask Why You Don't Want Me To Tell Her? Are You Sure She Doesn't Want To Know About Her Condition? Well, From Our Experience Years Ago, Its Best For The Patient To Know About Her Condition From The Start, This Will Give Her Some Sort Of Relief, Also To Comply Better With Treatment Or For Further Tests If Needed , And Don't Worry Mrs... , I Will Sit Beside Her , And Talk With Her To Know How Much She Knows And How Far She Wants To Know , And If She Wants To Know I Will Give Her Small Nuggets Of Information According To Her Ideas And Expectations , Don't Worry Mrs.. We All Care About Your Mum, We Are Beside Her, We Are Taking Care Of Her

A Patient Want To Fly To Her Mum Abroad But Can't Because Of Her Illness

I Understand Your Feelings Mrs. I Understand You Miss Your Mum And You Care About Her, But Its Better To Postpone It Until You Are Ok, I'm Afraid If You Go You Might Face ...... , So Its Better To Stay Here And Start Treatment And Go When You Are Completely Okay , As For Now If You Can Give Me Her Contact Numbers You Can See Her Through The Internet , She Will Understand Your Situation

A Patient With Transmissible Disease Doesn't Want To Notify Husband

I Think Its Better To Tell Him, He Will Be Very Supportive To You And Also, He May be infected as well and will need help, If You Are Not Happy To Tell Him, I Can Tell Him.

When A Complication Of A Procedure Happens

Well Mr. Your Father Came To Us Complaining Of ..., The Doctors Advised To Do... Which Was A Life Saving Procedure / Very Important To Do .... Usually Its Done Many Times In Our Hospital With Very Remote Complications, But Unfortunately ...... Happened, But I Assure You That It Was Managed Appropriately. Even In The Best Experienced Hands Complications Do Occur, We Explained The Procedure To Him And He Accepted The Risks And Signed An Informed Consent.

(This Is Not An Error = No Incident Report)

I Want To Meet The Consultant

Sure, With Pleasure, If You Want A Second Opinion I Will Arrange For An Appointment With The Consultant

Cell Death explanation (MI , Stroke)

Some Cells Have Lost Its Function

Drugs Better To Avoid In Pregnancy (Warfarin)

Well Its Better To Change Your Blood Thinner In It To An Injection Form Of Another Medication Because The Pills May Harm Your Baby; Heart Defects , Bleeding , Or You May Even Lose Your Baby

Non-Curable Disease

Unfortunately It Has No Cure Till Now, But Researches Are Still Going On, Hoping One Day We Will Find A Solution For That Problem , So You Will Have To Take This Palliative Treatment In Order To Keep You In A Good Shape So That You Will Be A Candidate For Any Future Form Of Curative Treatment.

Mrsa Infection Relatives Are Worried

I Assure You That The Hospital Team Observe A Strict Code Of Hand Washing , And Wearing Gloves To Protect Patients Form Infections , This Kind Of Bug Is A Weak Bug So Alcohol Rub Is Sufficient And I Will Revise Again With The Nurses (Nurses Are Not Changing Gloves With Patients Just Rubbing By Alcohol), I Assure You This Kind Of Bug Lives Harmlessly In Our Body

, In Our Nose , Throats , On Our Skin , But Under Certain Situations When We Are In A Low Defense Mechanism As Your Mother's Condition , It Can Flare Up , But Now , She Is Getting Better , She Is Ambulant And Can Walk , So It Will Resolve Hopefully , And We Will Give Her Antibiotics To Kill This Bug , This Bug Will Not Influence her Condition Negatively , If You Are Concerned About Yourself And Kids , Don't Worry It Is Not Transmitted By Breathing (Skin Infection) , If You Are Still Concerned You Can Make Some Protective Procedures Like Wearing A Mask , Gloves, Aprons (Respiratory Infection) , And We Can Let A District Nurse Come To Your Home To Make The Dressing Daily For Her, And If You Are Still Worried We Can Contact The Hospital Infection Control To Take Some Swab From Your Throat And If It Is Positive We Can Start Treatment.

IF PATIENT DOESN'T LIKE THE PAIN OF A REPEATED CANNULA INSERTION
We Can Do A PICC Line That Would Last Longer And Avoid Multiple Skin Pricking.

ADVICE FOR EPILEPSY PATIENT
Avoid Being At Home Alone, Avoid Locking The Bathroom From Inside, Avoid Flashes Of Light, Avoid Watching TV Late At Night, Avoid Driving, Practice Swimming Whilst Being Observed.

DISCUSSING PERCUTANEOUS ENDOSCOPIC GASTROSTOMY AFTER NASOGASTRIC TUBE FOR DISCHARGE IN A PATIENT STARTING TO REGAIN CONSCIOUSNESS.
Discuss Procedure (Anesthesia , Complications , Procedure) ,She Is Getting Better That's Why The Tube Is Irritating And Annoying For Her And Her Nose , And We Are Afraid She Try To Remove This Tube , And May Be The Food Enters In The Opposite Direction Which Might Cause Her Some Serious Conditions , So Our Consultant Decided To Try A Peg Tube (Do You Know Anything About It?) , We Will Feed Her Through A Tube In Her Tummy , It Carries Some Minor Complications With The Best Experienced Hands Of Our Doctors, Some Sort Of Minor Bleeding Or Infection Which Can Be Dealt With Very Easily , It Is A Minor Procedure , Will Be Carried Out In Outpatient Bases , With Local Anesthesia, A Small Gentle Flexed Tube With A Camera , The Gastro-enterologist Will Introduce It Gently To Visualize The Food Sac , And This Tube Will Reach Up Through Her Skin , It Will Be Carried Out With Some Local Anesthesia ,And PEG Tube Insertion Is A Very Simple Procedure , And She Can Go Home Safely , And I Will Arrange With The Social Worker To Arrange For Her A District Nurse Who Can Take Care Of Your Mum & Teach You How To Clean This Tube , And Feed Your Mum Through It

DISCUSSING TAKING MEDICATIONS IV
It Is Better To Take These Drugs Through Your Blood Conduits, Its Faster & More Effective, And You Will Get Better Sooner With It, I`M Afraid To Tell U That Its A Very Serious Condition For Which It's The Best Way To Kill These Bugs, But If U Stop Taking Them, I`M Afraid The Bug Might Flare And Spread Thru Ur Body And Might End Ur Life

PATIENT WORRIED ABOUT CONFIDENTIALITY OF A TEST (HIV):
I Assure You That It Will Be Done In A Strictly Confidential Way, We Are Using Some Sort Of Codes, Not Names, No One Will Know About The Results Except You, And We Will Inform You When The Test Results Are Back To Take The Results By Yourself , Not Over The Phone.

PATIENT DIAGNOSED WITH INHERITED DISEASE, NOT WANT TO TELL FUTURE WIFE
It Will Be Better Let Her Know, To See If She Accept To Have Kids Having Same Condition Like Their Father Or Not.

INHERITED DISEASES PRENATAL DIAGNOSIS BY CHRIONIC VILLOUS SAMPLING
Don't Worry, In Early Pregnancy With Advanced Research Of This Disease We Can Do Prenatal Screening To See If The Coming Baby Have The Same Problem Or Not, To Decide With Ur Wife Whether To Keep It Or Not

STOPPING THE MACHINES
Break The Bad News , We Were Hoping That He Would Regain His Consciousness , And We Did Every Thing To Improve His Condition , We Put Him On Machines To Support His Heart And Lungs , We Gave Him Drugs To Help His Heart To Function Better , We Were Hoping After These Maneuvers That He May Regain His Consciousness , So , What Do You Think We Could Do More For Him? , So In Such Situations After All This Time Of Maximum Support And He Didn't Regain Consciousness , So We Feel That It Would Be Extremely Unlikely That He Would Regain His Consciousness Again. The Team Decided It Is Unwise To Make Him Suffer More , And We Think Keeping Him On Machines Will Prolong His Days Of Suffering , Also He May Be Subjected To More Hazards Than Benefits, So This Decision Is For His Best Interest , The Team Decided To Leave Him In Peace And To Withdraw Him Of These Machines , I Can Arrange For You Another Chat With Our Consultant , I Can Give You Time To Contact Your Family Members To Come And Have A Last Look At Your Father , And If You Need To Have A Spiritual Guide For This Hard Time.

PERSISTENT VEGETATIVE STATE
We Are A Multidisciplinary Team Working For The Best Of Your Son , We Are Feeding Him, Drugs ,Hoping & Waiting , He Might Gain Or Regain His Normal State , I Assure You He Will Have All His Medical Care Unchanged For At Least 6 Months To 1 Year , And After That It Will Be Decided By The Court ,We Are Speaking In Advance Now , We Are Still Don't Know , So Be Sure For The Time Being His Medical Will Not Be Affected, I Know He Smiling And Making Some Movements With His Eyes , These Are Purposeless Movements , He Doesn't Mean Them (Court Order And Not A Medical Team Decision)

AMTS CHANGED FROM 1/10 TO 8/10 IN 75 YEARS OLD PATIENT, DECISION OF DISCHARGE IS TAKEN BUT HIS SON IS REFUSING
He Is Alert, Conscious, And Competent To Take His Own Decisions Now, And His Wish Is To Go Home, I Assure You. It Was A Reversible Condition , He Was Confused Because Of His Kidney Condition , And His Kidney Is Cured, He Is Improving , And The Health Team Has Decided It Is Safe To Go Home , As He Is Mobile And Was Assessed By Our Physiotherapists And Occupational Therapists And They Are Happy For Him To Go Home. You Feel That He Needs Help At Home, We Could Let You Meet Our Social Worker And We May Discuss Sorting A Care Package For Him.

A NEW DRUG THE PATIENT. HEARD ABOUT THROUGH THE INTERNET IN AN END STAGE CANCER, HE IS ANGRY HE WASN'T TOLD ABOUT IT, IT IS NOT LICENSED IN THE UK, AND HE WANTS TO TAKE IT
Well , We Have A Highest Level And Guidelines That We Follow , Which Is The NICE Guideline , And It Didn't Permit The Wide Use Of The Drug Till Now , Why They Didn't Tell You About It , I Don't Know , But I Will Raise The Issue To My Consultant , This Highest Level Didn't Approve This Drug Because Its(Yet Not Safe 100%/A Very Expensive Drug) , And Only Improve Survival For 6 Months (I Want These 6 Months , And I Can Afford It) , Ok I Will Discuss The Matter With My Consultant , And We Can Raise The Issue To The Authorities ,And Raise The Possibility Of A Drug Study For Example. If We Find Any Opportunity About That If They Can Afford This Drug, I Will Discuss This With My Consultant.

PATIENT. SENSITIVE TO A DRUG LEFT A NOTE ABOUT THAT , AND ONE OF YOUR HOSPITAL DOCTORS GAVE HIM THIS DRUG (CODIENE) , THE PT. RELATIVE IS ANGRY
I'M Deeply Sorry For What Happened , I Assure You, A Clinical Incident Report Has Been Completely And Actions Will Be Taken As Necessary , Also We Have Raised The Issue To The High Risk Managerial Team , And My Consultant , I Don't Know What Happened Exactly , May Be There Was Some Miscommunication Between The A&E Department And Our Unit , We Don't Know Exactly Where Is The Problem But Now It Is A Matter Of Investigation, And We Have Written On Her File With Bold Capital Letters(ALLERGIC TO CODEINE) And That Incident Should Not Happen Again , We Are Deeply Sorry Once Again , But You Know Your Mum Came In

A Very Critical Situation , She Came In An Advanced Stage Of Pneumonia , As Shown By The Tests Done Before Starting The Codeine ,So We Don't Know The Confusion Is From The Pneumonia Or From The Codeine , But Now She Is On Very Strong Antibiotics For Her Chest Infection And The Codeine Effect Should Be Transient. We Also Gave Her Some Medications That May Help Reverse The Sedative Action Of Codeine. If You Want To Make A Complaint I Could Help You Writing It And Sending It To The Legal Trust Department., I Assure You We Are Doing The Best For Your Mum , And We Are Waiting For Her To Improve Hopefully.

PROBLEMS WITH MARRIAGE
I Can Arrange For You A Meeting With A Marital Counselling To Help You Solve These Problems

ALL DISEASES HAVE A SOCIETY
You Can Join …. Society, And See How People Are Coping With Their Condition

Patient Discharge Pathways

- Not All Hospitals In The UK Provide All Services And Therefore Patient Care May Not Be Delivered At The Hospital Nearest To His Home. Care And Treatment Will Be Delivered At The Most Appropriate Location For The Patients' Needs With In The Same Trust. This Will Also Apply When The Patient Is Recovering From His Hospital Stay.
- Hospitals With Inpatient Beds Are Designed To Care For People With Acute Health Needs And Should The Patient Need To Continue With Non-Acute Care Such As Rehabilitation Or Recuperation Following His Acute Stay There Will Be The Need To Transfer Him To An Alternative Environment. This Environment May Be A Community Hospital, Intermediate Care Centre, Or Care Home Facility.

A) Going Home :

- The Patient Should Be Safe And Able To Manage If He Is To Be Discharged Back Home.
- Although Some People Need No Extra Help, It Is The Duty Of The Healthcare Multidisciplinary Team (Physicians, Nurses, Physiotherapists, Occupational Therapists And Social Services) To Assess The Patient's Needs And If Necessary They Can Aid To Organize Support From A Variety Of Services.
- If The Patient Is Assessed As Needing Help, This May Be Provided By Support Such As:
  o Intermediate Care Team (Nurses, Physiotherapists, Occupational Therapists)
  o Social Services
  o District Nurses
  o Community Matrons
  o Voluntary Agencies For Example The Red Cross.
- If The Patient Need Carer To Support Him At Home With Tasks Such As Getting Washed And Dressed, A Social Work Care Manager May Come To Talk To The Patient Whilst He Is Still In Hospital To Help Arrange The Right Help For Him.

B) Intermediate Care:

- There May Be Times When Although The Patient's Medical Condition Has Become Stable, He Still Needs A Little Longer To Recover From Being Unwell.
- In This Situation, He Should Be Transferred To An Alternative Setting, Usually Away From The Hospital, To Allow The Opportunity To Recuperate And Recover Before Returning Home.
- There Are A Variety Of Places Where People Can Recover And Recuperate After Being In Hospital, And These Are Located Around The Trust Area. However, As There May Not Be Space In The Place Nearest To The Patient's Own Home, We Would Expect The Patient To Be Flexible In Where He Stays To Receive This Treatment And Help.

I) Assessment Beds:
- If The Patients Require An In-Depth Assessment Into His Social Care Needs, Or Considering Whether It Would Be Appropriate To Move Into A Care Home, He Should Be Transferred To An Assessment Bed In A Care Home Setting.

II) Care Homes:
- It Is Sometimes Necessary To Arrange For The Patient To Be Cared For In A Care Home Setting Directly From The Acute Hospital. This May Happen If Illness Has Caused A Significant Change In The Patient's Ability To Do Things For Himself, Mobility Levels, Or If He Need The Care From Somebody To Remain Safe.
- Care Home Could Be A Residential Home (Offering Basic Care Only And Not Dealing With Medical Issues) Or A Nursing Home.

III) Continuing Healthcare:

- Those Patients In Need Of Ongoing Complex Healthcare And Support On Discharge From Hospital May Be Assessed For Provision Of Continuing Healthcare. This Is Provided Only When The Patient Is Considered To Have Challenging And Complex Needs Which Cannot Be Safely Provided By A Standard Level Of Nursing Care. The Assessment Process Is Undertaken By The Whole Clinical Team, And Will Involve The Patient And Their Next Of Kin (Or Other Identified Representative). Assessments And Decisions Around Continuing Healthcare Will Be Discussed With Patients And Their Family, By The Continuing Healthcare Team.

Common Pitfalls For Station II And IV

1-Being in a hurry, and forget to ask all the questions needed and cannot complete the task as asked.

2-Repeating; always try to rephrase.

3-Using medical jargon

4-Finishing the station before the 14 minutes are up

5-Forgetting to take social history in communication station, and station ii

6-Forgetting to take menstrual history from a female in station ii

STATION V

Brief Clinical Consultation

Introduction To Station V

You Have 5 Minutes Before Entering The Station.

You Have 2 Cases To Read And Think About During Your 5 Minutes Before Entering The Station.

Each Case Is 10 Minutes.

In Each Case You Have 8 Minutes To Take History, Examine The Patient Appropriately, Ask For Concern And Manage The Concern, Reaching A Diagnosis Or Differential Diagnoses And Deciding About The Management Plan.

The Rest Of The 10 Minutes (2 Minutes) Is A Case Based Discussion With The Examiner.

It's Tricky, You Only Got 8 Minutes To Figure It Out, So You Need To Practice, Practice, Practice....

Before Entering The Station, You Will Be Given 5 Minutes To Sort Out Your Ideas. Focus On The **Differential Diagnosis** And **Analysis Of The Main Complaint**, Then **Plot The Scheme** Mentioned In The Next Pages, In Order Not To Miss Any Item. Be Always Ready For Surprises In The Station, Which May Be Good Surprises Leading You To Your Diagnosis, Or Bad Surprises That May Mislead You, So Try Avoiding Bad Surprises And Deal With Them Appropriately. You Need To Be Lucky, Fully Concentrating, With Flexible Thinking.

Station V Outline Scheme

1. **Greeting**
2. **Introduce & Verify Yourself Clearly**
3. **Check The Patient Name & Identity.**
4. **Establish A Rapport**
5. **Explain The Aim Of The Appointment**
6. **Ask The Patient To Tell You More About The Problem** (Open Question)
7. **Take Short Targeted History Depending On The Major Complaint** (Only Relevant Questions/ No System Enquiry)
8. **By This Stage You Should Be Able To:**
   - *Plot A Provisional Diagnosis*
   - *Sort A List Of Differential Diagnosis*
   - *Complications*
   - *Causes*
   - *Risk Factors / Associations For The Condition.*
9. **Ask About These Issues.**
   - Quick Past Medical History
   - Medications
   - Family History If Relevant.
   - Social History
10.   **Address The Patient's** I C E
   - Ideas
   - Concerns
   - Expectations
11.   Relevant Examination Of The Patient Looking For:
   - *Confirming Your Diagnosis*
   - *Excluding Differential Diagnoses*
   - *Looking For Complications*
   - *Looking For Associated Conditions*
   - *Looking For A Cause If Appropriate.*
12.   **Explain The Condition** Briefly, And **Sort Out A Plan** (Bloods, Scans, Admission, Referral, Another Appointment, Driving Advice, Leaflets, Societies, Referrals Etc.)
13.   **Situation At Home**, And **Daily Life Activities** (If Relevant).
14.   **Recap**, And **Address Further Concerns** After Your Explanation + Manage It
15.   **End Of Appointment**

Station V Example

Good Afternoon I Am Dr....... SHO In .. Clinic, I Have Been Asked To Examine You/Mr... Is That Ok?

Am I Speaking To Mr...?

I Understand You Are Troubled By Some .... **Would You Like To Tell Me More About This?**

Let The Patient Speak For 1 Minute

Do A General Survey Of The Patient For Any Spot Diagnosis

Analyze The Complaint

- For How Long? Has It Started Suddenly Or Gradually?
- Getting Better Or Worse? What Makes It Better? What Makes It Worse?
- So You Have It All The Time? When Do U Have It Mostly?
- Is It Accompanied By Any Other Symptoms?
- Where Is This Pain? Does It Go Elsewhere? Describe How It Feels Like? Does It Radiate Any Where Else? Is It Associated With Any Other Symptoms?

Quick System R/V, PMH, FH, Social History According To Your Differentials:

- Have You Ever Been Diagnosed With Any Medical Condition, High Blood Pressure, And High Blood Sugar? Liver, Kidney, Heart & Chest Problems?
- Have You Done Any Recent Tests? Blood Tests & Imaging?
- Have You Ever Been Admitted To The Hospital Before? For What?
- Any Surgical Operations Or Minor Procedures?
- Are You Currently Taking Any Medication, Over The Counter Or Any Herbal Remedies For Any Condition? What? What Dosage? For What?
- Any Similar Conditions In The Family?
- Any Diseases Running In The Family?
- Do You Smoke? Drink Alcohol? Use Recreational Drugs?
- What Do You Do For Living? Can You Tell Me More About Your Job? Are You Coping Well Or On Sick Leaves?
- What Are Your Daily Activities?
- Do You Drive A Car?
- With Whom Do You Live?

Do A Targeted Examination & **Targeted History Taking** According To The _Main Complaint &_ _The Spot Diagnosis_ You Noticed On The Patient If Any, Looking For:

- Confirming The Diagnosis
- R/O Differential Diagnoses
- Looking For Complications
- Looking For The Cause
- Looking For Associated Conditions.

So What Are Your Concerns?

Manage The Concern

- Explain The Condition Briefly, And Sort out A Plan
- Diagnosis
- Investigations & Treatment
- Admission
- Referrals
- Advice
- Driving
- Prognosis If Applicable

Any Other Concerns?

Is There Anything Unclear You Need Me To Clarify?

Ok, I Will Be Around If You Need Anything Just Ask The Nurse To Give Me A Shout

Case Scenarios

Hand Shakes

Please Examine This Patient With Hand Shakes?

D.D Of Hand Shakes

- Thyrotoxicosis
- Parkinson's Disease
- Familial / Senile / Postural.
- B2 Agonists (COPD, Bronchial Asthma)
- Lithium (Bipolar Disorder)
- Cerebellar Disease (Alcohol, Ataxia Telangiectasia, MS)
- Anxiety
- Flapping Tremors:
  - CO_2 Retention
  - Chronic Liver Disease
- *Other Forms* Of Abnormal Hand Movements:
  - Dystonia
  - Hemi-Ballismus

Analysis Of Hand Shakes

- For How Long?
- Has It Occurred Suddenly Or Gradually?
- Is It Getting Better Or Worse?
- Anything That Can Increase It?
- Anything That Can Eases It Down?
- Is It At Rest Or When You Move Your Hands?
  - Static In Parkinson's
  - Intentional Tremors In Cerebellar Disease.
  - Familial Worse On Out Stretched Arms (Postural)
- Is It Fine Or Coarse?
  - Fine Means The Tremors Are Not Involving A Joint.
    - Parkinson's
    - Familial
    - Lithium Toxicity
    - Salbutamol Use.
    - Anxiety.
  - Coarse Means It Is Involving A Joint
    - Flapping Tremors.
    - Cerebellar Tremors.
- Any Associated Symptoms?
- Any Family History?
- Is The Patient On Medications?
- Any Past Medical History?
- Ask About S/S Of The Differentials Listed Above?

Once You Enter The Room Search For A Spot Diagnosis

(I Feel Lucky)

Lid Retraction + Exopthalmous + Enlarged Thyroid =

Graves` Disease

Analysis Of Hand Shakes

See Before

Targeted History:

Confirm Diagnosis, R/O Differential Diagnoses & Look For Associated Conditions

- Do You Have These Handshakes At Rest Or With Movement?
  - o All The Time
- Do You Experience *Abnormal Intolerance To Hot Whether* More Than You Used To?
  - o I Suppose It Is Difficult For Me To Tolerate Hot Weather Nowadays.
- Are You *Sweating* More Than Usual?
  - o I Believe So
- Any *Heart Racing*?
  - o More Or Less…
- Have You *Lost Weight*? *Normal Appetite*? (Thyroid Paradox)
  - o Oh Yes, I'm Losing Weight Although I Eat Normally And I Have Good Appetite
- Any *Lose Motions*, How Often Do You Open Your Bowels?
  - o No Lose Motions Doctor, But I'm Opening My Bowels More Frequent Than My Usual Habit
- Do You Feel Yourself More *Anxious* Nowadays?
  - o Yes, Doctor I'm So Nervous And It Is Affecting My Relationship With My Girl Friend
- *Sleeping Less*? *Night Mares*?
  - o Somehow Yes
- Do You *Smoke*? (Thyroid Eye Disease Is Worse With Smoking)
- Any Disturbances In Your Periods?
- **Complications:**
  - o *Shortness Of Breath*? (High Cardiac Output Failure/ Part Of Af/ Retrosternal Extension)
  - o *Change In Voice*? (Retrosternal Extension)
  - o *Difficulty Swallowing*? (Retrosternal)
  - o *Any Abnormality With Your Vision/Eyes*?
    - ▪ Diminution Of Vision (Optic Atrophy)

Targeted Examination

Examine Eyes:

- *Lid Retraction* (Apparent Upper Rim Of Sclera)
- *Proptosis* (Apparent Lower Rim Of Sclera)
- *Lid Lag Sign*: Look At My Finger, Follow It With Your Eyes, Fix Your Head (Your Finger Should Be At A Higher Level Than The Head, And Then Move It Downwards And Away From The Patient Like An Arch).
- *Eye Movement* (Opthalmoplegia)
- *Mobius Sign* (Failure Of Conversion).
- *Visual Acuity* (Counting Fingers).
- Visual Field & Fundus Examination (May I Examine His Fundus Sir?).

Examine Hands:

- *Acropachy* (Clubbing).
- *Onycholysis.*
- *Radial Pulse* (Tachycardia Or Atrial Fibrillation).
- Excessive Sweating.
- *Tremors* (Put Paper On The Back Of The Stretched Hands).
- *Palmar Erythema.*

Examine The Neck:

Inspect The Neck From The Front

Ask The Patient To Swallow A Sip Of Water; Looking For Moving Enlarged Thyroid.

Examine Neck From Back

- See Eyes For _Proptosis_.
- Palpate For _Lymph Nodes_.
  - o Could It Be Malignancy?
- Palpate _Thyroid Lobes & The Isthmus_.
  - o For Enlargement
  - o Consistency (Cystic Or Diffuse Enlargement)
  - o Thrills.
  - o Tenderness.
- Palpate _Lower Border Of The Thyroid Gland_ While Swallowing (For Retrosternal Extension) = (Take A Sip Of Water Please)

Percuss The Sternum (Retrosternal Extension)

- Normally It Should Be Resonant, Dullness Could Mean Retrosternal Extension

Auscultate The Lobes And Isthmus For Bruits.

- Bruits Means Increased Vascularity Which Could Occur With
  - o Graves` Disease.
  - o Malignancy.

Auscultate The Heart For Gallop Rhythm If In Heart Failure, Or Af.

Examine The Legs:

- _Proximal Weakness._
- _Lower Limb Edema_ (If In Heart Failure).
- _Pretibial Myxedema._
- _Brisk Reflexes._

Examine For Complications:

Do Pemberton Sign (For Retrosternal Goitre)

Search For Congested Face & Shortness Of Breath When Doing The Test

Raise Your Arms Up Above Your Head And Take A Deep Breath In For Me Please.

Comment On:

- The Gland Consistency, Surface, Tenderness, Thrill, Bruit, Retrosternal Extension,
- Thyroid Status Of The Patient (Euthyroid, Hyperthyroid, Hypothyroid), Any Complications Or Associations.
- I Would Like To Complete My Examination By Measuring Blood Pressure & Temperature.

_N.B:_

Graves` Disease Can Be Associated With Other Auto-Immune Disorders E.G. Vitiligo, Coeliac Disease, Type 1 D.M Etc…

Quick Discussion

Indications For Admission

- Congestive Heart Failure, Diminution Of Vision, Atrial Fibrillation, Pregnancy, Thyrotoxic Crisis.

Causes Of Thyrotoxicosis

- Graves` Disease (Exophtalmous, Opthalmoplegia, Acropachy, Pretibial Myxedema)
- Toxic Multinodular Goiter (Nodular Surface, No Eyes Signs ,No Nail Signs, No Pretibial Myxedema, Usually Older Age)
- Toxic Nodule (Palpable/Inpalpable Nodule, No Eye Signs, No Nail Signs)
- Thyroiditis
  o Dequervian (Tender Thyroid Gland)
  o Hashimotos Thyroiditis Initially
  o Amiodarone Induced Thyroiditis
  o Reidle Thyroiditis.
- Drug Induced (No Eye Signs)

Investigations

- T4, T3, TSH, U/S Scan Of The Thyroid, Thyroid Scan.
- FNAC (Fine Needle Aspiration Cytology) If Nodule Or Suspected Malignancy.
- Graves: Tshr Stimulating Abs.
- CXR/CT Scan Of The Chest For Retrosternal Extension.

Treatment

- **Stop Smoking** (Especially With Opthalmopathy)
- **Medical Treatment** (Usually Medical Treatment For 1.5 Years)
1) *Beta Blocker* (Symptom Control)
2) Carbimazole (Better Compliance Every 12 Hrs A Tablet , Inhibit T4 Conversion To T3 , & Anti Peroxidise, Immunomodulator Effect) Side Effects : Agranulocytosis
3) Propylthioracil (Preferred In Pregnancy)
- **Radio-Active Iodine**: Contraindications: Pregnancy , Lactation, Hypersensitivity , Eye Signs Complications: Thyrotoxic Crisis & Hypothyroidsim, Malignancy?
- **Surgery** Indications:
  o Failure Of Medical Treatment
  o Contraindication To Iodine.
  o Cosmetic.
  o Compression.
  o Cancer.
  o Patient Preference.

Expressionless Face + Infrequent Blinking + Static Tremors =

Parkinson`s Disease

Analysis Of Hand Shakes

See Before

Targeted History:

Confirm Diagnosis, R/O Differential Diagnoses & Look For Associated Conditions

You Need To Find Out, Is It Just Parkinson Disease Or Parkinson Plus Syndrome !!

- Problem With *Walking* (Shuffling)? Problems With *Writing* (Micrographia)? Problems With *Speech* (Monotonous)? Noticed To Be *Slower* Than Usual (Bradykinesia)? **(Symptoms Of Parkinsons)**
- Light Headedness When Suddenly Standing Up, Loss Of Control Your Water Works, Constipation? **(Shy Dragger)**
- Problems With Vision Or Falls During Walking Down Stairs? **(Supranuclear Palsy)**
- Memory Problems? See Unusual Things? Visual Hallucinations? Problems With Previous Medications? (**Lewy Body Dementia)**
- Do You Take Any Medications Regulary?

Targeted Examination:

You Need To Find Out, Is It Just Parkinson Disease Or Parkinson Plus Syndrome !!

- **Examine The Face** (Infrequent Blinking, Expressionless)
- **STATIC TREMORS** (Asymmetrical In Parkinson Disease, Increasing By Distraction And Decreases When Asked To Outstretch The Arms)
- **Monotonous SPEECH**
- **Cog Wheel RIGIDITY In Wrists** (If Tremors Are Present)
- **Lead Pipe RIGIDITY In Arms & Legs** (If Tremors Are Absent)
- **MICROGRAPHIA** (Write Your Name On This Paper)
- **BRADYKINESIA By Counting Fingers Test** (Count On Your Fingers, Faster)
- **+Ve Glabellar Tap Sign** (May I Tap On Your Forehead?)
  o Some Examiners Don`T Prefer You To Do This Sign.
- **Stooped POSTURE** (May I Ask You To Stand Up?)
- **Shuffling GAIT** (May I Ask You To Walk?)

Examine For Features Of Parkinson Plus Syndromes

- Quick Neurological Examination For Lower Limbs **(Pyramidal Lesion)**
- Cerebellar Signs **(Shy Drager)**
- Examine For Vertical Gaze Palsy **(Supranuclear Palsy)**
- Assess Mini-Mental State For Confusion / Dementia **(Lewy Body Dementia)**

Quick Discussion

Causes Of Parkinsonism

- Neurodegeneration Of Substantia Nigra.
- Dementia Of Lewy Body.
- Wilson`s Disease.
- Phenothiazines.
- Butrophenones.
- Metoclopramide (Extrapyramidal Manifestations)

Investigations

- CT, MRI To Exclude Other Conditions.
- Parkinsonism Is Mainly A Clinical Diagnosis.

Treatment

- Bromocriptine & Levo Dopa
- Ropinerol
- Apomorphine
- Anticholinergics (Tremors)
- Pramipexol
- Entacapone

What Are The Major Parkinson Plus Syndromes?

Multiple System Atrophy (Shy Dragger Disease):

Parkinsonism, Autonomic Failure, Cerebellar Dysfunction, And Pyramidal Signs That Are Poorly Responsive To Levodopa Or Dopamine Agonists.

Progressive Supranuclear Palsy:

Bradykinesia, Rigidity, Dysarthria, Dysphagia, And Dementia, As In Patients With Idiopathic PD. However, Tremor Is Rare, And The Patient Has Severe Postural Instability. Axial Rigidity Appears To Be More Prominent Than Limb Rigidity. Consistently, Patients Have Downgaze Ophthalmoparesis And Pseduobulbar Palsy.

Lewy Body Dementia:

Dementia, Depression, Auditory And Visual Hallucinations, And Paranoid Ideation May Occur. These Patients Are More Likely To Have Cognitive Adverse Effects With Levodopa Therapy In Early Stages Than Patients With Parkinson Disease.

Epistaxis

Please Examine This Patient With Epistaxis?

D.D Of Epistaxis

- **Unilateral**
  - Usually Local Causes.
  - Could Be Nasal Polyps.
  - Could Be Trauma.
- **Bilateral** (Usually Systemic Disease)
  Bleeding Disorders.
  - CLD (Chronic Liver Disease); See before
  - VWBD
  - Hemophilia.
  - Anticoagulants.
  - Aspirin Use.
  - ITP.
  - Hematological Malignancies.
  Blood Vessels Problems
  - Vasculitis Especially Granulomatosis With Polyangiitis.
  - HHT (Hereditary Hemorrhagic Telangiectasia)
  - Steroids.
  - Scurvy.
  Blood Pressure
  - Hypertension.

Analysis Of Epistaxis:

- For How Long?
- Suddenly Or Gradually?
- Getting Better Or Worse?
- Are You Bleeding From Other Parts Of Your Body? Bleeding From Your Gums? Coughing, Vomiting Blood, Bleeding With Your Bowel Motions?
- Any Rash? **(HHT)**
- Do You Take Any Blood Thinners? Steroids? Medications?
- Do You Feel Dizzy? Pallor? Any Chest Pains? And Falls Or Collapses? **(Anemia Symptoms)**
- S/S Of Differentials Above?

ONCE YOU ENTER THE ROOM SEARCH FOR A SPOT DIAGNOSIS

Multiple Telangiectasia =

Hereditary Hemorrhagic Telangectasia

Targeted History

Confirm Diagnosis, R/O Differential Diagnoses & Look For Associated Conditions

- Any Rash?
- Do U Bleed From Any Other Parts Of Your Body? Mouth, Nose? **(Recurrent Bleeding)**
- SOB, Racing Of Ht. Do You Look Paller Than Usual? **(Anemia)**
- Bleeding With Your Bowel Motions? **(Bowel A-V)**
- Any Blood With Your Water Works? **(Kidney A-V)**
- Any Weakness Or Clumsiness? **(Brain A-V)**
- Coughed Up Blood? **(Lung A-V)**
- Family History **(AD Condition).**

Targeted Examination:

Examine The NOSE For Local Problems

- Deviated Septum.
- Nasal Polyps.

Examine FACE, MOUTH, TONGUE, The Inside The MOUTH, The Inside Of The NOSE For Telangectasias.

Examine PALMS & SOLES For Telangiectasias.

NEUROLOGICAL EVALUATION If Weakness Is Present

Examine THE LIVER For Enlargement & Bruit (A-V Malformation)

Examine THE CHEST If Hemoptysis Is Present.

Quick Discussion

Causes

- Autosomal Dominant

Investigations

- FBC , Stool For Blood , Urine For Blood ,CT Head , Abdomen
- Angiography If Actively Bleeding.

Treatment

- Mild: No Treatment.
- Skin Lesions: Cautery
- Severe Cases: Estrogen Therapy

Recurrent Epistaxis + Depressed Nasal Bridge (Saddle Nose) + Other Symptoms (Below) =

Granulomatosis With Polyangiitis (Wegner's Granulomatosis)

Targeted History

Confirm Diagnosis, R/O Differential Diagnoses & Look For Associated Conditions

- Any Blocked Nose? Nose Bleeds? **(URT Affection)**
- Any Hearing Problems? **(Ear Affection)**
- Coughing Up Blood?
- Sore Eyes? Red Eyes?
- Any SOB? **(Pulmonary Infiltrates)**
- And What About Your Water Works? Change In Color? Decreased Amount? Are You Feeling Tired Nowadays? **(Renal Affection)**
- Are You Known To Have Any Kidney Problems?
- Any Joint Pains?
- Any Rash? (Palpable Purpra/ Skin Nodules)

Targeted Examination:

Examine The NOSE

- Perforated Septum.
- Saddle Nose.

Examine The EYES

- Conjunctivitis.
- Episcleritis.

Examine The Mouth

- Gingivitis.

Examine The Chest

- Crackles Of Pulmonary Hemorrhage.
- Crackles Of Pulmonary Congestion (If Associated Renal Failure).
- Cavitation Signs.
- Consolidation Signs.

Examine The Skin

- Skin Rash And Nodules.

Ask The Examiner For Temperature, Blood Pressure & Urine Dip Results, If Available Kidney Function Tests.

Quick Discussion

Causes

- Auto-Immune Condition.

Differential Diagnosis:

Here You Must Mention The Differential Diagnosis Of Pulmonary Renal Syndromes If The Patient Is Having Associated Hemoptysis + Urinary Symptoms Like Oliguria & Hematuria:

- Good Pasture Syndrome.
- SLE.
- Henoch-Schonlein Purpura.
- Severe Chest Sepsis.
- Rheumatoid Arthritis (RA).

Investigations

- FBC (Anemia, Unexplained Leukocytosis).
- CrP & ESR (Usually Raised).
- Kidney Function Tests (Might Be Deranged).
- Urinalysis.
- CT Scan Of The Chest If Hemoptysis.
- In Some Cases Might Need Lung Biopsy/Kidney Biopsy.
- ANCA (Usually C-ANCA +ve With High PR3 Titres).
- Anti GBM (To R/O Good Pastures Syndrome).
- Bronchoscopy If Hemoptysis.

Treatment

- Urgent Renal R/V If Kidneys Are Affected
- Urgent Respiratory R/V If Lungs Are Affected.
- Steroids
- Immunosupression (Cyclophosphamide, Mycophenolate Mofetil, Rituximab)
- Might Need Plasma Exchange.

Weight Gain

Please Examine This Patient With Weight Gain

<u>**Differential Diagnosis Of Weight Gain:**</u>

1) ***Intentional.***
2) ***Unintentional:***

- *Endocrinal Causes:*
  - Cushing Syndrome.
  - Hypothyroidism.
  - Insulinoma.
  - PCO (Polycystic Kidney).
- *Drugs*
  - Steroids.
  - Sodium Valproate.
  - Insulin, Sulphonylurea.
  - SSRIs.
  - OCPs.
  - Other Drugs.
- *Fluid Overload*
  - Heart Failure.
  - Renal Failure.
  - Nephrotic Syndrome.
  - Chronic Liver Disease.
- *Others*
  - Pregnancy, Smoking Cessation, Hypothalamic Tumors.
  - Familial Hyperlipidemia.

<u>**Analysis Of Weight Gain:**</u>

- How Much Weight?
- Have You Noticed Your Clothes Are Getting Tighter?
- Over How Much Period Of Time?
- Intentional Or Not?
- Where Exactly Did You Gain This Weight?
  - Local Site Or General Weight Gain
- What About The Appetite? Diet Habits (Detailed)?
- Any Family History?
- Are You Pregnant? Any Menstrual Periods Problems?
- Any Drugs?
- S/S Of Differentials Above?

ONCE YOU ENTER THE ROOM LOOK FOR A SPOT DIAGNOSIS

Facial Fullness + Plethora + Hirsutism + Acne+ Central Obesity + Multiple Striae + Purpura+ Supraclavicular Pad Of Fat =

Cushing Syndrome

Targeted History:

Confirm Diagnosis, R/O Differential Diagnoses & Look For Associated Conditions

- Where Exactly Did U Gain This Weight? **(Central Obesity, Facial Fullness, Interscapular)**
- Excessive Hair Growth? **(Hirsuitism)**
- Recurrent Skin Infections?
- Any Bruises? **(Easy Bruising)**
- Any Weakness In Your Arms Or Legs? **(Proximal Weakness)**
- Are U Passing More Urine Than Usual? Drinking More Than Usual? **(Diabetes Mellitus)**
- Any Striae?
- Any Recent Fractures Or Bony Pains? **(Osteoporosis, Avascular Necrosis)**
- What About Your Mood? **(Depression)**
- What About Your Periods? **(Menstrual Irregularities)**
- Do You Have High Blood Pressure? **(HTN)**
- Are You Taking Steroids? If Yes, For What?
- Headaches? Throwing Up? Blurred Vision? **(Cushing Disease)**

Targeted Examination:

Examine The Face

- Facial Fullness (You Cannot See The Ear Lobules Whilst Looking At The Patient Face From The Front)
- Facial Plethora
- Hirsutism
- Acne

Examine The Trunk For

- Supraclavicular Pad Of Fat
- Hirsutism
- Poor Wound Healing

Examine The Hands

- Thin Skin
- Purpura
- Bruises

Examine The Arms For Proximal Myopathy

Examine The Back For Inter-Scapular Pad Of Fat

Examine Visual Fields If Appropriate.

Look For Signs Of Diabetes

- Diabetic Dermopathy
- Necrobiosis Lipoidica
- Peripheral Neuropathy
- Mono-Neuritis Multiplex

Examine For The Cause If Drug Induced:

- Sarcoidosis (Examine Chest For Fibrosis, Lupus Pernio, HSM)
- SLE (Examine Chest For Lung Fibrosis , Pleural Effusion, Butter Fly Rash , Joint Pains)
- Polymyositis (Proximal Weakness)
- Dermatomyositis (Proximal Muscle Weakness, Heliotrope Rash, Gottron Papules)

- Transplanted Kidney Signs With Immunosupression
  - Rt. / Lt. Iliac Fossa Scar
  - Previous Hemodialysis Signs
  - Palpable Dull Mass Under The Scar
- COPD Signs.

Quick Discussion

Investigations

- Low Dose Dexamethasone Suppression Test To Confirm Diagnosis.
- 24 Hrs Urinary Cortisol May Be Used.
- High Dose Dexamethasone Suppression Test To R/O Pituitary Adenoma.
- Blood Glucose.
- Serum Ca For MEN I.
- MRI Looking For Pituitary Adenoma.
- Measure Other Pituitary Hormones.
- CRH , ACTH.

Treatment

- Surgery For Pituitary Adenoma.
- Adrenalectomy If Primary.
  - Surgical
  - Medical: Ketoconazole & Metyrapone

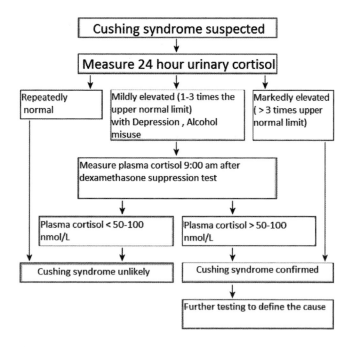

Multiple Xanthomata =

Familial Hyperlipidemia

Targeted History:
Confirm Diagnosis, R/O Differential Diagnoses & Look For Associated Conditions

- Where Exactly Did You Gain This Weight?
- Do You Have High B.P?
- Do You Have High Blood Sugar?
- Any Chest Pains? SOB? Heart Problems? **(IHD)**
- Weakness Or Clumsiness? Any Previous Strokes? **(Stroke)**
- Leg Cramps During Walking? Pain In Your Tummy? Problem With Intimate Relations? **(Vascular Disease)**
- Any PH Of Problems With Speech, Loss Of Consciousness, Sudden Loss Of Vision? **(TIA)**
- Have You Done Any Recent Tests? **(High Cholesterol Or Triglycerides)**
- Similar Conditions In The Family? **(Familial)**
- Any Deaths At Young Age In Your Family?
- FH Of Heart Or Brain Problems?

Targeted Examination:
Examine Skin Lesions

- **Tendon & Tuberous** (Over Bones) = High Cholesterol
- **Eruptive** (Not Over Tendons Or Bones)= High Triglycerides
- **Palmar Xanthomas** = Type III = Abeta-Lipoprotinemia Ask About:
  - Problems With Walking & Balance *(Ataxia)* **Examine Neurologically**
  - Problems With Vision (*Retinitis Pigmentosa)* Examine **Fundus**
  - Any Loose, Pale Motions? *(Malabsorption)*

Auscultate The Carotid Artery For Bruits

Palpate Abdomen For Organomegaly

Auscultate Abdomen For Mesenteric Or Renal Bruits

Quick Discussion
Investigations:

- Cholesterol > 4 mmol Or LDL > 2 mmol
- Serum Triglycerides.
- ECHO
- ECG
- Carotid Dopplers
- Doppler U/S If You Hear Any Bruits.
- See History taking station for classifications

Treatment:

- HIGH CHOLESTEROL =Statins , Ezetemibe, Cholectyramine
- HIGH TRIGLYCERIDES =Fibrates , Omega 3 , Ezetemibe , Niacin
- Cardiovascular Disease Prevention
  - Stop Smoking.
  - Weight Loss.
  - Refer To Dietician.
  - Control Blood Sugar.
  - Control HTN.

Coarse Hair + Facial Puffiness + Puffiness Around Eyes + Loss Of Outer 1/3 Of Eye Brow + Obese =

Hypothyroidism

Targeted History

Confirm Diagnosis, R/O Differential Diagnoses & Look For Associated Conditions

- Do You Feel The Cold More Than You Used To? Do You Feel Your Skin Is Dry? Any Problems With Hair? Are You Constipated? Problems With Memory And Concentration? Sleeping More Than Usual? Hoarse Voice? **(Symptoms Of Hypothyroidism)**
- What About Your Periods? Regular? Any Excessive Bleeding? Increased Frequency Of Your Periods? **(Menorrhagia)**
- Any Pins And Needles Sensation In Your Hands? **(Carpal Tunnel)**
- Excessive Tanning Of Your Skin? **(Addison)**
- Loss Of Normal Skin Color? **(Vitiligo)**
- Any SOB? Difficulty Swallowing? Change In Voices? **(Retrosternal Extension)**

Targeted Examination:

Examine The FACE

- Characteristic Facies
- May Be Associated With Other Auto-Immune Disorders You Might Find:
    - Vitiligo
    - Alopecia Areata
    - Alopecia Totalis.
    - Adissonian Features.

Examine The HANDS

- Puffy
- Coarse Dry Skin
- May Be Vitiligo
- Bradycardia
- Carpal Tunnel Syndrome Examination:
    - Wasting Of Thenar Eminence.
    - Weakness Of Thumb Abduction And Opponence.
    - Sensory Loss Of Lateral 3.5 Fingers.
    - Phalen`s Sign: Can You Bend Your Hands Like This?
    - Tinnel`s Sign: May I Tap On Your Wrist, Do You Feel Any Pain?

Examine The ARMS (Proximal Weakness)

Examine The NECK

- Thyroid Examination (See Before)
- Look For Thyroidectomy Scar

Examine The CHEST (Pleural, Pericardial Effusion)

Examine The ABDOMEN For Ascites.

Examine The LEGS For:

- Non Pitting Edema Of Legs
- Delayed Relaxation Of Reflexes **(Ankle Reflex)**

Quick Discussion

Causes

- Hashimoto Thyroiditis (Goitre Is Present)
- Primary Atrophic Thyroiditis (No Goitre)

- Endemic Goitre Due To Iodine Deficiency
- Radio-Active Iodine Treated Thyrotoxicosis.
- Multi-Nodular Goiter (Non-Toxic)
- Surgical Removal
  - No Goitre
  - Thyroidectomy Scar

Investigations

- Basic Investigations
- TSH, T3, T4, U/S Scan.
- Hashimoto: Anti Thyroglobin , Antimicrosomal Abs

Treatment

- L-Thyroxine, Taken First Thing In The Morning.
- Clinical Improvement Is Delayed After Lab Improvement.

Neurological Manifestations Of Hypothyroidisim

- Deafness, Delayed Relaxation Of Reflexes, Peripheral Neuropathy, CTS (Carpal Tunnel Syndrome) , Proximal Myopathy , Dementia , Psychosis.

N.B:

Hypothyroidism Can Be A Part Of Poly-Glandular Autoimmune Syndrome Commonly Type II

What Are The Polyglandular Autoimmune Syndrome?

Type I:

- Addisons Disease
- Muco-Cutaneous Candidiasis
- Hypoparthyroidism

Type II:

- Addison`s Disease
- Either Type 1 D.M Or Hypothyridisim
- Pernicious Anaemia
- Caeliac Disease
- Hypogonadism
- Primary Biliary Cirrhosis

What Are The Clinical Differences Between 1ry Hypothyroidism & 2ry Hypothyroidism (Pituitary Failure) Clinically?

	1ry hypothyroidsim	2ry hypothyroidism
Periods	Menorrhagia	Amenorhhea
Goitre	+ / −	−
Autoimmune disorders	+	−
Weight	gain	loss
Myxedema	+	−
Depigmentation of areola	−	+

Pins & Needles In Hands

Please Examine This Patient With Pins & Needles In His Hands?

D.D Of Pins & Needles In Hands

- *Sensory Peripheral Neuropathy*
  - Diabetes Mellitus
  - Amyloidosis
  - Alcohol
  - Sub-Acute Combined Degeneration (B12 Deficiency)
  - Hypothyroidism
  - Uraemia
  - Drugs:
    - Chemotherapy
    - Metronidazole
- *Carpal Tunnel Syndrome*
  - Hypothyroidsim
  - Acromegaly
  - Rheumatoid Arthritis
  - Amyloidosis (Ankylosing Spondylitis , Bronchiectasis)
  - Vibration Tools
  - B2 Microglobulinaemia (Dialysis Patients)
  - Pregnancy
- *Hypocalcaemia* (May Or May Not Be Accompanied By Tetany)
  - Hyperventilation (Respiratory Alkalosis)
  - Hypo-Parathyroidism
  - Renal Failure

Analysis Of Pins & Needles Sensation In Hands:

- How Long?
- Suddenly Or Gradually?
- Getting Better Or Worse?
- What Increases It? What Decreases It?
- Where In The Hands? (Distribution)
  - Peripheral Neuropathy In Glove & Stock Distribution
  - Radicular Pain (Dermatomal Distribution)
  - Nerve Compression E.G. Carpal Tunnel Affecting Lateral 3 ½ Fingers.
- Unilateral Or Bilateral:
  - Bilateral Pins & Needles In Hands Could Be Due To Peripheral Neuropathy.
- Any Pins & Needles In Legs?
  - If Legs Are Affected Could Be Peripheral Neuropathy.
- Any Weakness?
- Any Joint Pains?
- Any Rash?
- S/S Of Differentials Above?

ONCE YOU ENTER THE ROOM SEARCH FOR A SPOT DIAGNOSIS

Prominent Supraorbital Ridge + Large Nose + Large Lips + Prognasthism + Wrinkled Forehead =

Acromegaly

Targeted History:

Confirm Diagnosis, R/O Differential Diagnoses & Look For Associated Conditions

- Vision Problems? Do You Bump Into Objects Whilst Walking? Any RTA?
  - o **Bitemporal Hemi-Anopia**
- What About Shoe And Ring Size, Do They Fit? **(Enlarged Hands & Feet)**
- Any Excessive Sweating?
- Any Weakness In Your Arms Or Legs?
- Problems With Intimate Relations? **(Impotence)**
- Any Pain In Your Knees? **(Osteoarthritis Of Knees)**
- Drinking More Water Than U Used To? Passing More Urine Than Usual? **(Diabetes Mellitus Symptoms, Hypercalcaemia)**
- Pins & Needles In Hands? **(Carpal Tunnel Syndrome)**
- SOB? Swollen Legs? **(Heart Failure)**
- Constipation? Weight Loss? Bleeding With Bowel Motions? **(Cancer Colon)**
- Do You Have High Blood Pressure?
- Do You Drive ?
- Ask About Etiology?

1. **Raised Intracranial Pressure**
- Any Headaches? Vomiting? Blurring Of Vision? (Usually Macro-Adenoma)
2. **Part Of MEN I**
- Are You Passing More Urine Than Usual? (Hypercalcaemia)
- Watery Diarrhea? (Pancreatic Tumor?)

Targeted Examination:

Examine FACE (Facies As Above)

SKIN TAGS On Neck & Axilla

ACANTHOSIS NIGRICANS

Enlarged HANDS & FEET

Examine For Carpal Tunnel Syndrome

Proximal MUSCLE WEAKNESS

Examine The THYROID For Enlargement

Examine The ABDOMEN For Enlarged Organs

Examine KNEES For OA Signs

- Pain & Tenderness
- Crepitus
- Painful Limited ROM

Examine EYES

- **Acuity**
  - o Counting Fingers
  - o Hand Motion
  - o Light Perception
- **Field** (Bi-Temporal Hemianopia)
- **Fundus** (D.M, HTN, Papilledema, Optic Atrophy)

I Would Like To Complete My Examination By Measuring B.P, Blood Sugar And Do Urine Dipstick.

Clinical Signs Of Activity Of Acromegaly

- Sweating.
- Progressive Enlargement Of Hands & Feet.
- Skin Tags.
- Worsening Synmptoms.

Menomonic For Acromegaly Presentation:

A Acanthosis

B Blood Pressure (High)

C Carpal Tunnel Syndrome, Calcium ??

D Diabetes Mellitus

E Enlarged Organs

F Field Defect

G Goitre

H Heart Failure, Headache

I Insulin Like Growth Factore Is High

J Joint Pains (OA)

K Kyphosis

L Libido Loss

M Myopathy, Macroglossia

N Neuropathy

O OSA (Obstructive Sleep Apnea), Old Photo Check, Optic Atrophy

P Papilloedma , Prognathism

Q Query MEN I

R Ring Size

S Shoe Size, Stones (Renal)

T Tags Of Skin

U Undesirable Complications (Colon Cancer)

Menomonic For Acromegaly Investigations

S Supression Test

C Calcium In Serum, Colonoscopy If CA Colon Suspected

R Radiology (MRI Sella Tursica)

I ILGF-1 (Insulin Like Growth Factor 1) For Follow Up

P Perimetry For Visual Field

T Target Organ (TSH , FSH , LH , ACTH, Prolactin)

E Echo , ECG

Quick Discussion

Indications For Admission

• Sweating, Skin Tags , Worsening Symptoms ,Uncontrolled HTN , Uncontrolled D.M ,
  Progressive Visual Field Defect

The Cause Of Death

• CVS (IHD) , Malignancy (Colon) , Apoplexy

Investigations

• OGTT With Measuring Serum GH , Blood Sugar , IGF1 (Screening & Follow Up)
• Serum Prolcation
• MRI Sella Turcica
• NCV For Carpal Tunnel ,CPK For Myopathy
• Echo: Dilated Cardiomyopathy
• Perimeter (For Visual Field)

- Calcium For MEN1
- Colonoscopy (Above 40 Every 3-5 Years If Active Disease)

Treatment:

SURGICAL REMOVAL

- Trans-Sphenoidal Hypophysectomy, Trans-Nasal Hypophysectomy, Trans-Labial Hypophysectomy.
- First Line Of Treatment.
- Side Effects : Panhypopituitarism, Hemorrhage, Infection, CSF Rhinorrhea & Meningitis , Recurrence

OCTEREOTIDES

- Somatostatin Analogue
- Decreases The Size Of The Tumors.
- Side Effects: Gall Stones, Steatorrhea, Abdominal Pain, Diabetes Mellitus.

PEGVISOMENT

- Growth Hormone Receptor Antagonist
- S/C Once/Weekly
- Side Effects: Hepatitis, Doesn't Affect The Size Of The Tumor.

CAUSES OF ACROMEGALY:

- Pituitary Adenoma (Usually Macro-Adenoma)
- Ectopic GH Secretion (Very Rare)

Symmetrical + Deforming Arthropathy Sparing DIP + Ulnar Deviation =

Rheumatoid Arthritis

Targeted History:

Confirm Diagnosis, R/O Differential Diagnoses & Look For Associated Conditions

- Any Pain, Stiffness Of Your Joints? For How Long You Have This Stiffness (1 Hour) ? And When Do You Have It Mostly (Early Morning)? **(Morning Stiffness)**
- Where? Both Hands? Same Fingers? **(Bilateral Symmetrical)**
- Any Swellings? Any Bumps On Your Arms? **(Rheumatoid Nodules)**
- Any Pins & Needles In Your Hands? **(Carpal Tunnel Syndrome/ Peripheral Neuropathy)**
- Any Pain In Your Eyes? Do You Feel It Dry? **(Sicca Syndrome)**
- Any SOB, Coughing? Do You Feel Your Chest Is Noisy? **(Pulmonary Fibrosis)**
- Any Pain In Your Neck? **(Atlanto-Axial Sublaxation)**
- Passing Frothy Urine? Pins & Needles In Arms Or Legs? **(Amyloidosis)**
- Any Blackish Discoloration Of The Tip Of Your Fingers? **(Digital Infarcts)**

Targeted Examination:

Examine THE HANDS RHEUMATOLOGICALLY

Inspection

- Scars , Swelling , Wasting Of Small Muscles Of The Hand
- Digital Infarcts
- Deformities (Swan Neck , Boutonniere, Z Shaped, Ulnar Deviation)
- Palmar Erythema
- Signs Of Inflammation (Redness , Hotness , Tenderness)
  o Inflammation Of Joints In Rheumatoid Arthritis Should Be Bilateral Symmetrical Sparing DIP.

Palpation (Any Pain In Your Hands? Where?)

You Should Palpate Each Joint Independently Of Both Hands And Palpate The Wrist As Well Looking For:

- Hotness, Tenderness Of Joints (Bilateral Symmetrical)
- Crepitus Of Wrist, MCP Joints.
- Palpation Of Swellings (Usually Soft In RA)
  o Tenderness
  o Hotness
  o Consistency
  o Fluctuant Or Not

Range Of Motion Of Joints

- Examine ROM Of Wrist
- Examine ROM Of Small Joints Of The Hands.

Assess Functional Status

- **Power Grip :** (Can You Squeeze My Fingers Please)
- **Precision Grip:**
  o Ask The Patient To Botton Or Unbutton His Shirt.
  o Ask The Patient To Hold A Coin Between Fingers.
- **Key Grip**: Ask The Patient To Hold A Key & Pretend To Use It.

Examine For Carpal Tunnel Syndrome

- Wasting Of Thenar Eminence.
- Weakness Of Abduction & Oponence Pollicis

- Lost Sensation On Lateral 3.5 Fingers
- Phalen Sign
- Tinnel Sign (May I Tap On Youur Wrist, Any Pain?)

Examine The Hands NEUROLOGICALLY

Examine Arms For RHEUMATOID NODULES

Examine EYES For

- Scleromalcia (Bluish Discoloration Of Sclera)
- Scleritis (Painful Red Eye)
- Episcleritis (Painless Red Eye)

Examine LUNGS For

- Bibasal Fibrosis
- Brochiolitis Obliterans

Examine The HEART For Pericarditis

Examine The ABDOMEN For Splenomegaly ? Feltys Syndrome

- Neutropenia + Splenomegaly + RA = Feltys Syndrome

LOOK FOR ANY MONO-NEURITIS MULTIPLEX

LOOK FOR SIGNS OF NEPHROTIC SYNDROME

Quick Discussion

Complications

- Hand Deformities
- Atlanto-Axial Sublaxation → Quadriplegia
- Carpal Tunnel Syndrome.
- Kerato-Conjunctivitis Sicca.
- Pulmonary Fibrosis.
- Ischemic Colitis Part Of Vasculitis
- Amyloidosis
- Mononeuritis Multiplex
- G.N (Penicillamine , NSAIDS ,Amyloidosis)
- Complications Of Medications.

Investigations:

- Basic Blood Tests
    o Anemia (Chronic Illness, NSAIDS Induced, Bone Marrow Suppression By Medications, Pernicious Anemia, Part Of Renal Failure)
    o Neutropenia With Feltys Syndrome
    o Platelets May Be Raised (Reactive Thrombocytosis)
- ESR, CrP Are Raised With Activity.
- RF (Rheumatoid Factor) Is +ve But –ve In Felty`s Syndrome.
- X-Ray (Soft Tissue Swelling , Narrow Joint Space , Periarticular Osteopenia)
- Anti CCP

Treatment:

- NSAIDS
- DMARD (Methotrexate + Hydroxychloroquine + Sulphasalazine)
- Anti-TNF Alpha : Infliximab (<u>S.E:</u> Flare Of T.B) & Etanercept (<u>S.E:</u> Demylination)
- IL-1 Antagonist: Anakinra
- Steroids May Be Used With Severe Articular Symptoms But It Is Not A Corner Stone Of Treatment.
- Physiotherapy

- Surgical Intervention Of Deformities

Signs Of Activity

- Signs Of Inflammation In Joints
- Raised Inflammatory Markers
- Raised Titers Of RF (> 3 Folds)
- DAS 28 Score

Diagnostic Criteria Of RA

(2010 ACR/EULAR CRITERIA):

RA Is Based Upon The Presence Of Synovitis In At Least One Joint, The Absence Of An Alternative Diagnosis That Better Explains The Synovitis, And The Achievement Of A Total Score Of At Least 6 (Of A Possible 10) From The Individual Scores In Four Domains. The Highest Score Achieved In A Given Domain Is Used For This Calculation. These Domains And Their Values Are:

Joint involvement	Score
• 1 medium-large joint	0
• 2-10 medium-large joints	1
• 1-3 small joints	2
• 4-10 small joints	3
• More than 10 small joints	5
Serology	
• RF (-) and anti-CCP (-)	0
• RF (+) or anti-CCP (+)	2
• High RF (+) or anti-CCP (+)	3
Duration of symptoms	
• < 6 weeks	0
• ≥ 6 weeks	1
Acute phase reactants	
• CRP and ESR within normal	0
• elevated CRP or ESR	1

Side Effects Of Medications Used In RA Treatment:

NSAIDS:

PUD, Renal Failure, Salt & Water Retention.

Steroids:

PUD, Osteoporosis, Thinning Of Skin, Slat & Water Retention

Methotrexate:

Pulmonary Fibrosis, Hepatitis, Neutropenia

Sulfasalazine:

Rash, Hypersensitivity, Bone Marrow Failure

Anti-TNF:

Rash, Opportunistic Infections R/O T.B& Viral Hepatitis Before Use

Anti CD20 (Rituximab):

Opportunistic Infections, Malignancy If Used For Long Time

Penicillamine & Gold:

Not Used Any More However, Can Cause Nephrotic Syndrome, Thrombocytopenia And Rash

Tanning Of The Skin

Please Examine This Patient With Tanning Of His Skin

D.D Of Tanned Skin:

- Familial, Racial
- Addisons Disease
- Haemochromatosis
- Cushing Disease (Pituitary Adenoma)
- Chronic Hemolytic Anemia (2ry Hemochromatosis)
- Renal Failure
- Nelson Syndrome (Bilateral Adrenalectomy)
- Bronchogenic Carcinoma (Ectopic ACTH Secretion)
- Drugs (Minocycline, Phenothiazines, Anti-Malarials, Amiodarone)

Analysis Of Tanned Skin:

- For How Long?
- Suddenly Or Gradually?
- Getting Better Or Worse?
- Can I See An Old Photo Of Yours?
- Do You Take Any Medications Regularly?
- S/S Of Differentials Above?

ONCE YOU ENTER THE ROOM SEARCH FOR A SPOT DIAGNOSIS

Generalized Tanning + Pigmentation Of Knuckles & Palmar Creases +
Pigmentation Of Buccal Mucosa + Thin Patient =

Addison`s Disease

Targeted History:

Confirm Diagnosis, R/O Differential Diagnoses & Look For Associated Conditions

- Where Is It Exactly? **(Specific Distribution)**
- Have You Lost Weight?
- Any Pain In Your Tummy? Vomiting? Lightheadedness? Diarrhoea? **(Symptoms)**
- Faints Or Blackouts Whilst Standing Up From Sitting Position? **(Orthostatic Hypotension)**
- Are You Feeling Tired All The Time? **(Asthenia)**
- Sweating, Feeling Cold, Shaking, Irritability, LOC? **(Hypoglycemia)**
- Any Neck Swellings? Do You Tend To Feel The Hot Or Cold More Than Usual? Handshakes? Constipation? Sweating Excessively Or Dryness Of Your Skin? Anxious Irritable? **(Thyroid Disorder As Part Of APS)**
- Any Parts Of Your Skin Became Lighter/ Lost Color? **(Vitiligo)**
- Any Loss Of Hair? **(Alopecia Areata / Totalis)**
- SOB, Racing Of Your Heart, Looking Paller Than Usual? **(Pernicious Anemia)**
- PH Of **HIV, T.B, Meningitis**?
- DH Especially **Steroids,** If Patient Is On Or Used To Take Steroids Ask For The Reason , Dosage , Duration And Gradual Withdrawal.

Targeted Examination:

- **Examine Knuckles & Palmar Creases** For Increased Pigmentations
- **Examine New Scars** For Pigmentation(Old Scars Are Lighter)
- **Examine Buccal Mucosa** For Pigmentations Inside The Mouth
- **Examine The Nape & Axilla**
- **Look For Vitiligo**
- **Examine Thyroid** (Schmidt`s Syndrome)
- **Examine Abdomen** To Exclude Hemochromatosis (HSM)
- **I Would Like To Complete My Examination By Examination Of B.P, L/S (Lying/Standing) B.P, And Blood Sugar.**

Quick Discussion

Investigations

Basic Investigations:

- FBC (Eosinophilia)
- Serum K (High Or Upper Limit Of Normal)
- Serum Na (Low)
- Blood Glucose Could Be Low Or Low Normal
- Serum Ca (Increased)

Basal Tests:

- 9:00 Am Serum Cortisol (Usually Low)
- 9:00 Am ACTH (High If Primary Adrenal Insufficiency)

Dynamic Tests:

- Short Synacthen Test (Diagnostic)
- Long Synacthen Test If Short Synacthen Test Inconclusive

Tests For Etiology & Associations:

- Anti 21 Hydroxylase Ab (Autoimmune)

- Tfts
- CT Chest Abdomen (T.B)
- HIV Test

Treatment

- Oral Hydrocortisone 2/3 At Day Time & 1/3 At Night Is The Treatment Of Choice.
- Fludrocortisone If Postural Hypotension Is Resistant To Hydrocortisone (Primary Hypoaldosterolism) Using The Lowest Possible Dose Aiming For Plasma Renin Activity Of Upper Normal
- Treatment Is For Life.
- Cortisol Requirements Increase During Severe Illness And Surgery.
- Patient Has To Wear Steroid Bracelet Or Carry Card, & Carry Steroid Ampoule In His Pocket
- Follow Up Clinically & Lab.

Monitoring Of Therapy:

- Weight Gain
- Blood Pressure Improvement
- Avoid HTN Or Oedema (This Means Excessive Replacement)
- Serum Electrolytes & Plasma Renin.

What Do You Know About Addisonian Crisis?

- Vomiting, Diarrhea, Abdominal Pain, Hypotension, Hypoglycemia, Dehydration, Fever, Shock.
- Due To Stress =Infection Or Psychological Trauma
- Treatment Saline And IV Steroids

What Are The Causes Of Adrenal Insufficiency?

Primary

- Auto-Immune (Remember APS → Autoimmune Poly-Glandular Syndrome)
- HIV
- T.B
- Meningitis (Waterhouse Friedrichson Syndrome)

Secondary

- Hypopituitarism
- Long Term Steroid Use With Sudden Withdrawal.

Shortness Of Breath

Please Examine This Patient With SOB?

D.D Of SOB

Cardiac Causes:

- Congestive Heart Failure
- IHD
- Pericardial Diseases (Effusion/Tamponade)
- Valvular Heart Disease
- Cardiac Arrhythmias

Pulmonary Causes:

- COPD
- Asthma
- Pneumonia
- Pleural Effusion
- Pneumothorax
- Bronchiectasis
  - Kartagner`S Syndrome(Heart On Rt. + Bronchiectasis)
  - Cystic Fibrosis (Short Stature + Bronchiectasis + D.M + Malabsorption)
  - COPD
  - ABPA
- Pulmonary Embolism
- Bronchogenic Carcinoma
- Carcinoid Syndrome
- Lung Fibrosis
  - Asbestosis
  - Sarcoidosis
  - Ankylosing Spondylitis
  - RA
  - SLE
  - Scleroderma
  - Polymyositis
  - Dermatomyositis
  - Drugs (Amiodarone , Nitrofurantoin , Methotrexate , Bleomycin)
  - Idiopathic Pulmonary Fibrosis
  - Eosinophilic Pulmonary Fibrosis
  - Extrinsic Allergic Alveolitis (Hypersensitivity Pneumonitis)
    - Bird Fancier: Bird Droppings
    - Farmer's Lung: Aspergillus In Mouldy Hay
    - Bagassosis: Mouldy Bagasse (Sugar Cane)
    - Painters: Isocyanate
    - Compost Lung : Aspergillus
    - Hot Tub Lung: Hot Tubs Mist (MAC)
    - Tobacco Worker Lung : Mould
  - Viral Pneumonitis

Neuro-Muscular Disorders

- Guillian Barre
- MND (Motor Neuron Disease0
- Myasthenia Gravis
- Botulism

Others

- ARDS
- Sepsis
- Renal Failure (Fluid Overload, Metabolic Acidosis)
- DKA
- Thyrotoxicosis
- Anemia

Analysis Of SOB

- For How Long?
- Suddenly Or Gradually?
- Getting Better Or Worse? What Increase And What Decrease?
- Exertional Or At Rest?
- What Is The Patient`s Job?
- Associated With Coughing? If Yes Does The Patient Bring Up Any Phlegm? If Yes What Color Is It?
- Any Chest Pains?
- Coughing Up Blood?
- SOB On Lying Flat On Bed? (Orthopnea)
- Waking Up From Sleep SOB At Night? (PND)
- Swollen Ankles?
- S/S Of Differentials Above?

ONCE YOU ENTER THE ROOM SEARCH FOR A SPOT DIAGNOSIS

Lupus Pernio (Purple Rash On Cheeks Cross Nasolabial Folds Resembles Frost Bite) + Erythema Nodosum (Painful Red Nodules On Shins) =

Sarcoidosis

Targeted History:

Confirm Diagnosis, R/O Differential Diagnoses & Look For Associated Conditions

- SOB?
- Any Fevers?
- Coughing (Dry)?
- Pain In Legs?
  - ○ Pain Over Shins Due To Eryhtema Nodosum (E.N.)
  - ○ Pain In Joints Secondary To Sarcoidosis Itself.
- Dry Mouth? Dry Red Eyes? (Miculikz Syndrome).
- Painful Joints?
- Passing More Urine? (Diabetes Insipidus Secondary To Hypercalcaemia).
- Any Weakness In Face, Arms Or Legs? (Mononeuritis Multiplex).

Targeted Examination:

- **Examine The FACE For** Lupus Pernio, Red Eye, Parotid Enlargement.
- **Examine EYE MOVEMENTS** And Any Part With Focal Neurology Neurologically.
- **Examine The CHEST For** Lung Fibrosis.
- **Examine The PULSE & HEART For** Heart Failure Or Arrhythmias.
- **Examine The Abdomen For** HSM.
- **Examine The LEGS For** Erythema Nodosum.
- **Examine For L.Ns.**
- **Any Evidence Of Previous Use Of Steroids.**

Quick Discussion

What Are The Manifestations Of Neurosarcoidosis?

- Neuroendocrine Dysfunction.
- Focal Or Multifocal Encephalopathy.
- Myelopathy.
- Hydrocephalus, Aseptic Meningitis.
- Peripheral Neuropathy Or Myopathy.

What Are The Cutaneous Manifestations Of Sarcoidosis?

- Papules, Nodules, Plaques, And Atrophic Or Ulcerative Lesions.
- Lupus Pernio Is A Distinct Variant Of Cutaneous Sarcoidosis That Presents With Violaceous Or Erythematous Papules, Plaques, Or Nodules Predominantly Involving The Central Facial Skin. The Nasal Alae Are Often Affected. Patients With Lupus Pernio Appear To Have An Increased Risk For Sarcoidosis Involving The Respiratory Tract.
- The Development Of Sarcoidosis In A Scar Or Tattoo Site May Be The Initial Sign Of Sarcoidosis In Some Patients.
- Erythema Nodosum Is The Most Common Nonspecific Manifestation Of Sarcoidosis.

What Are The Manifestations Of Cardiac Sarcoidosis?

- Conduction Disease
- Arrhythmias
- Sudden Death
- Heart Failure
- Cardiomyopathy
- Valvular Heart Disease, And Myocardial Damage Simulating Infarction.

- Cardiac Sarcoidosis May Occur Alone Or Alongside Systemic Sarcoidosis But Is Frequently Clinically Silent.
- Findings On Electrocardiogram And Echocardiogram Are Nonspecific; Features On Cardiovascular Magnetic Resonance Imaging, And Positron Emission Tomography(PET) May Be Suggestive But Are Not Diagnostic.

Investigations:

- Basic Blood Tests To R/O Infections
- CXR: Reticulo-Nodular Shadows
- HRCT: Will Shows Pulmonary Affection In The Form Of:
  - Grade I: B/L Hilar Lymphadenopathy
  - Grade II: B/L Hilar L.N + Reticular Opacities
  - Grade III: Reticular Opacities With Shrinking Hilar Nodes
  - Grade IV: Reticular Opacities With Evidence Of Volume Loss, Predominantly Distributed In The Upper Lung Zones
- Serum ACE Usually Raised.
- Serum Calcium Raised In 30 % Of Cases
- Bronchoscopy & Biopsy For Histopathology
- CTKUB Might Show Nephrocalcinosis.
- Investigations For The Above Complications.
- Pulmonary Function Tests.

What Are The Causes Of Polyuria In Sarcoidosis?

- Could Be Central Due To Sarcoidosis Affecting Pituitary Gland
- Could Be Due To Nephrogenic DI Secondary To Hypercalcaemia.

Treatment:

Most Patients With Pulmonary Sarcoidosis Do Not Require Treatment, As A High Proportion Have Asymptomatic, Non-Progressive Disease Or Experience A Spontaneous Remission

Indications Of Steroids

- Neurosarcodidosis
- Bothersome Pulmonary Symptoms
- Deteriorating Lung Functions
- Hypercalcaemia
- Cardiac Sarcoidosis

Clear Lung Fields + Sinus Tachycardia + Either Hypercoagulable State Or Prolonged Immobility Or Long Flights Or Active Cancer =

Pulmonary Embolism

Targeted History:

Confirm Diagnosis, R/O Differential Diagnoses & Look For Associated Conditions

- Any Coughing? (Usually **No Coughing**)
- Sudden Or Gradual? (**Sudden**)
- Chest Pains? (**Pleuritic**)
- Hemoptysis? (**Could Occur**)
- **Ask About Risk Factors:**
  - Long Flights?
  - Cancers?
  - DVTs?
  - Pregnancy?
  - OCPs?
  - Prolonged Immobility?
  - Postoperative?
  - Hypercoagulable States?
    - Antiphospholipid Syndrome
    - Recurrent Abortion
    - Could Be Associated With SLE
    - Recurrent Arterial / Venous Thrombosis
    - Factor V Leydin
    - Homocysteinuria
    - Nephrotic
    - Paroxysmal Nocturnal Haemoglobinuria (PNH)
    - Myeloproliferative Disorders
    - Polycythemia
    - Protein C & S Deficiency
    - Behcet`s Disease

Targeted Examination

- **Examine PULSE** For Tachycardia
- **Examine NECK** For Raised JVP
- **Examine MOUTH** For Ulcers ? SLE ? Behcet`s
- **Examine The HEART** For Accentuated P2
- **Examine The CHEST** Usually Minimal Findings Or Findings Of Pleural Effusion.
- **Examine LEGS** For
  - Signs Of DVT
  - B/L L.L Edema Of Heart Failure Or Nephrotic Syndrome

Quick Discussion

Investigations:

- *Basic Blood Tests* To R/O Other Causes Of SOB
- *CXR:* Usually Clear Or Pleural Effusion
- *D-Dimers:* Usually Raised , Highly Sensitive
- *ECG:* Sinus Tachycardia, RBBB, Inverted T In V1 , RVH , SI QIII TIII Sign
- *CTPA:* Diagnostic
- *V/Q* If CTPA Cannot Be Done And Normal CXR.

- *Echo*: To Assess Right Ventricular Function And Look For Signs Of Pulmonary HTN, Pulmonary HTN Means Chronic Recurrent PE Rather Than Acute Massive PE Because Acute Massive PE Will Usually Cause Right Heart Failure

Treatment:

- Treatment Dose Enoxaparin 1.5 Mg / Kg If eGFR > 30
- Consider Warfarin Or NOACs

Loose Motions

Please Examine This Patient With Lose Motions

D.D Of Lose Motions:

GIT Causes

- Infective Causes
  - CDIF
  - Traveller`s Diarrhea
  - Bacterial
  - Viral
  - Gastro-Enteritis
- Malabsorption Syndromes:
  - Celiac (Dermatitis Herpitiform , Mouth Ulcers , Gluten Sensitive)
  - Whipple Disease
  - Tropical Sprue
  - Small Bowel Bacterial Overgrowth
  - Chronic Pancereatitis
- IBD (Pyoderma Gangrenosa , Mouth Ulcers)
- Irritable Bowel Syndrome
- Carcinoid Syndrome
- Overflow Diarrhea
- Ileal Resection
- Radiation Enteritis
- Acute Appendicitis.

NON-GIT Causes

- Medications
  - Laxatives
  - Antibiotics
  - Metformin
  - Colchicine
- Thyrotoxicosis
- Carcinoid
- Addison`S Disease
- Autonomic Neuropathy
- HIV

Analysis Of Lose Motions:

- How Long?
- Any Weight Loss?
- Is It Related To Meals Or Certain Kind Of Foods? **(Celiac/Chronic Pancereatitis)**
- Any Fevers? **(Infective / Inflammatory Bowel Syndrome)**
- How Many Times Do You Open Your Bowels A Day?
- Is It Getting Better Or Worse?
- Do You Wake Up From Your Sleep To Open Your Bowels? **(R/O Irritable Bowel Syndrome)**
- Any Itchy Rash? **(Coeliac)**
- Sexual History? **(HIV)**
- FH? **(IBD, Celiac)**
- Any Auto-Immune Diseases? **(Celiac)**
- Diabetes?
- Are You Taking Any Antibiotics?
- Any Blood Or Slime With Your Motions? **(Dysentery/Proctitis/Sigmoiditis)**
- Any Vomiting?

- Any Pains In Your Tummy?
- S/S Of Differentials Above?

ONCE YOU ENTER THE ROOM LOOK FOR A SPOT DIAGNOSIS

Itchy Erythematous Vesicles On Extensor Surface (DERMATITIS HERPETIFORM) =

Celiac Disease

Targeted History:

Confirm Diagnosis, R/O Differential Diagnoses & Look For Associated Conditions

- Any Lose Motions? Pale Offensive Floats Difficult To Flush? **(Steatorrhoea)**
- Is It Related To Meals? **(Related To Gluten Containing Food)**
  - o Wheat
  - o Barley
  - o Oats
- Any Heart Racing? SOB? Do You Look Pale?**(Anemia)**
- Do You Tend To Feel The Hot Or Cold More Than Usual? Constipations? Sleep? Handshakes? Memory Problems? **(Thyroid Disorder)**
- High Blood Sugar? **(Associated Diabetes)**
- Are You Bleeding From Any Parts Of Your Body? **(Vit. K Deficiency)**
- Any Pins & Needles In Hands Or Around The Mouth? **(Hypocalcaemia Secondary To Vit D Deficiency)**
- Any Skin Rash? Any Itching? **(Usually Elbows & Buttocks)**
- Any Family History?

Targeted Examination:

- **Examine Eyes For Pallor**
- **Examine Skin For Rash & Vitiligo**
- **Examine Abdomen**
- **Examine Thyroid**

Quick Discussion

Investigations

- Basic Blood Tests:
  - o Anaemia (Iron, B12 Deficiency)
  - o Raised Creatinine Secondary To Pre-Renal Failure Or Iga Nephropathy
  - o Hypokalaemia
  - o Hypocalcaemia
- Blood Film Will Show Target Cells Secondary To Hyposplenism Associated With Celiac Diseas.
- Blood Film Might Show Poikilocytosis.
- Urinalysis & Urine PCR To R/O Iga Nephropathy
- Stool Analysis, MC&S To R/O Infective Diarrhea
- Fecal Fat Will Be Raised
- Anti-Gliadin Abs
- Anti-Endomysial Abs
- Anti TTG
- Endoscopy With Duodenal Biopsy

Treatment

- Gluten Free Diet (Avoid Oats, Barley, Wheat).
- Maize & Rice Are Ok.
- Dapsone For Skin Rash.
- Renal R/V If Suspecting Iga Nephropathy.

Deep Ulcer Over The Shins + Violaceous Undermined Border + Painful
(PYODERMA GANGRENOSUM) =

Inflammatory Bowel Disease

Targeted History:

Confirm Diagnosis, R/O Differential Diagnoses & Look For Associated Conditions

- Do You Have Any Pains In Your Tummy?
- Any Lose Motions? Any Blood With Your Motions?
- Any Mouth Sores?
- Any Skin Rash?
  - o Pyoderma Gangrenosum
  - o Erythema Nodosum
- Any Weight Loss?
- Any Fevers, Sweats?
- Eye Problems?
- Back Pains?
- Any Family History?
- Have You Noticed Your Eye White Turned Yellow? (**Jaundice With PSC In UC)**
- Have You Had Any Previous Camera Tests?
- Analysis Of The **PYODERMA GANGRENOSUM**:
  - o How Did It Look Like At The Start (Small Lump Doesn't Respond To Antibiotics)?
  - o Is It Painful?
  - o Any Discharge? Bleeding?
- **EXTRA GIT MANIFESTATIONS:**
  - o Painful Joints?
  - o Peri-Anal Disease? (Crohns)
  - o Severe Abdominal Pain + SIRS + Distended Abdomen = R/O Toxic Megacolon

Targeted Examination:

- **Examine The BACK For Sacro-Ilieitis**
- **Examine The ABDOMEN For Scars And Tenderness & Rt.Iliac Fossa Mass**
- **Examine MOUTH For Ulcers**
- **Examine EYES For Pallor Or Jaundice**
- **Assess The Fluid Status Of The Patient** (JVP, Skin Turgor, Presence Or Absence Of L.L Edema, Sunken Eyes, Dry Mucous Membranes)
- **Examine Any SKIN RASH**

Quick Discussion

Investigations:

- ESR Is Raised
- Raised WBCs
- Stool MC & S To R/O Infection
- Colonoscopy With Biopsy
- AXR, Abdominal CT Scan To R/O Toxic Megacolon
- Swab Of The Ulcer MC & S

Treatment

UC

- Mild Localized Disease→ Mesalazine Rectal
- Pancolitis → Oral Mesalazine/Oral Glucocorticoids
- ? Surgery

Crohns

- Induce Remission By Glucocorticoids & Mesalazine
- Azathioprine To Maintain Remission
- Metronidazole For Peri-Anal Disease
- Infliximab For Fistulating Disease
- ? Surgery

Complications Of Ulcerative Colitis

Toxic Megacolon, Perforation, Strictures, And The Development Of Dysplasia And Colorectal Cancer, Primary Sclerosing Cholangitis.

Complications Of Crohn's Disease

Transmural Involvement Of The Bowel, Including Fistulas, Abscess, Perianal Disease.

Extraintestinal Manifestations, Such As Arthritis, Eye And Skin Disorders, Biliary Tract Involvement, And Kidney Stones.

Causes Of Pyoderma Gangrenosa

- IBD (Inflammatory Bowel Disease)
- RA (Rheumatoid Arthritis)
- MM (Multiple Myeloma)
- Vasculitis
- Seronegative Arthropathies

Quick History If Faced By A Case Of Pyoderma Gangrenosum:

- Any Pain In Your Hands? Joints? Stiffness? (RA)
- Pain In Chest? Frothy Urine? Back Pains? Bone Pains? (MM)
- Cough ? Coughing Blood? Problems With Your Kidneys? (Vasculitis)

Investigations For A Case Of Pyoderma Gangrenosum:

- Biopsy Of The Ulcer (Neutrophilic Dermatosis)
- CXR / CT Chest, Urine Analysis, Urine PCR, U & Es If Suspecting Vasculitis
- Protein Electrophoresis If MM Suspected
- Investigations For IBD If Suspected
- Investigation For RA If Suspected

Treatment Of Pyoderma Gangrenosa

- Treatment Of The Cause
- Wound Care
- Glucocorticoids If Extensive
- Immunosuppressant Agents Might Be Needed; Seek Expert Help

Tipped Nose + Skin Puckeringaround Mouth + Narowing Of Mouth + Telangectasia + Thin Stretched Shiny Skin + Sclerodactyly + Curling Of Fingers (Flexion Deformity) =

Scleroderma

Targeted History:

Confirm Diagnosis, R/O Differential Diagnoses & Look For Associated Conditions

- Joint Pain? Changes Of Your Skin? Skin Tightness? Heart Burn? SOB? Constipation Or Lose Motions (Bacterial Overgrowth) ? Difficulty Swallowing? Cold Blue Hands? Sores Or Wounds In Hands? Frothy Water?
- Any Weakness Climbing Up Stairs , Combing Your Hair? Any Rash On Your Nose Cheecks ? Sensitivity To Sun? (Mixed C.T Ds)

Targeted Examination:

- **Narrow Mouth** (Put 3 Fingers In Ur Mouth)
- **Examine The Hands For Stretched Skin** (Hand + Mouth Only = Limited, Look For PH)
- **Examine Upper Arms & Trunk If Involved With Hand & Face** = Diffuse =Fibrosis
- **Examine Chest For Basal Fibrosis & PH**
    - Decrease Breath Sounds
    - Fine End Inspiratory Crackles or
    - Palpable 2nd Sound
    - Elevated JVP
    - Accentuated P2
- **Features + Palpable Purpra** (Vasculitis)

Quick Discussion

Complications Of Scleroderma

- Renal Crisis (Malignant HTN, Azotemia, Microangiopathic Haemolytic Anemia) May Be dt. Steroids Treat with ACEIs
- Hand Curling &Deformities With Limitations
- Esophagus : Reflux, Dysphagia, Anemia, Barretts
- Ischemic Colitis And Pseudo-Intestinal Obstruction
- Pulmonary Fibrosis & Pulmonary HTN

Investigations

- ANA
- Anticentromere (Limited)
- Anti SCL 70 (Diffuse)
- Kfts
- Urine Analysis
- Echocardiography & CXR
- Differentiate Between Limited & Diffuse Scleroderma By Examining The Skin Involvement Of The Trunk And Shoulders

Treatment

- Pain : NSAIDS
- Raynauds: Nifidipine
- Skin Tightness : Methotrexate ??
- Kidney : Aceis, Dialysis
- Active Alveolitis : Cyclophosphamide (Not Steroids =Renal Crisis & Pneumonia)
- Pulmonary HTN :Bosentan (Endothelin Receptor Antagonist)

Cold Hands

D.D Of Cold Hands

- Hypothyroidism
- Raynaud`s Disease (Bilateral, Age <40, BBs, Ergots, OCPs, Chemo)
- Raynaud`s Phenomenon (SLE , Scleroderma)
- Peripheral Arterial Disease (D.M, HTN)

Painful Joints

Please Examine This Patient With Pain In His Joints?

D.D Of Painful Joints

Mono/Oligoarthritis	Polyarthritis
• Trauma	• RA
• Septic Arthritis	• SLE
• Crystals Arthritis	• Viral Infection
• Sero –Ve Arthritis	• Vasculitis
• Osteoarthritis	• Sero –ve Arthritis
• Lyme Disease	• Osteoarthritis
• Malignancy	• Sarcoidosis
	• Malignancy
	• Parvovirus B 19
	• Hemochromatosis

Unilateral	Bilateral (Sym/Assym)
• Trauma	• SLE
• Septic Arthritis	• RA
• Crystal Arthritis	• Sero –ve Arthritis
o Gout	o Enteropathic Arthrtitis
o Pseudogout	▪ Inflammatory Bowel Disease
• Sero –ve Arthritis	▪ Whipple`S Disease
• Osteoarthritis	o Reiter Syndrome
• Haemoarthrosis	o Psoriatic Arthropathy
• Gonococcal Arthritis	o Ankylosing Spondylitis
• Osteomyelitis	o HLAB27 +ve, RF -ve
• Osteosarcoma	• Osteoarthritis
• Rheumatic Fever	• Sarcoidosis
• RA	• Malignancy
	• Parvovirus B 19
	• Hemochromatosis

Sausage Shaped Fingers + DIP Affection +Nail Changes (Pitting, Onycholysis) + Erythematous Plaques Covered By Silvery Scales =

Psoriatic Arthropathy

Targeted History:

Confirm Diagnosis, R/O Differential Diagnoses & Look For Associated Conditions

- Any Rash? Where? Itching? Nail Changes? Back Pain? Pain In Legs ? Similar Conditions In Family?
- DH: Lithium , BBs ,CCBs, Captopril, INF, NSAIDs, Alcohol , Hydroxychloroquine
- Guttate Psoriasis (Small Numerous Plaques , Tear Drop Like) Preceeded By Strept Infection

Targeted Examination:

- **Examine Extensors Of Elbow , Knees , Scalp** (Hair Line), **Umblicus , Buttocks For Rash** (Auspitz Sign)
- **Examine Nails**
- **Examine Hands Rheumatologically**
  - o Assymetrical Joint Affection , DIP Affected
- **Examine Back For Sacroilitis**

Quick Discussion

Investigations

- HLA B27
- X-Ray (Pencil In Cup Sign , Narrow Joint Space , Distal Joint Affection)
- MRI Sacroiliac Joint

Treatment

- Skin: PUVA , Coal Tar , Topical Steroids , Dithranol ,Retinoids
- Arthritis: Methotrexate , Sulphasalazine (Never Hydroxychloroquine)
- Biological Therapy: Etanercept

Asymmetrical, Non-Deforming Joint Affection + PIJ Osteophytes (Bouchard) + DIJ Osteophytes (Heberden Nodule) =

Osteoarthritis

Targeted History:

- Pain In Your Knees? Back? Neck? What Do You Do For Living?
- Morning Stiffness? (<1 hour)
- Any Other Joints affected?
- FH
- Manual Worker?
- How Is That Affecting Your Job?

Targeted Examination

- **Examine The HAND RHEUMATOLOGICALLY**
- **NO NAIL CHANGES**
- **Tenderness affecting DIJ**
- **Might present without Nodules**
- **Look for Psoriatic rash → No Rash if rash is present think about psoriasis**
- **Examine other Joints → e.g. Knee OA**

Quick Discussion

Investigations:

Xray (Narrow Joint Space, Subchondral Cysts, Osteophytes)

RF to R/O RA

Treatment

NSAIDS Creams + Paracetamol

Multiple Tophi =

Chronic Tophaceous Gout

Targeted History

- Joint Pains?
- Kidney Problems?
- Passing Gravels With Urine?
- Any Lumps?
- Alcohol?
- History Of Tumors And Chemotherapy?

Targeted Examination

- **Examine Hand Rheumatologically**
- **Other relative examination according to the history**

Quick Discussion

Investigations:

- X-Rays
- Serum Uric Acid

Treatment Of Acute Attacks

- NSAIDS
- Colchicine
- Prednisolone
- Allopurinol

Short Stature

Please Examine This Lady With Short Stature

D.D Of Short Stature

- Familial
- Constitutional Delay Of Growth
- Malnutrition
- Chronic Illness.
  o Coeliac Disease
  o Renal Failure
  o Inflammatory Bowel
  o Congenital Heart Disease
  o Cystic Fibrosis
- Dysmorphic Syndromes
  o Turner
  o Noonan Syndrome
  o Down $
    ▪ Silky Hair, Low Hair Line
    ▪ Epicanthal Fold , Low Set Ear
    ▪ Macroglossia ,Flat Occiput
    ▪ VSD, Simian Crease
    ▪ Widely Spaced Big Toe
    ▪ Enlarged Colon
- Laurance Moon Biedel Syndrome
  o Retinitis Pigmentosa
  o Polydactyly
  o Obesity
- Endocrinal Disorders
  o Pan-Hypopituitarism
  o Cretinism (Hypothyroidism)
  o Precocious Puberty
  o Pseudo Hypoparthyroidism
  o Dwarfism (GH Deficiency)
    ▪ Empty Sella Syndrome
    ▪ Short Stature
    ▪ 1ry Amenorrhea
    ▪ No 2ry Sexual Characters (Small Breasts, Small Testis)
    ▪ Hypothyroidism
    ▪ Postural Hypotension, Soft Dry , Wrinkled Skin (Alabaster Skin)
    ▪ Gynecomastia Not Present Except If Sex Hormones Are Introduced
- Achondroplasia (Disproportionate Short Stature)

Analysis Of Short Stature

- For How Long?
- Any Similar Conditions In The Family?
- What About Your Parents & Siblings Height?
- Do You Have Any Children? Any History Of Chronic Disease?
- Is It Proportionate Or Disproportionate?
  ✓ Disproportionate Means Span & Height Are Not Equal,
  ✓ Proportionate Means Span Equals The Height
- S/S Of Differentials Above?

ONCE YOU ENTER THE ROOM SEARCH FOR A SPOT DIAGNOSIS

Webbed Neck + Multiple Pigmented Nevi + Shield Chest + Widely Spaced
Nipples + Cubitus Valgus + Low Hair Line + Proportionate Short Stature =

Turner`s Syndrome

Targeted History

- When Did You Notice This?
- I`m Sorry To Ask You Private Questions?
  - Have You Noticed Enlargement Of Your Breasts? And what about Your Periods?
  - Have You noticed Hair growing In Your Private Areas?
  - Are you Married? Any Kids?
- Any SOB? Leg Cramps During Walking? Chest Pain? Weakness Clumsiness? **(Co-arctation of the Aorta)**
- Do You Have Low Tolerance To Cold Weather? Constipation? Weight Gain? Sleeping More Than Usual? Problems With Memory & Concentration ? **(Thyroid Problems)**
- Any headaches? Photophobia? Blurred vision? Neck Stiffness? **(SAH)**

Targeted Examination:

- **Examine Span = Height** (Proportionate)
- **Webbed Neck & Low Hair Line**
- **Shield Chest , Widely Spaced Nipples**
- **Multiple Pigments Nevi , Cubitus Valgus**
- **Short 4th Metacarpal Bone**
- **Examine Pulse In Arms & Feet** (Weaker Pulse In Feet)
- **Examine Pulse In Radial & Femoral** (Radiofemoral Delay)
- **Auscultate Lt. Infraclavicular Area For Systolic Murmur Of Coarctation**
- **Auscultate The Heart**
- **Examine Thyroid**
- **Examine neurologically if any headaches**

Quick Discussion

Cause:

- 45 X (Non-Disjunction)

Associations:

- Hypothyroidism, D.M
- Horse Shoe Kidney
- Coarctation Of Aorta, Bicuspid Aortic Valve, Berry Aneurysm

Investigation:

- Chromosomal Analysis
- CT Head & LP is SAH suspected

Treatment:

- Height = GH Before Puberty
- Period =Estrogen, Infertility = Donor Eggs

Short Obese + Short 4th Metacarpal + Skin Scars + Normal Hair Line =

Pseudo-Hypoparathyroidism

Targeted History:

Confirm Diagnosis, R/O Differential Diagnoses & Look For Associated Conditions

- Noticed Breasts Getting Larger? Periods? Hair In Private Areas? **(R/O Turner)**
- Weight Gain? Sleeping More Than Usual? Feel Cold More Than Usual? Constipations, Memory & Concentration Problems? **(Thyroid Problem)**
- Any Cramps in Legs or Hands? **(Tetany)**

Targeted Examination:

- **Examine Span** = Height (Proportionate)
- **Examine Hair Line** (Normal = Not Turner)
- **Examine Short 4**th **Metacarpals**
- **Examine Scars**
- **Examine Thyroid Completely**
- **Chovsteck Sign** (Facial) , **Traussu Sign** (Carpopedal Spasm)

Quick Discussion

Causes: AD

Investigations: Eleveted PTH And Low Calcium Levels

Painful Knees

Please Examine This Patient With Painful Knee?

Targeted History

- Any Other Joints Affected? Any Stiffness? Any Lumps Or Bumps? (RA)
- Have You Injured Yourself? (Hemo-arthrosis)
- FH
- Are You on Any Blood Thinners?

D.D Of Painful Knee

- *RA*
- *Osteo-Arthritis*
  - Acromegaly Or Obese
  - Wasting Of Quadriceps
  - Tenderness Over Joint Line
  - Crepitus
  - Effusion
  - OA in other joints
  - Manual Worker
  - Family History
- *Haemo-Arthrosis*
  - Recurrent
  - Haemophilia A , B (X-L R)
  - FH
  - After Minor Trauma
  - Bleeding Tendency From Other Parts Of The Body
  - Swollen Joint
  - No Signs Of Inflamation
- *Meniscal Injury*
- *Reiter*
- *Septic Arthritis*
  - IV Drug User
  - Gonococcaal (Multiple Sexual Partners , Burning Water)
- *Gout*
  - Excessive Alcohol
  - Renal Failure
  - Lymphoma/Psoriasis/Metabolic Syndrome/Glycogen Storage Disease
- *Pseudogout*

Knee Examination

- INSPECTION
  - Swelling , Deformity , Scars
- PALPATION
  - Hottness , Tenderness , Crepitus , Effusion (Bulge Signs , Patellar Tap)
- ROM
- SPECIAL TESTS
  - ACL → Anterior drawer test
  - PCL → Posterior Drewer test
  - MCL , LCL
  - Apply Compression Test For Menisci
- NEURO-VASCULAR EVALUATION

ONCE YOU ENTER THE ROOM SEARCH FOR A SPOT DIAGNOSIS

Swollen Ankles

Please Examine This Lady With Swollen Ankles

Targeted History:

Confirm Diagnosis, R/O Differential Diagnoses & Look For Associated Conditions

- Does It Leave A Mark When You Press on It ? (Pitting Edema)
- Any Other Joints Affected? Any Pain Stiffness In Her Joints? (Rheumatological Problem)
- Is It Painful (DVT, Inflammation)   / Painless , Weakness , Problems With Walking D.M? (Charcoat`s Joint)
- Any Mouth Sores, Sores In Private Areas (Behcet`s, APS)? Have You Ever Been Diagnosed By Having Clot In Your Blood Channels? FH Of Clots In Blood Channels? (DVT)

D.D Of Swollen Ankles

- **DVT**
  - Behcet (Mouth Ulcers) , AP$ (Miscarriages) , Hypercoagulable State (Immobility , Fractures , Chemotherapy , Tamoxifen , HRT , Ocps)
  - Swollen Calf (Measure 10 Cm Below Tibial Tuberosity Both Sides)
  - Pitting Edema
  - Varicose Veins
  - Tender Calfs
- **Varicose Veins**
  - Pigmentation
  - Ulcer On Medial Malleolus
  - Itching
  - Dilated Veins
  - L.L Edema (Pitting)
- **CHF, RF, Nephrotic, Malabsorption, CLD**
- **Pretibial Myxedema**
- **Myxedema** (Non-Pitting)
- **Charcoat Joint**
  - Starts As Swelling (Neuropathic Joint)
  - Completely Deformed Joint
  - Painless Or Painful
  - Lost Peripheral Sensations
  - Weakness Of Movements
  - Lost Peripheral Pulsations
  - Sensory Ataxia (Abnormal Coordination With Closed Eyes)
  - Signs Of Diabetes (Dermopathy , Necrobiosis Lipoidica , Amputation)
  - Alcohol , HSMN , Syphilis , D.M

ANKLE EXAMINATION

- **INSPECTION**
  - Swelling (Pitting Or Non Pitting Edema)
  - Difference In Size Of Both Legs
  - Deformities
  - Scars
  - Amputations , Digital Infarcts
  - Diabetic Signs
    - Necrobiosis Lipoidica
    - Diabetic Dermopathy
- **PALPATION**
  - Tenderness , Crepitus , Edema
- **ROM**
- **SPECIAL TESTS**

- o Anterior Drawer
- o Posterior Drawer
- o Valgus Stress
- o Varus Stress
- **NEUROVASCULAR EVALUATION**
  - o Motor Power , Sensations , Reflexes , Dorsalis Pedis

Gynecomastia

Please Examine This Man Complaining Of Enlarged Breasts?

D.D Of Enlarged Breasts

- Klinfelter
- Hyperthyroidsim
- Cushing Disease
- Prolactinoma
- Bronchogenic CA
- Leydig Cell Tumour (Peutz Jegher Syndrome)
- CLD
- RF
- Drugs:
  - o Spironolactone, Cimetidine, Digoxin, Amiodarone

ONCE YOU ENTER THE ROOM SEARCH FOR A SPOT DIAGNOSIS

Tall +Wide Hips + Narrow Shoulders + Gynecomastia =

Klinefelter`s Syndrome

Targeted History

- Breasts Enlarged?
- Noticed Beared Growing ? Voice Changed? Sexual Desires?
- Any Problems With Your Intimate Relations?
- Are You Married? Any Children?
- Any Fractures?

Targeted Examination

- Tall
- Wide Hips
- Absent secondary Sexual characters
- Small Testis

Quick Discussion

Causes

- 47XXY

Treatment

- Testerone Replacement For 2ry Sexual Characters

Patches Of Oral Pigmentations =

Peutz Jegher`s Syndrome

Targeted History

- Any Pigmentations On Hands? Any Pain In Your Tummy? Any Blood With Your Bowel Motions?
- PH Of Surgery With Your Bowel (Intussusception)?
- FH Of Bowel CA? Pancreatic CA?

Targeted Examination

- Patches Of Pigmented Macules On Lips , Buccal Mucosa , Palms & Fingers

Quick Discussion

Cause:

AD = LKB1, STK11 On Chromosome 19

Investigation:

Colonoscopy , Endoscopy , CT , MRI , Barium Follow Through

D.D:

- Addison`s disease,
- Maccune Albright (Precocious Puberty , Café Au Lait, Polyostotic Fibrous Dysplasia)

Treatment:

Polypectomy

Back Pain

Please Examine This Patient With Back Pain

D.D Of Back Pain

- Ankylosing Spondylitis
- Psoriatic Arthropathy
- Paget Disease Of The Bone
- Enteropathic (Whipple)
- IBD
- Reiter
- Osteoporosis
- Metastatic Bone Disease
- Disc Prolapsed
- Vertebral Fracture

Analysis Of Back Pain:

- SOCRATES
- Any Lose Motions? Pale Offensive Floating Difficult To Flush? Blood With Motions? (IBD, Enteropathic,Reiter)
- Any Sudden, Abnormal Movements Of Your Back? (Mechanical Back Pain)
- Any Pain In Joints Of Your Hands? Nail Changes? (Psoriatic)
- Any Burning With Your Water Works? (Reiter)
- Any Rash? (Psoriasis, Reiter ; Keratoderma Blenorrhagica)
- Any weakness in the legs? (Cord Compression, Cauda Equina, L5/S1 Lesion)
- Loss of Bowel control, Urinary incontinence? (Cauda Equina)

ONCE YOU ENTER THE ROOM SEARCH FOR A SPOT DIAGNOSIS

Kyphosis + Limited Spine Flexion =

Ankylosing Spondylitis

Targeted History:
Confirm Diagnosis, R/O Differential Diagnoses & Look For Associated Conditions

- Any Stiffness In Your Back > 1h ? More in The Morning? Eye Problems?
- Any Racing Of Heart, Chest Pain? (AR)
- Pins & Needles In Your Hands? Pain In Your Hand Joints? Frothy Urine? (Amyloidosis)
- Any Shortness Of Breath? (Lung Fibrosis)
- Can You Control & Hold Your Bowel And Water Works?

Targeted Examination:

- **Inspect Back For Kyphosis , Scoliosis**
- **Palpate For Tenderness Over Spines & Sacro-Iliac Joints**
- **Measure Flexion Of Spine By Modified Schober Test** (Place A Point 5 Cm Below Dimples & 10 Cm Above And Ask Him To Flex If Limited < 5cm Inc. = Ankylosing)
- **Ask Him To Stand Against Wall** = Inc. Occiput Wall Distance (Normally Occiput Touches The Wall)
- **Neurological Evaluation Of Lower Limbs** (Straight Leg Raising Test For Sciatica)
- **Palpate Radial For Bradycardia (A-V Block) , Collapsing Pulse (AR)**
- **Auscultate The Lungs For Apical Fibrosis**
- **Auscultate Heart For Aortic Regurgitation , MVP , MR**
- **Examine Eyes For Uveitis , Scleritis**

Quick Discussion

Complications

- AR , MVP , MR
- Apical Fibrosis
- Deformity & Kyphosis
- Cauda Equina
- Uveitis, Achilis Tendinitis
- Amyloidosis (CTS ,HSM , Restrictive Cardiomyopathy)

Investigations

- ESR , CrP (High)
- HLA B27
- X-Ray (Sacroiliac Sclerosis , Narrowing Of Joint Space)
- ECHO
- CT Chest (Apical Fibrosis)

Treatment

- Stop Smoking
- Physiotherapy
- NSAIDs
- DMARD For Preipheral Arthritis
- Surgical Correction

Enlarged Head At Frontal & Occiput + Anterolateral Bowing Of Femur +
Anterior Bowing Of Tibia =

Paget Disease Of The Bone

Targeted History

- Changes Of Your Bones? Back Pain? Problems With Vision? Problems With Hearing? Problems With Closing Your Eyes, FH?
- Swollen Legs? SOB?

Targeted Examination

- **Examine Facial Features**
- **Examine Cr. Ns : II , V ,VII , VIII**
- **Acuity, Filed**
- **Sensations Of Face**
- **Masseter & Temporalis Power** (Clench on Your Teeth)
- **Jaw Deviation** (Open Your Mouth For Me Please)
- **Look Up , Close Eye , Show Me You Teeth , Whistle** (VII)

Quick Discussion

Causes:

Viral (RSV, Measles), Genetic

Investigations:

Inc. ALP, X-Rays, Bone Scan

Treatment:

Bisphosphonates

Recurrent Chest Pain

Please Examine This Patient With Recurrent Chest Pains

D.D Of Recurrent Chest Pains

- ISHD
- Reflux (SCLERODERMA)
- Recurrent Pleurisy (SLE)
- Mixed C.T Disease
- Recurrent Pneumothracies (MARFAN)
- MVP (Marfan , Ankylosing , Myotonia , ADPKD , Ehler Danlos , Pseudoxanthoma Elasticum)
- AS =HOCM (Friedrichs Ataxia) , Turner
- Recurrent Pulmonary Embolism (Normal Chest Examination)
  - BEHCET (Oral , Genital Ulcers , Swollen Legs)
  - APS (Recurrent Miscarriages , Swollen Legs , Butter Fly Rash , Mouth Ulcers)
  - PNH
  - Antithrombin III Defiency & Factor V Leyden

ONCE YOU ENTER THE ROOM SEARCH FOR A SPOT DIAGNOSIS

Butterfly Rash Sparing The Nasolabial Folds =

Systemic Lupus Erythematosis

Targeted History:

Confirm Diagnosis, R/O Differential Diagnoses & Look For Associated Conditions

- Any Pain In Your Joints? Stiffness? Sensitivity To Sun? Any Rash? Mouth Sores? Chest Pains? SOB? Frothy Urine ? Blood With Your Water Works? Fevers? Eye Problems? Loss Of Hair?
- Miscarriages? PH Of Clots In Your Blood Channels?
- Muscle Weakness During Climbing Stairs Or Combing Your Hair?
- Kidney problems? Neurological S/S?

Targeted Examination

- **Examine Rashes , Mouth Ulcers**
- **Proximal Weakness, Heliotope Rash, Gottron Sign (Mixed C.T.Ds)**
- **Examine Chest For Basal Fibrosis Or Pleural Effusion**
- **Examine Hand Rheumatologically**

Quick Discussion

Investigations

- **FBC:** Anemia (Hemolytic? Renal? Chronic Illness? Drug Induced), Leucopenia (Activity? Drug Induced E.G. Cyclophosphamide?), Thrombocytopenia (APLS)
- **U&Es:** Nephritis?, **Urine Dip And Urine PCR/ USS**
- **ESR** Usually Raised In Activity +/- CRP
- **Clotting :** Prolonged A PTT And Thrombocytopenia → APLS
- **ANA:** Almost Always Positive
- **ANTI Ds DNA :** Specific In 60% Of Patients
- **Anti C1q:** Most Specific
- **C3 &C4:** Consumed In Activity, Renal And Neurological Involvement
- **Renal Biopsy:** Different Types Of Lupus Nephritis
- **CXR:** Shrunken Lung Syndrome

Treatment

- Skin Involvement: Sun Screens, Anti Malarial Drugs (Hydroxychloroquine)
- Joint Involvement: NSAIDS, Hydroxychloroquine Steroids If Severe Pai
- End Organ Damage E.G Nephritis, Cerebritis : Pulse Steroids, Cyclophosphamide, Mycophenolate Mofetil (MMF), Plasma Exchange, Rituximab
- ESRD : Hemodialysis Or Renal Transplant
- Aspirin & Warfarin For Antiphospholipid Syndrome

DIAGNOSTIC CRITERIA

- 4 Out Of 11 Of The Following
  o Malar Rash
  o Photosensitivity
  o Oral Ulcers
  o Discoid Rash
  o Serositis
  o Arthritis
  o Blood (Anemia , Thrombocytopenia , Leucopenia)
  o Immunology (Antiphospholipid , Anti Dsdna, Anti-Smith)
  o Nephritis
  o Siezures, Psychosis
  o ANA

Tall + Long Fingers + Upward Lens Dislocation+ Scoliosis + Pes Planus + Hammer Toe + Pectus Excavatum Or Carinatum + High Arched Palate =

Marfan`s Syndrome

Targeted History

- Any Chest Pains? SOB?
- Double Vision? (Lens Dislocation)
- Any Lumps (Hernias)?
- Any Blood With Back Passage (Haemorrhoids)?
- Any Heart Problems? (MVP, AR)
- FH?

Targeted Examination

- **Features**
- **Examine Span > Height**
- **Examine For Thumb Sign & Wrist Sign**
- **Examine Chest For Pneumothorax**
- **Examine Heart For AR , MVP** (Mid Systolic Click) , (MR)
- **Examine Hernial Orifices**

Quick Discussion

Cause: AD, Defect In Fibrillin Gene On Chromosome 15

Wrinkled Skin + Pseudoxanthomas + Plucked Chicken Appearance+ Long Standing Visual Problems =

Pseudoxanthoma Elasticum

Targeted History

- Any Lumps Or Bumps (Hernias)?
- Chest Pain? Awareness Of Heart Beats? (MVP , AR)
- Blood With Bowel Motions? (Haemorrhoids)
- Swollen Legs (Varicose Veins)?
- Previous History Of Skin Resections

Targeted Examination

- **Features**
- **Examine Heart For AR , MVP , MR**
- **Examine Hernia Orifices**
- **I Would Like To Examine The Fundus** (Macular Degeneration)

Quick Discussion

Causes: AR On Chromosome 16

Treatment: Anti-Androgen Medications, Laser Photocoagulation For Macula

Myopia (Glasses) + Thin Skin + Hyper-extensibility Of Skin + Hyperlaxity Of Joints + Pseudo-tumors Of Knees & Elbows + Kyphoscoliosis + Flat Feet=

Ehler Danlos

- Examine Heart For AR, MVP , MR
- AD

Diminution Of Vision

Please Examine This Patient With Diminution Of Vision?

D.D Of Diminution Of Vision

- Diabetes (Retinopathy , Maculopathy , Cataracts)
- HTN
- Retinitis Pigmentosa
- Papilledema
- Optic Atrophy
- Retinal Artery Or Vein Occlusion
- TIA
  - Hypercholesterolemia (Xanthomata) , AF (Graves) , LV Thrombus
  - Behcet , APS , Factor V Leyden
- Field Defects

Targeted History

- Can You Explain It To Me?
- Do You See Things Double And/Or Any Pain While Moving Your Eyes (Opthalmoplegia) ?
- Can You See The Sides Of The Road (Biteporal Hemianopia)?
- Can You See Well At Night? (Retinitis Pigmentosa)
- Blurring Of The Centre Of Your Visual Field (Distorted Images)? (Maculopathy)
- Headaches, Cramps Of Jaw During Eating, Pain In Head & Scalp (Temporal Arteritis)?
- Weakness Clumsiness, Pain With Moving Eyes (MS)?
- Problems Seeing At Night, Similar Conditions In Family (Retinitis Pigmentosa) , Problems With Hearing (Usher)?
- Any Headaches, Throwing Up, Blurred Vision (Inc. Cranial Pr.)? Shoe & Ring Size, Sweating (Acromegaly)? , Breast Discharge, Problem With Periods (Prolactinoma)? Weight Gain, OCPs, Vit A, Retinoids (BIH)? Mouth Ulcers, History Of Blood Clots In Your Blood Channels (Behcet, AP$, Family History Of Thrombophilia =Sinus Thrombosis)?
- Central Or Peripheral? Can You Watch TV Properly? Do You Bump In Surroundings While Walking?
- Change In Colour Vision? With MS Or Optic Neuritis In General
- Unilateral Or Bilateral?
- Any Accompanying Hearing Loss?
- Trauma?
- HTN?
- D.M? If You Suspect Diabetic Retinopathy ask about other complications of D.M.? ; Frothing Water Works? Pins & Needles In Legs, Hands? Walking Problems?
- Do You Drive?

Targeted Examination

- **General Survey For The Patient**
  - Cushing =D.M , HTN , Papilledema , OA
  - Acromegaly =D.M , HTN , Papilledema , OA
  - Mouth Ulcer=Papilledema
  - Grave`S= D.M , HTN , Papilledema
  - Walking Aid=OA (MS)
  - Hearing Aid =Retinitis Pigmentosa (Usher)
  - Signs Of D.M.= Preprolefrative , Prolefrative , Maculopathy
    - Amyotrophy
    - Necrobiosis Lipoidica
    - Charcoat Joint / Amputations

- **Acuity**
- **Field**
- **Fundus**
- **Eye Movements**
- **Clinical examination of the Cause & Its complications e.g.:** if diabetic retinopathy examine for peripheral neuropathy and do urine dip stick for proteinuria

---

Visual Acuity Examination

- Counting fingers 1 m apart
- If can`t see count fingers 30 cms
- If he can`t see do hand movement
- If can`t see do perception of light
- Ideally it should be done by Snellen`s Chart

Visual Field Examination

- Examine it 1 meter apart on the same level with the patient
- Remove Your eye glasses
- Sit at a level where your eyes & the Patient`s eyes are on the same level
- Test each eye individually
- He close the RT.eye And You the Lt.eye with your left hand
- Examine temporal field from upper quad , middle , lower
  (When You see my waggling finger tell me)
- Then change hands with closing Your eyes
- Then examine nasal from upper quad , middle , lower
- Then repeat with other eye
  - ❖ Pit.Tumours→ Bitemporal Hemianopia
  - ❖ Pit tumours→Enlarged blind spt
  - ❖ Papillaedema → Enlarged blind spot
  - ❖ Optic Atrophy →Central scotoma, Disturbed color vision
  - ❖ Occipital cortex→ Homonomous hemianopia
  - ❖ PITS Quadrantanopia (Cortex)

Fundus examination

- Remove your glasses and adjust the opthalmoscope on Your vision
- great the pt., take permission
- Sit The Patient Up & and stand at his level
- Ask the examiner : (May I ask to dim the light sir?)
- Turn on Your opthalmoscope
- Ask the Pt. To fix his eyes on light straight ahead
- With Your **Rt. Hand** , **Rt. Eye** , examine patient **Rt. Eye**
- Examine **Red reflex** first
- Get the **Vessels** , **The disc** , and **Move on all quads**
- Ask the patient to look directly at the light for the **Macula**

Comment on

- Red reflex (Any cataracts)
- **OPTIC DISC & CUP**
    - Normal
    - Well defined , pale
    - ILL defined , Swollen . with congested veins & Patton lines
- **VESSELS**
    - Normal
    - Dot hemorrhage
    - A–V nipping , Silver wiring
- **ADDED COMMENTS**
    - Exudates (soft & hard)
    - Hemorrhages (dot , blot , flame)
    - Pigmentations
    - Laser photocoagulation
    - New vessels formation

Always Palpate the <u>Radial Pulse for AF</u> , <u>Carotid</u>
pulse and Listen for its Bruit in all cases of

During Fundoscopy Look For

VESSELS

- **Normal** (veins size >arteries)
- **Silver wiring**
- **A-V Nipping**=HTN
- **Congested Tortous vessels** (Papilledema)
- **New vessel formation** =Prolefrative D.M (in Trabeculae or mesh)

HAEMORRHAGES

- **DOT haemorrhage**=D.M
- **Blot haemorrhage**=D.M , HTN
- **Flame shaped Haemorrhage** = HTN

EXUDATES

Hard Exudates	Soft Exudates
Very small	Large
Shiny	Not shiny
Yellow	White /Pale yellow
Muliple when found	Lower in number
More common with D.M	More common with HTN

RETINITIS PIGMENTOSA
LASER PHOTOCOAGULATION
OPTIC DISC

Normal	Papilledema	Optic Atrophy
Yellow Or Pink	Pink	White Or Pale Yellow
There Is Hyperaemic Rim	Increased Hyperaemic Rim	No Hyperaemic Rim
Cup May Be Normal , Inc. Dec.	Swollen No Cup	No Cup
Well Defined Border	ILL Defined Border	Well Defined Border

Preprolifrative Diabetic Retinopathy

- Dot Hemorrhage (Aneurysm Of Vessels)= (Specific For D.M)
- Blot Hemorrhage
- Hard Exudates (Yellowish, Shiny, Well Circumscribed , Small , Multiple) Fat Deposition
- Soft Exudates (Cotton-Wool Spots) (Fluffy White , Well Or Ill Defined, Not Shiny, Large, Few) = Ischemic Nerve Fibers
- Necrobiosis Lipoidica, Dermopathy, Ulcers , Charcoat`s Joint , Diabetic Amyotrophy
- To Differentiate Hard Exudates It From Light Reflex=It Doesn't Move With When U Move The Light

Treatment:

- Stop Smoking
- Maintain Blood Pressure 130/80 With ACEIs
- Insulin Use=Tight Control Of D.M= HBA1c
- Routine Referral To Ophthalmologist
- Urine Analysis , U&Es

"You Have Changes In The Back Of Your Eyes Due To Long Standing High Blood Sugar"

Proliferative Diabetic Retinopathy

- Same Findings As Pre Proliferative + Neovascularisation (New Vessel Formation) In Mesh Or Trabeculae

Treatment:

- Urgent Referral To Ophthalmologist
- Laser Photocoagulation
- Viterectomy
- Intraocular Steroid Injection

Diabetic Maculopathy

- Macular Edema , Exudates , Hemorrhage

Treatment:

Needs Urgent Referral To Ophthalmologist

"You Have Changes In The In The Back Of Your Eye In The Centre Of Vision Due To Long Standing High Blood Glucose "

Papilledema

BILATERAL, Blurred Disc Margin, Venous Engorgement, Swollen Optic Disc, Patons Lines (Radial Retinal Vessels Cascading The Disc), Loss Of Cup , May Progress To Post-Papilledemic Optic Atrophy

Causes Of Papilledema:

- Malignant HTN (Flame Hge ,Soft Exudates)
- Raised Intracranial Pressure
  - Tumors
  - Cerebral Sinus Thrombosis (Hypercoagulable State)
  - Cerebral He
  - Idiopathic Intracranial HTN (Obese, OCPs, Vit A, Tetracyclins)
- Respiratory Failure
- Chiari Malformation
- Field Defect=Enlarged Blind Spot=Perimetry

Investigations

- FBC,
- ESR
- MRI Brain
- MR Venography = (Sinus Thrombosis)

Treatment

- Acetazolamide , Weight Reduction , Lumbar Puncture , Shunt If BIH
- Steroids=Inflammatory Causes
- The Head Of The Electric Cable Supplying Ur Eye Is Swollen , Which Is Usually Due To Increase In The Pressure Inside The Brain

Hypertensive Retinopathy

- Grade 1= Attenuation Of Vessels + Silver Wiring
- Grade 2= Same + A-V Nipping
- Grade 3= Same + Soft Exudates , Hard , Flame He
- Grade 4= Papilledema (Swollen, Ill-Defined Disc, With Congested Veins)
- Macular Star= Hard Exudates In Form Of Star In Macula =Urgent Referral

N.B: Soft Exudates Are More Common Than Hard Exudates In HTN

Retinitis Pigmentosa

Mottling Of Retinal Epithelium With Black-Bone Specule Epithelium Pallor Of Optic Nerve May Be Seen (Degenerative Changes In Rods & Cons) , Optic Atrophy

Causes:

- **Primary**
- **Secondary**
  - Usher Syndrome (HEARING LOSS) =Genetic Disorder , TTT :Gene Therapy
  - Kearns-Sayre : Ataxia,Opthalmoplegia,Cardiac Conduction Defects,Dysphagia)=Mitochondrial Disease
  - Abetalipoprotinemia (Steatorrhea , Peripheral Neuropathy)
  - Laurance-Moon-Biedle: (Retardation , Ataxia , High Arched Palate , Syndactyly / Polydactyly ,Obesity)
  - Refsum Disease (HEARING LOSS) (Inc. Phytanic Acid)
  - Alport (HEARING LOSS)

Field Defect = Funnel Vision & Night Blindness

Frequency =1 Million Worldwide, 50% AD , 25% AR , 25% XL

Investigations: Electro-Retinogram

Treatment: No Definitive Treatment, Vitamin A Reduces Progression

There Is Increase In The Pigmentations In The Back Of Your Eye, Which Is The Sensor Of Our Visions , These Pigmentations Obscure Its Ability To Sense Normally

Optic Atrophy

(Axonal Degeneration In Retino-Geniculate Pathway)

- WELL DEFINED, PALE DISC
- If You Find Optic Atrophy In One Eye Look For Papilledema In Other Eye = FOSTER KENNEDY SYNDROME (Optic Nerve Compression , Increased Intracranial Pressure)

Causes:

Commonest Cause =MS

- P=Increased Intracranial Pressure (Tumours) , Glaucoma (IOP)
- A= Ataxia (Friedrichs)
- L= Leber`s Optic Atrophy
- E
- D= Degenerative= Retinitis Pigmentosa,/Dietary (Vit. B12)
- I= Ischemia (Giant Cell Arteritis , Wegner, Churg Strauss)
- S= MS
- C= Cyanaide Poisoning ,Ethambutol , Methanol , Ethylene Glycol
- 1ry = Well Defined Pale Disc , Disappear Of Cup , Attenuated B.Vs
- 2ry= Ill-Defined Or Well Defined Pale Disc, Cup Preserved , Normal B.Vs

Field Defect= Central Scotoma , Disturbed Color Vision

Investigations: CT Or MRI Brain , Orbital U/S , Vit. B12

Treatment: Idebenone In Leber OA

The Head Of The Electric Cable Of Your Eye Is Starting To Lose Its Function

Branched Retinal Vein Occlusion

Retinal Hemorrhage, Retinal Edema + Cotton Wool Spots , Respecting Horizontal Raphe With, Papilledema

Causes: Thrombophilia, Sarcoidosis

Treatment: Steroids Intra Ocular, Vascular Endothelial Growth Factor Inhibitor

Branch Retinal Artery Occlusion

Pale Retina, Attenuated Vessels

Examine The Pulse For AF & Listen To Carotids For Bruits

Causes: D.M, HTN, TIA , Smoking , Cholesterol Emboli

Treatment: Clopidogrel, Aspirin, Warfarin If In AF

Bloody Diarrhea

Please Examine This Patient With Bloody Diarrhea

- HHT (Telangectasia Of Hands And Mouth)
- IBD (Pyoderma Gangrenosa , Mouth Ulcers)
- Ischemic Colitis (RA , SLE , Scleroderma , Henoch Shenolien, Behcet`s disease)
- Bleeding Disorders & Anticoagulants
- Haemorrhoids (Marfan , Ehler Danlos , Pseudoxanthoma Elasticum)

Skin Rash

Please Examine This Patient With Skin Rash?

- Where Exactly? Any Other Parts Of Your Body? What Did It Look Like In The Beginning? Have It Changed Since Onset? Flitting? Bleeds? Itchy? Painful? Other Rash?

ONCE YOU ENTER THE ROOM SEARCH FOR A SPOT DIAGNOSIS

Differential Diagnosis Of Skin Rash

a) **Primary Dermatological Condition**
   - Eczema
   - Bullous Pemphigoid
   - Pemphigous Vulgaris
   - Lichen Planus
   - Vitiligo
   - Alopecia (Areata, Totali)
   - Primary Skin Infections E.G Tenia, Cellulitis, Erysiplas
   - Steven Johnson Syndrome, TEN
   - Parasitic Infestations: Scabies, Warts

b) **Secondary To Systemic Disease**
   - All Previous Primary Dermatological Disorders Could Be Secondary To Other Diseases
   - Drug Related : Erythema Multiform (Target Lesions)
   - Erythema Nodosum: Streptococcal Infection, Sarcoidosis, Inflammatory Bowel Disease, T.B.
   - Pyoderma Gangrenosum: RA, Inflammatory Bowel Disease
   - Vasculitic Rash
   - Hypersenstivity Rash
   - Parasitic Infestations: Cutaneous Larva Migrans
   - Malignancy: Necrolytic Migratory Erythema (Glucagonoma)
   - Collagen Disorders
     - **SLE:** Butterfly Rash, Discoid Lupus
     - **Dermatomyositis:** Heliotrope Rash, Gottron Sign
     - **Rheumatoid Arthritis:** Digital Infarcts
     - **Rheumatic Fever:** Erythema Marginatum
   - Diabetes Mellitus: Infections, Necrobiosis Lipodica, Dermopathies
   - Renal Failure: Uremic Frost, Itching Marks, Perforating Collagenosis

Loss Of Hair With No Signs Of Scarring Or Inflammation + Nail Pitting + At The Periphery Small Tiny Hair =

Alopecia Areata Or Totalis Or Universalis

Targeted History

- Have You Lost Hair From Other Parts Of Your Body? Do You Live Stressful Life?
- Any SOB ? Heart Racing? Do You Look Paller Than Usual?
- Feeling The Hot Or Cold More Than Usual? Sweating Or Dryness Of Skin? Lose Motions Or Constipations? Sleep? Neck Swelling?
- Loss Of Normal Skin Color Or Increased Tanning? High Blood Sugar?

Targeted Examination

- **Examine The Whole Body Hair**
- **Examine The Thyroid**

Quick Discussion

Treatment:

Topical Steroids , Minoxidil

Discrete Areas Of Loss Of Pigmentations + No Loss Of Sensations =

Vitiligo

Targeted History

- Exclude Any Associated Autoimmune Disorders
- any Other Rash? Loss Of Sensations?
- Heart Racing? SOB? Does He Looks Paller Than Usual?
- Tend To Feel The Hot Or Cold More Than Usual? Constipation , Loose Motions? Sleep? Sweating Or Dry Skin? Neck Swelling?
- Any Areas Of Increased Tanning?
- High Blood Sugar?

Targeted Examination

- **Examine The Lesion Sensations** (Not Leprosy)
- **Examine Thyroid**

Quick Discussion

Treatment:

Steroids / Sun Screens / PUVA /PUVB / Camouflage Creams

Purplish Itchy Flat Topped Papules + White Wickman Striae On Surface & Buccal Mucosa + Longitudenal Nail Ridges =

Lichen Plannus

- Itching? Any Other Rash? Change Of Voice, SOB (Larynx)?
- Difficulty, Painful Swallowing (GIT affection)?
- Burning With Your Water (Renal affection)?
- Redness Of Eyes (Conjunctival affection)?
- <u>DH:</u> Beta blockers , Thiazides , Antimalrials , Metfromin

Quick Discussion

Tretment:

Topical Steroids

Sharply Demarcated Thin Shiny Atrophic Area, With Yellowish Waxy Centre, Telangiectasia On The Surface (Asymptomatic May Be Tender With Central Ulcers) =

Necrobiosis Lipoidica

Targeted History

- D.M? For How Long? Controlled?
- What Medications Do You Take?
- Passing More Urine? Frothy Urine (Renal Affection)?
- Pins & Needles In Legs Or Hands (P.N)?
- Blurring Of Vision Or Problem Of Vision (Retinopathy)?

Targeted Examination

- **Examine The Fundus** (May I Examine The Fundus?)
- **Examine For P.N**
- **Examine Hand Rheumatologically If Any Pain In Hands** (RA)

Quick Discussion

Investigations:

Biopys: Mixed Inflammatory Cells Infiltrates

Treatment:

- Steroid Cream Or Injection (Might Help)
- Caring Of Ulcers
- Tight Glycemic Control Will Not Reverse It
- Excision & Skin Grafting

Capillary Hemangioma Respecting The Midline =

Port Wine Stain

Port Wine Stain + Weakness/Fits = STURGE WEBER SYNDROME

- Any Fits? Weakness (Brain Hemangiomas)?
- Pain In Eyes Or Decrease Of Vision (Glucoma)?
- **Examine Any Weak Limb Neurologically**
- Examine Fundus (May I Examine The Fundus?)
  - o Glaucoma , Chorodial Hemangioma

Quick Discussion

Investigation:

CT Scan & MRI Brain

Cause:

Congenital

Treatment

- Skin: Laser Therapy
- Radiation :Choroidal Hemangiomas
- Glaucoma :Medical (Acetazolamide, BB) , Surgical

Thickened Area Of Skin, Indurated Adherent To Underlying Tissue, Multicolored (Initially Violaceous Then Ivory) + No Hair Follicles + Loss Of Sensations + Depressed Areas =

<u>MORPHEA (Localized Scleroderma)</u>

- Usually No Systemic Symptoms Of Scleroderma
- Do You Have Any Pain In Joints? Cold Hands? Heart Burn? SOB? Other Skin Problems? Constipation?

Investigations:

o ANA, RF, Anti Histone Ab, Anticentromere Antiphospholipid Are +Ve
o Inc. IgM, IgG
o MRI For Depth Of Lesion
o Skin Biopsy: Sclerotic Changes (Thickening, Homogiznation Of Collagen) In Lower Reticular Dermis

Treatment:

Spontaneous Resolution In 3-5 Yrs ,Topical , Intralesional , Systemic Steroids , Antimalrials ,Methotrexate

Inflamed Wheeping Skin = Acute Eczema
Inflamed Lichenified Skin =

<u>Chronic Eczema</u>

- Itching? Bleeding? Noisy Chest? Asthma ? Hay Fever?
- Any Sort Of Allergies? Jewellery? Metals? Allergies To Fish? Peanuts? Fragrances?
- What You Do For Living (Latex, Hair Dyes)?
- Can You Attribute It To Anything You Were Exposed To?
- Any Difficulty Swallowing? (Eosinophilic Esophagitis)
- SOB? Cough? (Eosinophilic Pneumonia)

<u>Quick Discussion</u>

Investigations:

- Eosinophilia , Inc. IgE , Skin Prick Test , Patch Test , RAST

Treatment:

- Avoid Allergen Calamile Lotion , Antihistaminics For Itching ,
- Steroids , Treat Infections

Multiple Neurofibromas (Soft & Firm, Sessile, Mobile, Along The Course Of Peripheral Nerves) + Café Au Lait Patches +Axillary Freckles + Lisch Nodules=

Neurofibromatosis

- Problems With Chewing Food (V) ?
- Do You See Things Double (VI)?
- Does Soap Enters Your Eyes During Washing Your Face (VII)?
- Problems With Hearing Or Balance (VIII)? Balance Problems? (Acoustic Neuroma)
- Do You Cough Normally (IX, X) ? Turn Your Head Normally (XI)? (Jugular Foramen $)
- Headaches , Sweating (Pheochromoyctoma MEN II) ? Neck Swellings? (MEN II)
- Any Weakness Or Clumsiness? (Spinal Cord Lesion)
- **Examine Sensation Of Face**
- **Palpate Masseter & Temporalis** (Clench Your Teeth)
- **Opening Jaw For Any Deviation**
- **Eye Movements** (Fix Your Head Look At My Finger Move With Your Eyes Only)
- **Elevate Eye Brow , Close Eyes , Blow Mouth**
- **Examine Hearing**
- **Examine Uvula Movement (IX , X)** (Open Your Mouth And Say Ahhh)
- **Examine Power Of Trapezius & Sternomastoid (XI)** (Shrug Your Shoulders , Resist Me , Turn Your Head Right , Left Resist Me)
- **Auscultate Abdomen For Renal Bruits**

Quick Discussion

Causes:

AD NF1 Chromosome 17, NF2 Chromosome 22

Diagnosis:

Genetic Screening, MRI

Treatment:

Surgical Removal

Anti-epileptics

Multiple Bullae Arising From Normal Skin Or Red Skin Filled With Clear Or Yellow Or Hemorrhagic Fluid =

Bullous Pemphigoid

- ITHCHING?
- Fevers? Wt.Loss? Throughing Up? Difficulty Swallowing? Throughing Up Blood? Lumps? (Malignancy)
- PH Of Any Skin Rash? Exposure To UV Rays Or Radiations?
- Any Pain Stiffness In Your Joints? (SLE) Feeling Hot Or Cold More Usual?
- <u>DH:</u> Captopril, NSAIDs (Ibuprofen), Frusemide , Antibiotics
- **Examine L.Ns**
- **Examine Abdomen**

Quick Discussion

Causes:

- Auto-Immune, Drugs, Radiations Hidden, Malignancy, SLE

Investigations:

- Immunoflurescence Deposition Of Igg C3 In Dermo-Epidermal Junction
- Not Fatal As Pemphigus
- Nikolsky Signs Is -Ve

Treatment: Steroids & Azathioprine

NB: Nikolsky Sign:
The Top Layers Of The Skin Slip Away From The Lower Layers When Slightly Rubbed.

Flaccid Thin Roofed Blisters Containing Serous Fluid , & Arising Over Normal Skin (Axilla , Trunk) + Most Of Blisters Burst Leaving Red , Exuding Areas Which Are Tender + Red Denuded Patches In The Mouth, Pharynx & Eyes =

Pemphigus Vulgaris

- PAINFUL
- Any Mouth Sores?
- Any Loss Of Weight? Fevers? Sweats? Lumps? (Non Hodgkin Lymphoma)
- Any Weakness Combing Hair? Climbing Stairs? (MG)
- Any Drugs?
- **Examine L.Ns**
- **Axillary**
- **Cervical**
- **Inguinal**
- **Examine For Proximal Weakness**
- **Nikolski Sign Is +Ve**
- Fatal

Quick Discussion

Causes:

Captopril, Penicillamine, Rifampicin, MG, Lymphoma

Investigations:

- Immune-Florescence Biopsy: Epidermal Deposition Of IgG & C3
- Anti Desmogliein Abs

Treatment:

High Dose Corticosteroids & Azathioprine

Erythematous Rash Around Eyes (Heliotrope) , Over Knuckles (Gottron) =

Dermatomyositis

- Weakness Climbing Stairs, Combing Hair? (Proximal Weakness)
- Fevers, Weight. Loss? Difficulty Swallowing, Throwing Up Blood? (Malignancy)
- SOB ? Cough? (Lung Fibrosis)
- Painful Hand Joints? Rash On Cheecks, Sensitivity To Sun? (Mized connective tissue disease)
- **Examine For Proximal Weakness**
- **Examine Chest**
- **Examine Abdomen For Malignancy + L.Ns**

Quick Discussion

Investigations:

- Anti Mi2 Ab
- CPK
- Anti Jo1 Ab
- EMG
- Endoscopy

Treatment:

- Steroids
- Hydroxychloroquine
- Azathioprine

Waxy, Discolored Induration Of The Skin, Peau D'Orange + Thyroid Eye Signs=

Pretibial Myxedema

- **Ask About Symptoms of Graves` disease**
- **Examine Thyroid Gland and eyes**
- **Associated With Graves Disease**

Quick Discussion

Biopsy: Mucin In The Mid- To Lower- Dermis. There Is No Increase In Fibroblasts

Treatment:

- Regress Spontaneously After Months Or Years
- Local Steroids
- NO Surgery As It May Increase The Dermopathy
- Compression Wraps Or Stocking

Mouth Ulcers

Please Examine This Patient With Mouth Ulcers

- Behcet's Disease; See Before
  - DVT
  - Cerebral Sinus Thrombosis= Headaches , Papilledema
  - PE
- SLE; See Before
- Celiac Disease; See Before
- Pemphigus; See Before
- Steven Jonson Syndrome
- IBD; See Before
- Trauma
- Infections

Transient Focal Neurological Deficit

Presentations

- LOC
- Weakness of Limbs
- Slurred speech
- Transient loss of vision
- Facial asymmetry

Differential Diagnosis

- TIA
- Hypoglycemia
- Sudden Hypotension
- Acute Coronary Syndrome

Transient focal neurology resolved within 24 hours, no LOC, normal Blood sugar =

TIA

Targeted History

- How many times?
- Age?
- Onset ?
- Course?
- Duration?
- What was the focal neurology?
  - ○ Slurred speech
  - ○ Or Limb weakness
- Risk Factors for atherosclerosis?
  - ○ Smoking
  - ○ D.M.
  - ○ HTN
  - ○ Family history
  - ○ Previous strokes
  - ○ IHD
  - ○ Limb Ischaemia
- Cardiac arrhythmias?
  - ○ AF
  - ○ Atrial flutter
  - ○ Calculate CHA2DS2VASC score & HASBLED
  - ○ Ask specifically about anticoagulation
- Any metallic heart valve?
  - ○ Ask about anticoagulation
- Any constitutional symptoms suggestive of IEC

Targeted Examination

- **Examine pulse for AF**
- **Examine carotids for bruits**
- **Examine heart for metallic heart valve or valvular heart disease or signs of IEC**
- **Ask to measure B.P**
- **Measure Blood Sugar**
- **Calculate ABCD2 score**

Quick Discussion

How Would You Manage This Patient?

- Give aspirin 300 mg stat & Clopidogrel 75mg OD afterwards
- Consider admission if ABCD2>4
- If ABCD2 < 4 then TIA clinic referral within 1 week
- If crescendo TIAs (2 or > 2/week) then admit for Inpatient stroke team R/V
- Carotid Doppler
- ECG
- ECHO
- Treatment of the cause
- CT head if weakness hasn't completely resolved

Transient Focal Neurology/LOC/ Symptoms of low blood sugar which completely resolved after taking a sugary drink =

Hypoglycemia

Differential Diagnosis

- Insulinoma
- Drugs
  - Insulin & Sulphonylureas
  - Either increased dose or Renal Failure development
  - Metformin doesn't cause hypoglycemia
- Adrenal insufficiency
  - Sudden withdrawel of Steroids
  - Primary adrenal insufficiency

Specific History

- Ask about symptoms of *Whipple`s Triad?*
  - Sweating, feeling cold, Palpitations, Shaky, Blurred vision and light headedeness
  - Low blood sugar < 3 mmol/L
  - Symptoms resolved after replacing sugar
  - Ask if the patient is aware when he has hypoglycemia.
  - Causes of hypoglycemic Unawareness:
    - Beta Blockers
    - Autonomic Neuropathy
    - Tightly controlled blood sugar
    - Diabetes for long time
- Is he *Diabetic?*
- Is he *on Insulin/ Sulphonylureas?*
- Any Predisposing factors for Hypoglycemia?
  - Decreased Eating & Drinking
  - Increased doses recently?
  - Any Kidney disease?
- S/S of *Kidney disease?*
- Any predisposing factors for kidney disease?
  - Analgesics
  - Dehydration
  - Nephrotoxics
  - D & V
  - Glomerulonephritis
- S/S of insulinoma
  - Weight gain
  - Hypoglycemia after prolonged fasting
  - Other signs of MENI

Quick Examination

- **Examination For Signs Of Diabetes Including Fundi**
- **Examination For Signs Of Addison`s Disease**
- **Examination For Signs Of Renal Failure**
- **Measure Blood Sugar**

Quick discussion

How Will You Manage This Patient?

- B.M chart
- Reduce insulin dose
- DSN R/V / Endocrinology R/V
- Measure C-peptide & serum insulin
- Prolonged fasting test for insulinoma
- Kidney functions

- Short synacthen test for Addison`s
- Treat The Cause

Recurrent Falls

Differential Diagnosis

- **Infectious causes**
  - Any infection in elderly people can cause falls especially if causing delirium
  - UTI
  - LRTI
- **Polypharmacy**
- **Cardiac causes**
  - ACS
  - Postural hypotension
  - Carotid sinus hypersensitivity
  - Complete heart block
  - Aortic Stenosis
  - Tachy-arrhythmias (e.g. AF)
  - Cough/Micturation/ defecation Syncope
  - Sick Sinus Syndrome
  - Vasovagal Syncope
- **Neurological causes**
  - Stroke
  - MND
  - Peripheral neuropathy
  - Proximal Muscle Weakness
  - Vitamin D deficiency
  - Hypothyroidism
  - Thyrotoxicosis
  - Paraparesis
  - Seizures
  - Polymyositis
  - Dermatomyositis
  - Parkinson`s disease due to
    - Bradykinesia, Rigidity & gait abnormalities
    - Postural Hypotension
    - Cerebellar affection if Parkinson`s Plus
- **Neuropsychiatric/Cognitive causes**
  - Dementia
  - Depression
  - Psychosis
  - Delerium
  - Alcohol
- **Musculoskeletal causes**
  - Knee OA
  - Hip OA
  - RA
- **Visual Problems**
- **Vestibular problems**
- **Social & Environmental causes**
  - Accidental Trip
  - Slippery floor
- **Endocrinal causes**
- **Hypoglycemia**
- **Drugs**
  - Statins → Proximal weakness
  - TCA/SSRI → Postural hypotension
  - Antihypertensive→ Postural drop
  - Insulin/Sulphonylureas → Hypoglycemia
  - Beta-blockers → Bradycardia
  - Donepezil→ Fits/Cardiac conduction problems

Analysis & Assessment of Recurrent Falls

1. How Many Falls In The Last 6 Months?

By this question you will determine if the patient is a frequent faller, thus, you will need a comprehensive assessment of the patient and physiotherapists, occupational therapists input.

2. How Does He Usually Walk? Stick? Frame? Bed Bound?

This back ground information is extremely important when taking further decisions regarding patient management e.g; resuscitation decisions.

According to this information you might get an obvious reason why the patient had a fall e.g.: tripped whilst walking with his frame.

3. Circumstances Of The Fall?

- What was the patient doing whilst he fell down?
- Was he trying to *stand up from sitting position?*
  - o Proximal muscle weakness
  - o Postural drop
- Did he feel *dizzy* whilst walking?
  - o Postural drop
- Did he feel his *heart racing* and suddenly collapsed?
  - o Tachyarrhythmia
- Was he *tying his tie* for an outdoors dinner?
  - o Carotid hypersensitivity
- Was he *Coughing? Micturition? Defecation?*
  - o Cough/micturition/defecation syncope
- Has he had any *Crushing Chest Pains, Sweating, Nausea And SOB?*
  - o ACS
  - o Aortic Stenosis
  - o ACS can present with falls without any chest pains.
- *LOC*
  - o Cardiac→ AS , Postural drop , tachyarrhythmia , Brady arrhythmia , vasovagal
  - o Fits → wet himself , bite his tongue , post ictal state , Tods paresis
- *Any head injuries? Is he on anticoagulants? Does he need a CT scan?*
- Any *Pains Anywhere?*
  - o Injuries
  - o Fractures or dislocations
- *Ask About S/S to R/O D.D Above?*

4. Systemic R/V?

- Any chest symptoms → LRTI
- Any Urinary symptoms→ UTI
- Any Fits→ Seizures
- D & V → dehydration & postural drop
- Neurological symptoms→ Stroke , Meningitis , Encephalitis
- Is he bleeding→ hypovolaemic
- Weakness in arms or legs → Stroke/Osteomalacia/Paraparesis

5. Past Medical History?

- D.M→ Dehydration, ACS, Neuropathy, postural drop, hypoglycemia secondary to medications
- HTN→ Stroke, ACS
- Neurological problems→ Parkinson's (Parkinson's causes falls because of bradykinesia, static tremors, rigidity & postural drop), stroke, MS
- Addison's → postural drop
- Hypo/Hyperthyroidism → proximal weakness
- Dementia→ recurrent falls secondary to cognitive impairment.

6. Medication History?

- Sinemet→ postural drop
- Donepezil→ Fits, Cardiac arrhythmias
- Diuretics→ postural drop
- SSRIs, TCA → postural drop
- Antihypertensive → postural drop
- Insulin & Sulphonylureas → hypoglycemia

7. Social History?

- Alcohol→ coordination problems , subdural hematomas, Delerium, anemia
- Smoking → ACS
- Stair lift?

8. Assess The Patient`s Cognitive Function; Is He Confused? Is He Known To Have Dementia?

- Asses his AMT if < 8 this means confusion; collateral history needed to diagnose acute or chronic confusion.
- Acute confusion is an important cause of falls.

9. General Examination

- Look for pallor → Anaemia
- Resting tremors→ Parkinson`s
- Cataracts→ visual problems
- Proximal muscle wasting→ proximal weakness
- Dermatomyositis rash

10.   Feel The Pulse

- Is he tachycardic/Bradycardic? Is he in AF?
- Does he have a weak pulse→ shocked, dehydrated

11.   Auscultate The Heart

- Does he have Aortic stenosis?

12.   Examine The Chest; Any Signs Of Chest Infection?

13.   Examine Patient Neurologically

- Proximal muscle weakness → malignancy, polymyositis, statins , hypothyroid, hyperthyroid , vit. D deficiency .
- Peripheral neuropathy →D.M
- Impaired coordination? MS? Alcoholic? Any previous strokes?

14.   Assess The Patient Rheumatologically; Knee/Hip OA?

15.   Assess Visual Acuity? And Visual Fields?

16.   Measure L/S B.P? Is There A Postural Drop?

17.   What Is His ECG Like? Any Arrhythmias?

18.   Urine Dip; Does The Patient Have UTI

19.   CXR & Basic Blood tests

20.   Monitor Blood Sugar

Quick Discussion

How Would You Manage This Patient?

1-Treat The Cause

- Replace any fluid loss
- Stop antihypertensive if postural drop and reintroduce cautiously
- Treat infections with antibiotics
- Treat seizures
- CXR if suspected chest infection
- Urine dip if suspected Urinary infections
- ECG→ ACS , Arrhythmias
- CT head if acute confusion
- ACS protocol for suspected ACS with further management regarding PCI if applicable.
- Treat arrhythmias
- Pace maker if indicated rhythm problem.
- Osteoporosis Protection medications to prevent fractures

2-Look For Complications

- CT head if head injury
- X-rays if suspected fractures

3- The Timed Up And Go Test (TUG)

Is a simple test used to assess a person's mobility and requires both static and dynamic balance.

It uses the time that a person takes to rise from a chair, walk three meters, turn around, walk back to the chair, and sit down. During the test, the person is expected to wear their regular footwear and use any mobility aids that they would normally require. The TUG is used frequently in the elderly population, as it is easy to administer and can generally be completed by most older adults.

One source suggests that scores of ten seconds or less indicate normal mobility, 11 – 20 seconds are within normal limits for frail elderly and disabled patients, and greater than 20 seconds means the person needs assistance outside and indicates further examination and intervention. A score of 30 seconds or more suggests that the person may be prone to falls.

4-Multidiscplinary Team Approach

- Physiotherapists and occupational therapist input.

Common Pitfalls In Station V

1-Overlooking one or more of patient's symptoms; either by not analyzing this symptom or by not examining the patient regarding this symptom

2- Many candidates concentrate only on the patients complaint in examination, and forget related, associated conditions, causes and complications.

3-Overlooking one or more of the patient`s concerns because of the stress of the examination; you have to manage all the patients concerns

4-Forgetiing to refer the patient to the appropriate specialist

5-Failure to admit the patient when needed.

6- Admitting the patient inappropriately.

Printed in Great Britain
by Amazon